Department of Social Policy and Social Work
University of Oxford
Barnett House
32 Wellington Square
Oxford OX1 2ER
England

Contents

Foreword

There is nothing quite like this gem of a book, which provides much the best introduction to child psychiatry that has been written. It is succinct, very easy to read, and immensely practical in the guidance it provides on conceptual isues, on diagnosis and on treatment. Most introductory textbooks achieve accessibility for practitioners at the cost of a lack of scientific rigour and questioning; this splendid volume shows well that this price need not be paid. It is thoroughly up to date in its distillation of research findings and it conveys, with both interest and clarity, how modern clinical work is being shaped by the products of scientific investigation. Quite appropriately, the details of the research are not described but the spirit of scientific inquiry pervades the whole of the book. References to a well selected short list of key review papers and chapters are provided, so that readers may both extend their understanding and also assess the evidence for themselves. The account given here, however, does a remarkably good job of selecting from an immense literature the research findings that are of greatest clinical relevance now. I would be surprised if reading this book does not stimulate most people to read further. Equally, I am sure that they will be astonished to discover how little that is important has not already been well covered in this volume. Quite a feat!

Both the authors are experienced clinicians and their wealth of practical knowledge, together with their 'feel' for clinical issues and for patients' needs, comes through on every page. All the major varieties of mental disorders are covered but the approach taken is distinctive in four main respects. To begin with, the book provides very helpful guidance on the details of *how* to do what is needed. This is as evident in the first chapter on assessment as in those dealing with different forms of treatment. Indeed, the description of how clinicians need to think about the questions involved in assessment is masterly despite (or perhaps because of) its brevity. Second, there is a particularly insightful description of the different kinds of risk and protective factors and of how they might operate. Third, the discussion of clinical issues involves an explicitly developmental focus with an accompanying consideration of just how overt disorders relate to the variations in normal development. Finally, the book is skilfully organised to be most helpful to those preparing for professional examinations (with a useful list of 200 multiple choice questions). Remarkably, it achieves this organisation without the drawback of unwarranted dogmatism that mars so many introductory texts. My only regret is that I did not write this excellent book!

Professor Sir Michael Rutter
Honorary Director
MRC Child Psychiatry Unit, Institute of Psychiatry

From the reviews

'The outstanding achievement of this . . . book is that it is comprehensive. . . All clinicians who have the care of children should have some understanding of child psychiatry. This book provides us with an opportunity to review and refresh our knowledge. I hope the book is a great success. It deserves to be.'

Professor Sir David Hull
Paediatrician and Past President of the
Royal College of Paediatrics and Child Health

'A comprehensive but clearly written and accessible text which summarises the major developments in clinical child psychiatry. . . This text will meet the needs of not only trainee child psychiatrists but also trainees in all other disciplines relevant to child mental health.'

Professor William Yule
Clinical Psychologist and Chair of the
Association for Child Psychology and Psychiatry

'The time has come for paediatricians and other members of the child health team to place their rather superficial and disorderly approach on a more systematic base. *Child Psychiatry* fills this need and provides the theoretical background as well as the practical approach.'

Professor Otto Wolff
Paediatrician
Great Ormond Street Hospital, London

Preface

We nearly called this volume *My First Book of Child Psychiatry*. Aware that this may well be a reader's only book on the subject, we have aimed to get straight to the heart of child and adolescent psychiatry. Our goal has been to be brief, clear, practical, thoughtful, up-to-date, scientifically accurate, clinically sound, and relevant for examinations. We have been very encouraged by the exceptionally positive response so far from trainees and senior colleagues from a variety of disciplines.

The chapters are grouped into four sections. Firstly, an introductory section on assessment, classification and epidemiology. Secondly, a section covering each of the main specific disorders and presentations. Thirdly, a section on the major risk factors predisposing to child psychiatric disorders. Finally, a section on the main methods of treatment. Each chapter presents the key facts, concepts and growing points in the area, drawing on clinical experience as well as the latest research findings.

It has been our good fortune to work alongside a diverse and talented group of clinicians and researchers at one of the world's leading child psychiatric centres. We hope we have communicated some of the excitement of being at the 'cutting edge' of a discipline that is increasingly benefiting from advances in subjects as varied as developmental psychology, neurobiology, genetics, social anthropology, linguistics and ethology. As practising clinicians, we have also been keen to make this a book about working with children and families as well as theory. Because successful practitioners need to master techniques as well as concepts, we have included plenty of 'how to' tips on assessment and treatment.

To make the book read as easily as possible, we have not interrupted the text with references. Instead, each chapter ends with suggestions for further reading, providing convenient entry-points into the current literature.

The book has been written with several groups of readers in mind. Trainees in psychiatry, paediatrics and general practice should find it useful to them as an accessible introduction to the subject when they are first working with troubled children; as a continuing source of practical and conceptual guidance when assessing and treating children with unfamiliar disorders; and as a comprehensive textbook when preparing for professional examinations. Trainees from other disciplines – psychology, nursing, social work and education – should find this book meets their needs when working with troubled children, and also helps them to understand psychiatric perspectives on problems that often require interdisciplinary working. Finally, for established professionals in many fields, this book should be an easy way to keep abreast of current thinking, and a convenient source-book for preparing teaching sessions and for reference.

Two hundred multiple choice questions (MCQs) and answers have been provided for trainees approaching professional examinations, as well as for other readers who enjoy quizzes as a way of consolidating their knowledge. Our MCQs are modelled on Membership questions set by the various Royal Colleges, particularly emphasising the examiners' favourite topics.

This book has been greatly strengthened by the comments and suggestions of many colleagues and trainees from a range of disciplines; we are extremely grateful to them all. We are keen to go on improving this book and look to you, our readers, for help. Please do write to us telling us what you liked and what needs changing. What should be cut and what should be expanded? How could we make the book more useful to you? We hope that your advice to us will benefit future readers and, through them, troubled children and their families.

Robert Goodman and Stephen Scott

We dedicate this book
to all children and parents,
especially our own

Child Psychiatry

Robert Goodman

PhD, FRCPsych, MRCP
Reader in Brain and Behavioural Medicine,
Institute of Psychiatry, Honorary Consultant, Maudsley and
Great Ormond Street Hospitals

Stephen Scott

MRCP, MRCPsych, DCH
Senior Lecturer, Institute of Psychiatry,
Consultant, Maudsley Hospital

b

Blackwell
Science

© 1997 by
Blackwell Science Ltd
Editorial Offices:
Osney Mead, Oxford OX2 0EL
25 John Street, London WC1N 2BL
23 Ainslie Place, Edinburgh EH3 6AJ
350 Main Street, Malden
  MA 02148 5018, USA
54 University Street, Carlton
  Victoria 3053, Australia
10, rue Casimir Delavigne
  75006 Paris, France

Other Editorial Offices:

Blackwell Wissenschafts-Verlag GmbH
Kurfürstendamm 57
10707 Berlin, Germany

Blackwell Science KK
MG Kodenmacho Building
7–10 Kodenmacho Nihombashi
Chuo-ku, Tokyo 104, Japan

First published 1997
Reprinted 1998

Set in 10.5/13 Ehrhardt
by DP Photosetting, Aylesbury, Bucks
Printed and bound in Great Britain by
MPG Books Ltd, Bodmin, Cornwall

DISTRIBUTORS

Marston Book Services Ltd
PO Box 269
Abingdon
Oxon OX14 4YN
(Orders: Tel: 01235 465500
         Fax: 01235 465555)

USA
Blackwell Science, Inc.
Commerce Place
350 Main Street
Malden, MA 02148 5018
(Orders: Tel: 800 759 6102
                781 388 8250
         Fax: 781 388 8255)

Canada
Login Brothers Book Company
324 Saulteaux Crescent
Winnipeg, Manitoba R3J 3T2
(Orders: Tel: 204 837 2987
         Fax: 204 837 3116)

Australia
Blackwell Science Pty Ltd
54 University Street
Carlton, Victoria 3053
(Orders: Tel: 03 9347 0300
         Fax: 03 9347 5001)

A catalogue record for this title is available from
the British Library

ISBN 0-632-03885-3

Library of Congress
Cataloging-in-Publication Data
Goodman, Robert, MRCPsych.
    Child psychiatry/Robert Goodman,
Stephen Scott.
      p. cm.
    Includes bibliographical references and
index.
    ISBN 0-632-03885-3
    1. Child psychiatry. 2. Adolescent
psychiatry. I. Scott, Stephen, MRCPsych.
II. Title.
    [DNLM: 1. Mental Disorders–in infancy
& childhood. 2. Mental Disorders–in
adolescence. WS 350 G6535c 1997]
RJ499.G665 1997
618.92'89–dc21
DNLM/DLC
for Library of Congress   97-7393
                                               CIP

For further information on Blackwell Science,
visit our website:
www.blackwell-science.com

Part I
Assessment, Classification and Epidemiology

1 Assessment

For the beginner, a child psychiatric assessment can all too easily become a long and dreary list of topics to be covered and observations to be made – turning the occasion into an aversive experience for all concerned. It is far better to start with a clear idea of the goals and then pursue them flexibly. Ends and means are different: this first part of the chapter deals with ends; the second half of the chapter deals with means, providing some 'how to' tips with suggestions about the order in which to ask things.

FIVE KEY QUESTIONS

A full assessment focuses on five key questions, given in the following list, and remembered by the mnemonic SIRSE, while also engaging the family and laying the foundations for treatment. Carrying out a comprehensive assessment on the first visit is a good target to aim for, unless it results in such a pressured interview that it puts the family off coming again. As long as you are able to engage the family, it is not a disaster if the assessment is incomplete after the first session *provided* you recognise the gaps and fill them in during subsequent sessions. Indeed, all assessments should be seen as provisional, generating working hypotheses that have to updated and corrected over the entire course of your contact with the family. Just as it is a mistake to launch into treatment without an adequate assessment, it is also a mistake to forget that your assessment may need to be revised during the course of treatment. Consider the need for a reassessment if treatment does not work.

- Symptoms   What sort of problem is it?
- Impact   How much distress or impairment does it cause?
- Risks   What factors have initiated and maintained the problem?
- Strengths   What assets are there to work with?
- Explanatory model   What beliefs and expectations do the family bring with them?

Though child psychiatrists and their colleagues may be involved in many types of assessment, these five key questions will be relevant in nearly all cases, albeit with variations in emphasis and approach. Most of the rest of this chapter focuses on an approach that seeks, where possible, to explain the presenting complaint in terms of the child having one or more disorders – leading on to a fuller formulation involving aetiology, prognosis and treatment. For some referrals, however, it may be more appropriate to focus on parenting problems or on the problems of the family system as a whole rather than on the problems of the presenting child.

Symptoms

Most child psychiatric syndromes involve combinations of symptoms (and signs) from four main areas: emotions, conduct, development and relationships. As with any rule of thumb, there are exceptions, most notably schizophrenia and anorexia nervosa. The four domains of symptoms are:

(1) Emotional symptoms
(2) Conduct problems
(3) Developmental delays
(4) Relationship difficulties.

(a) The *emotional symptoms* of interest to child psychiatrists will be very familiar to most mental health trainees. As with adults, it is appropriate to enquire about anxieties and fears (and also about any resultant avoidance). Ask too about misery and, if relevant, about associated depressive features including worthlessness, hopelessness, self-harm, anhedonia, poor appetite, sleep disturbance and lassitude. Classical symptoms of obsessive–compulsive disorder can be present in young children, even preschoolers. One difference in emphasis from adult psychiatry is the need to enquire rather more carefully about 'somatic equivalents' of emotional symptoms, e.g. Monday morning tummy aches may be far more evident than the underlying anxiety about school or separation.

Parental reports are the primary source of information on the emotional symptoms of young children, with the child's own account becoming increasingly important for older children. Somewhat surprisingly, parent and child reports of emotional symptoms often disagree. When faced with discrepant reports, it is sometimes straightforward to decide who to believe. Perhaps the parents have described in convincing detail a string of incidents in which their child's fear of dogs has resulted in panics or aborted outings, while the child's own claim never to be scared of anything seems to be due to a mixture of bravado and a desire to get the interview over with as soon as possible. Alternatively, a teenager's own account may make it clear that she experiences a level of anxiety that interferes with her sleep and concentration even though her parents are unaware of this because she does not confide in them and spends much of her time in her room. In other instances, it is harder to know who to believe – and perhaps it is more sensible to accept that there are multiple perspectives rather than a single truth.

(b) The *conduct problems* that dominate much of child psychiatric practice are less familiar territory for most mental health trainees, as adults with comparable symptoms are more likely to be in prisons than hospitals. Enquiry should focus on three main domains of behaviour: defiant behaviour, often associated with irritability and temper outbursts; aggression; and antisocial behaviours such as stealing, fire-setting and substance abuse. Reports from parents and teachers are likely to be the main source of information on conduct problems, though children and teenagers sometimes tell you about misdeeds that their parents or teachers do not know about. There is only limited value in asking children about their defiant behaviours since children (like adults) often find it hard to recognise when they are being unreasonable, disruptive or irritable, however good they are at recognising these traits in others.

(c) Evaluating *developmental delay* can be particularly hard for new trainees who do not have children of their own or a background in child health. Development complicates what, in adults, would be a simple assessment. Consider a physical analogy. An adult height of one metre is small, whereas a childhood height of one metre may be small, average or large; it obviously depends on the age of the child and, unless you have a growth chart handy, you could easily fail to spot children who were unusually small or tall for their age. The same problem is even more pronounced in the psychological domain. What are you going to make of an attention span of five minutes at different ages? Are you missing children whose speech is immature or excessively grown up for their age? How long should a five-year-old sit still without fidgeting? In the absence of good published norms, you will mostly have to rely on experienced colleagues until you 'get your eye in'. Remember, too, that experienced parents or teachers are rarely concerned without good reason.

The areas of development that are of particular relevance to child psychiatry are: attention and activity regulation; speech and language; play; motor skills; bladder and bowel control; and scholastic attainments, particularly in reading, spelling and mathematics. When judging current levels of functioning, you will be able to draw on direct observations of the child as well as reports from parents and teachers. Asking parents about developmental milestones can tell you about the child's previous developmental trajectory.

(d) Assessing children's *difficulties in social relatedness* is another taxing task, partly because children's relationships change with development. In addition, it is not always clear whether a child's problems getting on with other people reflect primarily on the child or on the other people. For example, if a child with cerebral palsy is unable to make or keep friends, how far does this reflect the child's social ineptness, and how far does it reflect the prejudice of other children?

The most striking impairments in relatedness are seen in the autistic disorders, generally taking one of three forms: an aloof indifference to other people as people; a passive willingness either to play alone or to interact provided others take the initiative and tell them what to do; and an awkward and rather unempathic social interest that tends to put others off because of its gaucheness. Disinhibition and lack of reserve with strangers are prominent in some autistic, hyperkinetic and attachment disorders, and may be accompanied by a pestering, importuning style. In small doses, some of these traits can seem quite charming – after a few minutes acquaintance, you may judge the child to be delightfully frank or open or eccentric. The charm generally palls with longer acquaintance, however, and the history usually makes it clear that the child's manner soon becomes very wearing for the children and adults in regular contact with the child.

Some children have difficulty relating to most social partners, whether adults or children, strangers or friends. Other children have problems with specific types of social relationship, e.g. with attachment or friendship relationships. The problems may even be specific to one important social partner. Thus, most children are specifically attached to a relatively small number of key people, and the quality of a child's attachment – secure, resistant, aloof, disorganised – may vary depending on which of these key people the child is relating to. For example, the attachment may be insecure with the main caregiver but secure with the other caregivers (see Chapter 27). Similar specificity can be seen in sibling relationships.

You can gather information on a child's social relationships from several sources. Observing the family interactions in the waiting room or consulting room can be very helpful. See how the child relates to you during the physical and mental state examinations. If your assessment follows a fairly standardised pattern for all children, it is all the more striking that one child is shy and monosyllabic throughout while another child of the same age greets you as a best friend and wants to climb onto your lap. Also note what might in other circumstances be called the countertransference, e.g. did you find the child irritating? Does the interview leave you feeling exhausted? These are often valuable clues to the feelings the child evokes in many other people. Direct observation is supplemented by the history. Parents can often tell you a lot about their child's relationships from the early years onwards. It is worth getting a teacher's report on the child's peer relationships – but remember that teachers are not always aware of peer problems, even when these are fairly substantial, perhaps because teachers do not usually supervise the playground.

Most patients have symptoms from more than one domain

Only a minority of patients have symptoms restricted to just one domain, but such children do exist. Thus, children with *generalised anxiety disorder* may have pure emotional symptoms, children with *socialised conduct disorder* may have pure conduct problems, and children with *disinhibited attachment disorder* may have pure relationship difficulties. Though many children have pure developmental delays, such as primary enuresis, receptive language disorder or specific reading disorder, these children are not usually seen by child psychiatrists in the absence of other symptoms. Some hyperactive children seen by child psychiatrists do seem to have fairly pure delays in the development of attention and activity control.

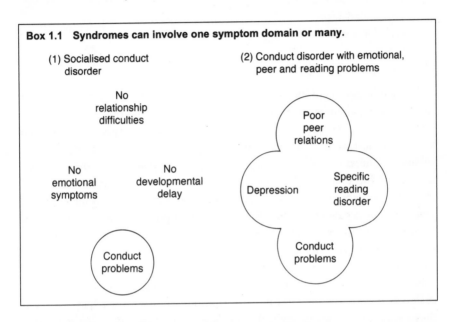

Box 1.1 Syndromes can involve one symptom domain or many.

(1) Socialised conduct disorder

(2) Conduct disorder with emotional, peer and reading problems

Most child psychiatric patients have symptoms from two or more domains. For example, children with conduct disorder also commonly have emotional symptoms, peer problems, and developmental delays, such as specific reading disorder or hyperactivity (Box 1.1).

Autism provides another illustration of symptoms in multiple domains. The core symptoms of autism span two domains, with characteristic patterns of relationship problems and developmental delays (as well as developmental deviance and rigidity). In addition, autistic children commonly display some conduct problems, such as marked temper tantrums, and some emotional problems, such as unusual phobias.

Impact

Judging whether symptoms add up to a disorder rather than a normal variant involves a consideration of the symptoms' impact. In general, you should only diagnose a disorder if the symptoms are having a substantial impact. DSM–III criteria for psychiatric disorders did not include impact; the result is illustrated by a study that found that half of a large representative sample of Puerto Rican children had a psychiatric disorder. This is a ridiculously high rate since most of these children were not considered 'cases' on clinical grounds. This has since been rectified: DSM–IV and the research diagnostic criteria of ICD–10 generally include impact criteria. Impact is judged from:

(1) Social impairment
    (a) family life
    (b) classroom learning
    (c) friendships
    (d) leisure activities
(2) Distress for the child
(3) Disruption for others.

The main measure of impact should be whether the symptoms result in significant social impairment, substantially compromising the child's ability to fulfil normal role expectations in everyday life. The main areas of everyday life to consider are family life, class work, friendships and leisure activities. Two subsidiary measures of impact are also important: distress for the child and disruption for others. Like their adult counterparts, anxious or depressed children are sometimes able to fulfil normal role expectations while experiencing considerable inner anguish. Equally, conduct problems can sometimes lead to substantial disruption for others without resulting in much apparent distress or social impairment for the child. For example, the parents and siblings of children with severe physical or intellectual problems are sometimes remarkably stoical in the face of marked defiance, tantrums, and destructiveness – suffering themselves but making sure that the child does not 'pay for it'. In these instances, it may be clinically sensible to diagnose a disorder as present, and treat it, even though the child is not really socially impaired by the symptoms. Is this a slippery slope to labelling all 'deviants' as psychiatrically ill? We hope not.

Risk factors

Why does the child you are assessing have his or her particular constellation of psychiatric problems? Though the world is full of people who think they do know *the* cause of particular child psychiatric disorders – dietary allergy, lack of discipline, bad genes, poor teaching, hypothalamic damage, unresolved infantile conflicts, etc. – the identification of a single cause for a child psychiatric disorder is rarely scientifically justifiable. There are exceptions. Thus it seems reasonable to say that the compulsive self-biting behaviour in Lesch-Nyhan Syndrome (which can lead to affected children severing their own fingers and extensively damaging their lips and tongue) is caused by a specific genetic deficit resulting in complete deficiency of one of the enzymes involved in purine metabolism. The presence of this inborn error of metabolism seems to guarantee the characteristic behaviour, irrespective of other genetic or environmental factors.

By comparison, most of the 'causes' in child psychiatry are best thought of as risk factors that increase the likelihood of a particular disorder without guaranteeing that it will occur. Thus although exposure to a high level of parental conflict is a risk factor for conduct disorder, many children who are exposed to marital conflict do not develop conduct disorder. Perhaps we need to explain child psychiatric disorders in terms of particular combinations or sequences of risk factors. One such scheme invokes three types of risk factors: predisposing, precipitating and perpetuating factors. The window has a hole in it because the glass was particularly thin and brittle (the predisposing factors), it was hit by a piece of gravel (the precipitating factor), and no one has subsequently replaced the broken pane (the perpetuating factor). A child who has always been rather clingy and has never had many friends (the predisposing factors) refuses to return to school after a row with a friend and a few days off sick with a cold (the precipitating factors). His parents are so worried about his level of distress that they feel it would be harmful to force him to return to school, but every day off makes it harder for him to go back since he falls further behind with his school work and his former playmates find new people to play with (the perpetuating factors). The presence of a disorder can be explained in terms of:

- Predisposing factors
- Precipiating factors
- Perpetuating factors

and the absence of:

- Protective factors.

Even if you do train yourself to think in terms of multiple interacting causes, you will still need to remember how incomplete our present knowledge is. Our current understanding of aetiology will probably look ridiculously simplistic or misguided in a hundred years time (or much sooner). It often helps to admit this to parents: dogmatic insistence that you know the whole truth about causation may be less well received than the more defensible claim that you probably know enough about causation to provide some useful pointers to treatment.

In gearing your assessment to look for or ask about known risk factors, you will have to cover many areas. The traditional focus on family factors is partly justified since our family provides us with our genes and an important part of our environment. Thus a family history of Tourette's syndrome may be of genetic relevance, while a history of parental friction may be of environmental relevance, and a history of parental mental illness could be either. Most children inhabit three rather different social worlds: family, school and peer culture. Do not confine your interest in environmental factors to the social world of the family – school factors such as scapegoating by a teacher and peer factors such as bullying may be at least as important. Adverse life events and more chronic social adversities should also be questioned. Physical and psychological examinations may also unearth previously unrecognised risk factors for psychiatric problems. For example, an adequate history and physical examination may suggest that the child has a dementing disorder, mild cerebral palsy, complex seizures or fetal alcohol syndrome – warranting referral to a specialist for a more definitive view. Psychometric assessment can detect low IQ and specific learning problems – risk factors for various psychiatric problems that may, sadly, have gone undetected in school.

Strengths

If you asked only about symptoms, impact and risk factors, your focus would be almost exclusively negative, dwelling on what is wrong about this child and family. It is also important to establish what is right about this child and family. Identifying protective factors may make it clearer why this child has a mild rather than a severe disorder. It may also be possible to identify protective factors that apply to siblings but not to the referred child that help to explain why only one child in this family has developed a disorder. Relevant protective factors include a sense of worth stemming from being good at something, a close supportive relationship with an adult, and an easy temperament.

Your treatment plan needs to build on the child and family's strengths (and also on the strengths of the child's school and wider social network). Though the *aim* of treatment is determined by what is wrong, choosing the *mode* of treatment often depends on what is right. You should design the treatment to harness the strengths in the child, such as the ability to make friends or respond to praise, and the strengths in the parents, such as an openness to trying new approaches in the family.

If you dwell exclusively on the negatives in a child's life, the child and the family may leave the assessment feeling emotionally battered – and be correspondingly less willing to return. We live in a society that generally blames parents for their children's problems. If a child has a tantrum in the supermarket, most of the bystanders will look reproachfully rather than sympathetically at the accompanying parent. Parents stand accused, and often feel uncertain in their own minds whether they are to blame or not. On the one hand, they are likely to share society's view that parents cause children's problems and most parents can identify many ways in which their child-rearing has been less than perfect. On the other hand, most of the parents you see in clinic will also feel that they are neither better nor worse than many other parents they know whose children seem fine. Many parents are frightened that you will judge them 'guilty as charged' and may be defensive and prickly in anticipation of this. One of your key tasks is to convey that you see them not as fundamentally deficient people but as individuals who, like the rest of us, have strengths as well as weaknesses. An interview presents plenty of opportunities for registering the positive things they and their child do whilst avoiding being patronising. If parents come to feel that you are not against them, they are much more likely to accept the treatment plan you recommend, including suggestions for change on their part. If you ally yourself with the child against the parents – which is a common temptation for beginners – you will probably only succeed in redoubling the parents' criticisms of the child and losing the family from the clinic.

When you meet parents who seem to have particularly glaring weaknesses, it is vital that you put even more effort into identifying their strengths. This is not to say that you should be blind to their problems in parenting – they may need to be the focus of treatment or even the grounds for initiating care proceedings – but you need to remember (for your own sake as well as theirs) that they have their own strengths, often despite harrowing personal backgrounds of their own. Parents have usually put a great deal of effort into parenting. Though successful parents may put in more effort, they also generally get much more back from their children, so failing parents may be putting in more effort per unit reward than successful parents!

It is sometimes helpful to identify the presenting problem as the opposite side of the coin to a valuable strength. For example, a strong-willed child who is seen at the clinic because of defiant and disruptive behaviour at home and at school may also show an admirable determination to succeed in the face of adversity. Similarly, a sensitive child who is prey to all manner of anxieties may show admirable empathy and consideration for others. In each case, identifying a trait as both good and bad rather than as entirely bad may make the trait easier to live with. In addition, the therapeutic task is redefined: it is not to abolish the trait – which is likely to be impossible anyway – but only to reduce the trait's troublesome consequences.

The family's explanatory model

The way we construe children's emotional and behavioural difficulties will depend on our cultural and professional backgrounds. This book draws on a set of *explanatory models* derived from current academic child psychiatry that is empirically orientated. Other professionals, such as social workers, educational psychologists or psychotherapists, may apply a different set of explanatory models, leading to radically different formulations even if they see the same child and family. It is easy to forget that colleagues from other disciplines have different explanatory models – an oversight that can hamper communication no end. The same can be said of communication between professionals and families since professionals are often unaware that families may have distinctive explanatory models of their own, assuming instead that all right-thinking members of the public hold similar, albeit less detailed, views to their own.

Little is yet known about the range of explanatory models that structure the ways in which families from different social and cultural backgrounds think about children's emotional and behavioural difficulties. Nevertheless, it is clear that members of the public often have complex explanatory models that differ substantially from those of doctors and other professionals – as regards aetiology, phenomenology, pathophysiology, natural history and treatment. In other words, families come to clinics with expectations that may differ radically from your own. You should not guess a family's views on the basis of your stereotypes about their class and culture; the only sensible way to find out what they believe is to ask them open-ended questions and listen carefully to their replies.

After you have asked the family about the presenting complaint, it flows naturally to enquire what they make of the problem; what they think it is due to; and how they think it might be investigated or treated. Some families will look puzzled and say that they don't know, that's for you to tell them. Many others will tell you things you could not easily have guessed. You may learn, for example, that the parents of a child with poor concentration fear he has a brain tumour, or think he needs a brain scan, or believe that you will be able to cure the symptoms with hypnosis. If you had not asked them, they might never have told you and they might have gone away disappointed, never to return again. It is also worth asking the parents whether other important people, including grandparents, friends, neighbours, teachers, have expressed strong opinions about causation, investigation or treatment. The child's mother may tell you, for instance, that her mother-in-law has been very insistent that the child's problems have arisen because the mother has always worked and has not spent enough time with her child.

Knowing about people's explanatory models gives you a chance at the end of the assessment to present your views in the way that will be most relevant to them. You can explain that the symptoms are not at all like those of a brain tumour; that a scan would not alter management; and that although you are not a trained hypnotist, even a professional hypnotist would be unlikely to be of much help in this instance. You can also mention that the quality of the day care that they have arranged for their child gives no reason for concern, and there is no scientific basis for linking hyperactivity to working mothers when the quality of alternative care is good. You can say too that you would be very happy to discuss this further with the child's grandmother if the family want you to. Some families hold to their explanatory models with great tenacity, but most families are willing to update their explanatory models if you take the time to present the facts. At the end of a careful assessment in which the family may have invested considerable hope, it would be a great shame if failure to explore the family's explanatory models left you and them at cross-purposes and mutually dissatisfied.

SOME 'HOW TO' TIPS

What means will you employ to answer the five key questions and engage the family? There are no hard and fast rules to suit all clinics, all clinicians, all families and all presenting complaints. This is where good clinical supervision is particularly helpful. Sitting in on assessments carried out by a range of senior colleagues can be very instructive. The rest of the chapter is taken up with a variety of 'how to' suggestions that are guides rather than fixed recipes.

How to: take the history from parents

As a trained clinical interviewer, you should not simply be a speaking questionnaire. If you only want the parents' answers to a fixed series of predetermined questions, a questionnaire would be quicker and easier for them to complete, unless they are poor readers. One style of interviewing, which is known as 'fully structured' or 'respondent-based' interviewing, amounts to little more than a verbally administered questionnaire. The wording of questions is predetermined, and the style of questioning is 'closed', calling for a limited range of possible responses: often a yes–no answer, or a rating of frequency, duration or severity. Questionnaires and fully structured interviews are widely used as research and clinical tools, since they are quick, cheap and easy to administer in a standardised fashion. Their main limitation is that the parents' answers sometimes tell you more about the parents' beliefs (or misunderstandings of the terms used) than about the child.

A different style of interviewing, know as 'semi-structured' or 'interviewer-based', can help you get beyond the parents' *views* to the *observations* on which they are basing their views. The interviewer is expected to ask whatever questions are needed to elicit from parents the information needed for the *interviewer* to decide whether a particular symptom (or impairment or risk factor, etc.) is present or not. In order to do this, the interviewer will often need to use 'open' questions that offer the parents the chance to make a wide range of possible responses. Obtaining detailed descriptions of recent instances of the behaviour in question is usually very helpful.

An example may make this clearer. One of the questions in a questionnaire or fully structured interview might be 'Does your child have concentration problems?' If the parents answered 'Yes', you would still not know whether the child's concentration was objectively poor or whether the parents were setting unrealistically high standards (or had misunderstood the question). A semi-structured approach would use a mixture of open and closed prompts to get the parents to describe, using recent examples, how long the child has been able to persist with specific activities without switching from one thing to another: playing alone, playing with friends, watching television, looking at a book, and so on. You could then make up your own mind from this evidence whether the child's concentration at home was age-appropriate or not.

Similar methods can be used to explore irritability, fearfulness or any other reported area of problems. It is also sometimes relevant to explore why parents are not concerned. For instance, if teachers report major problems with concentration but parents do not, it is important to explore whether the child really does concentrate adequately when out of school, or whether the parents simply have unusually low expectations.

Semi-structured interviewing is a valuable technique but you do have to be careful not to overdo it or the interview will go on for hours! One option is to use questionnaires or fully structured interviews to get an overall view and then use semi-structured interviewing to obtain more details about the most relevant aspects of the case. Finding the time to get parents to describe their child's typical day, perhaps yesterday, can often be a particularly illuminating window, not only on symptoms and any resultant impairment but also on family life, child-rearing tactics and expressed emotion.

Here is one possible scheme for taking a history from parents:

(1) *Presenting complaint*
    When did it begin? When was he last completely well or not doing it? How does it show itself? How often? When? Always get specific examples rather than accept general statements. What is going on just before it happens? After? How do you respond? What's the result? What effect is it having on the rest of the family? Why are you coming about it now?

    • Review of other symptoms: emotions, conduct, attention and activity, somatic – sleeping, eating, bladder and bowels, pains, tics.

(2) *Current functioning*
    • Typical day's activities: Dressing and eating, play and leisure, going to bed, sleeping.

    • Social relationships:
      Friends: Got any? What exactly do they do together? Do they go to each other's house? How often? Shy? Able to take turns? Leader or follower? Sexuality?
      Adults: How does child get on with each parent? With other carers? How do they feel about the child? Any good times? When?
      Siblings: Who does she spend time with? Like? Dislike? Jealous?

(3) *Family history*
    • Composition: Draw a family tree ('genogram'). Ask a few details about each relative, including medical and psychiatric problems. For members of the immediate family, record age, occupation, what they are like.

    • Relationships: How do the parents get on together. Do they support each other? What are their expectations for the child? What were their own childhoods like? Do they agree on rules and how discipline should be applied? Arguments? How do the children get on together? Who is close to whom? Who gets into most trouble? Who least? How are they treated differently?

- Circumstances: Housing. Debt. Have circumstances changed recently? Has there been contact with social services?

(4) *Personal history*
- Birth and infancy: Planned and wanted? What sort of baby was he or she? Milestones – were these earlier or later than siblings or friend's baby.

- Schools: Names and dates. Difficulties in classroom, playground or small groups? Academic functioning: their position in class, whether they are underachieving, whether they are receiving, or ought to be receiving, special help. Social functioning: friends, type of play.

- Physical health: Fits and faints, illnesses, hospital or psychiatric contact.

How to: see the child alone

Do not rush into difficult topics – it is obviously best to engage with the child first by focusing initially on pleasant and neutral topics or activities. Equally, do not become so focused on making the interview fun that you avoid difficult topics entirely (though you may want to postpone some difficult topics for a second interview).

- Children over five: You should both sit down. It is often helpful to ask the child to do a drawing. Chat and use directed questioning.
- Children under five: Observe play, play too, chat, use fewer directed questions.

Aims

(1) This is a useful opportunity to observe:
  (a) Activity and attention. Is the child squirmy and fidgety? Does he or she keep getting out of the chair and wandering about? Is it hard to get him or her to persist in a task? Is he or she easily distracted by extraneous stimuli?

  (b) Quality of social interaction. Does he or she show too much or too little anxiety about coming with you initially? Is the child interested in social interaction? Does he or she make good eye contact? Does he or she talk to you or at you? Is he or she inappropriately friendly, overfamiliar or cheeky? What feelings does the interaction evoke in you?

  (c) Developmental level. Consider complexity of language, ideas, drawing and play.

(2)   You can enquire about emotional symptoms. It is not unusual for older children to be experiencing considerable anxiety or misery without their parents being aware of this. Children rarely volunteer information on their obsessions and compulsions unless asked directly – they are often ashamed to admit to such 'mad' symptoms. Much the same applies to symptoms of post-traumatic stress disorder.

(3)   Ask about friends, teasing and bullying; the child's account may differ significantly from the parents' and teachers' accounts.

(4)   It is often worth asking a general question about undisclosed abuse or traumas. 'Sometimes nasty or frightening things happen to children, and they find it difficult to tell anyone about it. Has anything like that ever happened to you?' Sometimes it is also necessary to ask about abuse more directly.

(5)   What does that child make of his or her biography and current life situation? What account can the child give of the problems that led to referral? In a first interview you will only be able to explore a few themes, but this will often give you a better feel for the child. It is sometimes helpful to ask the child for a blow by blow description of a typical day, or for a detailed account of the last episode of 'problem behaviour'. 'What happens when you are naughty?' 'How does mummy react when you do that?' It is often revealing to get a child's view of potentially significant life events such as the death of an uncle or grandparent (even if the parents have previously told you that the child was unaffected).

(6)   The assessment may lead on to direct work with the child. This is your first opportunity to engage the child. At the very least, the interview should allay a child's fears that seeing a professional is bound to be unpleasant. Many children come to the clinic with all sorts of frightening expectations, sometimes because their parents have used referral to the clinic as a threat. They may fear, for example, that they will be told off, taken into care, admitted to the ward, or have painful things done to them. Remember to explain what will happen and allay fears whenever possible.

How to: observe the family as a whole

Are the parents supervising the children and setting limits if necessary? How sensitive and supportive are the parents if the child shows signs of anxiety or distress? How much warmth and criticism do the parents express in relation to the child? (NB warmth and criticism are independent, not the opposite sides of the same coin).

Is there overt marital friction? Do they countermand or back one another up? Who does the talking? Do they notice if they disagree? If so, do they reach a consensus?

How do siblings relate to one another? How do the parents treat the children differently from one another? Are there particular alignments within the family? For example, a mother's child or a father's child.

How does the child behave in relation to the parents? Possibilities include exploring from a secure base, interrupting their conversation, ignoring or challenging their requests, and watching them at a distance.

What does the child do with the available toys? What can you note about the form of play? Is it imaginative? What developmental level does it suggest? Are there any notable themes in the content of the play (e.g. sexualised doll play)? Beware of overhasty interpretation of small snatches of play.

How to: obtain information from teachers

Children's behaviour in school is often markedly different from their behaviour at home. Although parents can often tell you if teachers have relayed any complaints or concerns about their child, it is best to get the information first hand from the school if at all possible, provided parents are willing to agree to your contacting the school.

Having identified someone to contact, you can write and ask for their comments and a copy of a recent school report. Asking the teacher to complete a brief behavioural screening questionnaire is often helpful. Since teachers have considerable experience of what to expect of children of any given age, their views are generally accurate. Whereas parents' answers to questionnaires often need to be explored through semi-structured interviewing, it is usually appropriate to take teachers' answers at face value. It is sometimes helpful, though, to get back to the teacher by 'phone to explore one or two particular issues in greater depth. Though teachers are generally excellent observers, they may miss or misconstrue some symptoms. In a busy classroom, disruptive behaviours are generally a lot more obvious than emotional symptoms. Consequently, teachers may miss anxiety or depression unless these have resulted in a dramatic decrease in the quality or quantity of the child's work. Subdued children may even seem better behaved than before. Thus in one study, the rate of problems reported by teachers on a standardised questionnaire went down in the aftermath of a disaster. Recognising hyperactivity in the classroom can also pose problems if the child has learning difficulties or dislikes academic work. If children are unable to do the work or lack any interest in the work, they will often seem inattentive or distracted in class. Imagine how any child would behave if placed in a class taught in a language they did not understand – they too might well appear distracted or wander round the room at any excuse! What you really want to know to make a diagnosis of hyperactivity is whether children are also restless and inattentive when engaged in tasks that are within their capability and that interest them. Sadly, some children are never engaged in any such tasks at school. Finally, as noted earlier, teachers are sometimes unaware of problems in peer relationships because children who seem averagely popular with their classmates in class may be isolated or victimised on the playground without teachers necessarily spotting this.

How to: do a physical examination

Systematic observation of the child's physical features and skills is an *essential* part of a complete child psychiatric assessment. You are primarily looking for:

(1) Evidence of a physical disorder that definitely or probably affects the brain. Recognising that there is a 'hardware fault' is important – characterising the type of disorder is less important provided the child is referred to an expert. Relevant evidence includes abnormal neurological signs, dysmorphic features, and cutaneous stigmata of a neurocutaneous syndrome.

(2) Signs of neglect or abuse. Observing, weighing and measuring the child, and plotting the values on an appropriate growth chart, can provide evidence of injury and growth failure.

Medical trainees should not discard their hard-won medical skills; if the child is present at the assessment, you should always set aside some time for observing the child with a 'medical hat' on. Even if you never lay hands (or tendon hammer or stethoscope) on the child, there is much that you can learn just by looking at the child's face, hands, gait and play. So during the time you see the child – in the waiting room, in the family interview, or in the individual interview – take some time off from thinking about family relationships or psychiatric symptoms and consciously concentrate on the child's physical state. Do they have a dysmorphic syndrome? (If you do not spot this soon after you first set eyes on them, you will be so used to the way they look that you will probably never notice.) Do they have a neurological syndrome? Are they peering at things or straining after sounds? Are there any visible bruises, burns, bites or other possible signs of abuse?

Which children need neurological examinations?

Ideally you should examine all children, if only to practice your technique and learn the range of normal variation. If time constraints prevent this, you should at least examine children with one or more of the following features:

(1) History of seizures or regression
(2) Developmental delay or mental retardation
(3) Abnormal gait
(4) Does not play well using both hands
(5) Dysmorphic features
(6) Skin signs of a neurocutaneous disorder
(7) Other suspicious features, e.g. dysarthria.

A basic neurological examination

Though some items will be impossible with very young children, aim to include the following in your neurological examination:

(1) Measure head circumference and plot on chart.
(2) Observe walk, run, 'walking a tightrope', hop.
(3) Observe standing with feet together, arms outstretched, eyes closed.
(4) Check eye, face, and tongue movements.
(5) Move and shake all four limbs (as part of a game) to assess tone.
(6) Test strength: pyramidal weakness is most evident from testing abduction at shoulder, extension at wrist, abduction of fingers, dorsiflexion of ankle and big toe.
(7) Test reflexes.
(8) Test coordination: finger–nose, finger–thumb, rapid tapping or 'piano playing', put cap on pen or thread a bead.

If you find an abnormality (and asymmetries are often easier to detect than bilateral changes), the child probably needs further evaluation by a paediatrician or paediatric neurologist. Similarly, if you suspect visual or hearing problems, it is essential to ensure that the child is referred to an appropriate clinic.

Congenital syndromes

There are hundreds of these, only some of which have known chromosomal, genetic or environmental causes. When should you suspect one? The best clues are dysmorphic features, such as funny looking facial features or fingers, and extreme values for height, weight and head circumference (below 3rd or above 97th centile). They should also be sought whenever mental retardation is present. Three examples:

(1) *Fragile X syndrome*. Probably the most common cause of inherited mental retardation. Although once said to affect about 1 in 1000 births, more recent estimates based on DNA analysis suggest that the rate may be closer to 1 in 5000. It affects both males and females, though the degree of intellectual impairment tends to be greater in males. Physical characteristics are highly variable, but may include a long face, prominent ears, wide jaw, hyperextensible joints and large testes after puberty. Equally, physical appearance may be normal. Fragile X is associated with gaze avoidance/social anxiety and hyperactivity, but the link with autism remains controversial. It is due to an excess of trinucleotide repeats at a specific site on the long arm of the X chromosome and may be detected by direct DNA analysis.

(2) *Fetal alcohol syndrome*. Affects up to 1 in 300 births. May cause up to 10% of mild mental retardation. Low height, weight and head

circumference from birth onwards. Short palpebral fissures, hypoplastic philtrum. Associated with hyperactivity.

(3) *Sotos syndrome* ('Cerebral gigantism'). Sporadic. Excessive height, head circumference and bone age, particularly when young. High forehead with frontal bossing, prominent jaw, hypertelorism, and downslanting eyes. Clumsy. Most have mild or borderline mental retardation. Associated with hyperactivity and autistic problems.

The neurocutaneous disorders

These disorders involve characteristic combinations of brain and skin abnormalities (reflecting their shared ectodermal origins). Recognising the skin signs allows you to infer a 'hardware' defect. The commonest three neurocutaneous syndromes are:

(1) *Tuberous sclerosis.* This is an autosomal dominant disorder with variable penetrance and expression. It is often a new mutation. Skin lesions include: hypopigmented leaf-shaped patches from birth, best seen with UV light (Woods light); the adenoma sebaceum butterfly rash on face, rarely evident before two years, but present in half by five years; a rough irregular 'shagreen' patch over lumbar area; and lumps (periungual fibromata) in and around finger and toe nails. There is a high rate of severe mental retardation, infantile spasms, and other seizures. Autistic and hyperactive features are common in affected children, particularly if they have had infantile spasms.

(2) *Neurofibromatosis-1* is transmitted as an autosomal dominant with variable expression. Skin lesions include café au lait patches which increase in size and number with age (so that by adulthood the presence of over five patches of over 1.5 cm diameter is highly suggestive); axillary freckling; and cutaneous and subcutaneous nodules in the distribution of cutaneous nerves appearing in later childhood. Various neuropsychiatric manifestations are reported but unconfirmed.

(3) *Sturge-Weber syndrome* is usually sporadic. There is a port-wine naevus from birth, involving the forehead and variable amounts of the lower face. It is usually unilateral but can be bilateral. The ipsilateral hemisphere is affected, resulting in seizures, hemiplegia, and mental retardation, plus variable neuropsychiatric features.

Subject reviews

Cox, A.D. (1994) Interviews with parents. In *Child and Adolescent Psychiatry: Modern Approaches*, 3rd edn (M. Rutter, E. Taylor and L. Hersov, eds) Blackwell Science, Oxford, pp. 34–50.

Angold, A. (1994) Clinical interviewing with children and adolescents. In *Child and Adolescent Psychiatry: Modern Approaches*, 3rd edn (M. Rutter, E. Taylor and L. Hersov, eds) Blackwell Science, Oxford, pp. 51–63.

2 Classification

DIAGNOSTIC GROUPINGS: THE PRINCIPLES

Making it useful

Classification should be an aid to communication and research rather than a 'train spotting' exercise conducted for its own sake. Classifying a child's disorder should be more than a mere 'naming of parts'; it should provide helpful pointers to: aetiology; associated problems (thereby directing further enquiries and investigations); choice of treatment; and prognosis. Ideally, the same classification would be useful for all these purposes. In practice, however, this is not always the case. For example, schizophrenia and schizotypal personality disorder are most sensibly classified separately as far as choice of treatment is concerned. From the perspective of genetic aetiology, however, a combined category of 'schizophrenia spectrum disorder' arguably makes more sense.

How do we decide whether a diagnostic scheme is following nature or imposing arbitrary divisions, whether it is 'carving nature at the joints' or hacking blindly through bones? To start with, a diagnostic category is unlikely to be useful unless individuals with that diagnosis differ significantly from individuals with other diagnoses. These differences must extend well beyond the defining characteristics of the diagnostic group. In the case of conduct disorder, for example, we need to know that children with conduct disorder differ from children with other psychiatric disorders not just in having more conduct problems (which is simply a consequence of the definitions used) but in other respects as well, e.g. sex ratio, age of onset, socioeconomic status, or association with scholastic problems. Furthermore, at least some of the validating features that distinguish children with different diagnoses should be clinically relevant. Thus if the children with two diagnoses differ only in sex ratio and socioeconomic status, the two diagnoses should be merged rather than kept separate. Demographic variables are certainly worth examining, but some of the differences between diagnostic groups should be more immediately relevant to aetiology, associated problems, treatment response, or prognosis.

It is possible to have satisfactory diagnostic categories but an unsatisfactory overall classification. This is true when too many cases fail to meet the criteria for any category, or have to be fitted into 'atypical' or 'miscellaneous' categories.

An ideal classification is as valid *and* as comprehensive as possible, but these two aims sometimes pull in opposite directions.

Phenomenology above all

The classification of both child and adult psychopathology has increasingly focused on the presenting features of each disorder rather than on the supposed aetiology or pathogenesis. When disorders are defined in this way, it is possible to study aetiology and pathogenesis with an open mind. Diagnostic categories based on pathogenesis, such as 'minimal brain damage' or 'reactive psychosis', have generally impeded rather than facilitated clinical and research progress. For similar reasons, recent classifications of epilepsy have also emphasised presenting features rather than the supposed organic underpinnings, e.g. 'complex partial seizures' rather than 'temporal lobe epilepsy'. Although most child psychiatric disorders are now defined on the basis of phenomenology alone, a few disorders such as 'reactive attachment disorder' and 'post-traumatic stress disorder' are defined both in terms of phenomenology and the supposed cause.

Dimensions or categories?

Some aspects of childhood psychopathology seem to reflect extreme values on a continuum that extends into the normal range, with many (or all) children exhibiting lesser degrees of the same features. Is the imposition of a cut-off between normality and abnormality simply an arbitrary but convenient way of converting a dimension into a category? Sometimes this is so. In other cases, though, individuals with extreme values are genuinely a case apart. There are three possible indications of discontinuities between normal and extreme values. Firstly, the distribution may be bimodal, e.g. with a subsidiary hump in the tail of the main distribution (as for severe mental retardation). Secondly, there may be a threshold effect. In the case of behavioural inhibition, for example, marked inhibition as a toddler predicts continuing shyness whereas moderate inhibition has no such predictive value. Finally, individuals with extreme and less extreme values on some particular scale may differ qualitatively in other important respects. Thus mild mental retardation is often associated with social disadvantage and is not commonly associated with neurological abnormalities – whereas severe mental retardation is less commonly associated with social disadvantage and much more often associated with neurological abnormalities.

To complicate matters further, dimensional and categorical classifications of the same phenomenon are sometimes both valuable, but for different purposes. Blood cholesterol provides a convenient example. There is a dose-response relationship between cholesterol level and the risk of ischaemic heart disease, with most of the attributable risk in the population being due to the large number of individuals with 'high normal' values rather than to the small number of individuals with extremely high values. In this respect, high cholesterol is best treated as a dimensional rather than a categorical disorder. At the same time, individuals with extremely high levels of cholesterol are a distinctive category from an aetiological point of view, having a Mendelian rather than a multifactorial–polygenic disorder.

Identifying dimensions and categories

Multivariate statistical techniques now exist to help identify dimensions and categories of disorder. Though complex in detail, the general principles underlying factor analyses and cluster analyses are relatively easy to understand without having to go into the mathematics (see Boxes 2.1 and 2.2). Factor analyses are used to identify dimensions while cluster analyses identify categories. Whereas factor analyses classify *attributes* of an individual, cluster analyses classify the *individuals themselves*.

Box 2.1   A do-it-yourself factor analysis.

Look at the following list of measures that could be made on a sample of adults. Group these measures in such a way that they correspond to two dimensions:

- Height
- Shoe size
- Size of vocabulary

- Ability to complete puzzles
- Shoulder-to-elbow length
- Skill at mental arithmetic.

You will have had no difficulty in grouping height, shoe size, and shoulder-to-elbow length as highly correlated measures that tap an underlying dimension that could be labelled 'linear growth'. The remaining three measures are also highly correlated with one another and tap the underlying dimension we normally label 'intelligence'. The two dimensions are almost independent – you do not expect much of a correlation between the two groups of variables, e.g. between height and size of vocabulary. Congratulations – you have carried out a factor analysis using your intuitive knowledge of correlated and uncorrelated measures to identify the underlying dimensions.

Pervasive or situational?

For hyperactivity problems, and perhaps for other types of problem too, diagnostic schemes increasingly emphasise the distinction between pervasive and situational disorders. Pervasive disorders are evident in a wide variety of everyday settings (e.g. at home and at school), whereas situational disorders are only evident in a restricted range of settings (e.g. at home but not at school). Pervasiveness suggests that constitutional factors in the child are paramount, while situation specificity suggests that it is more important to establish what is special about that particular environment (or that particular informant).

Unfortunately, the term 'pervasive' is used in two very different ways in discussions of child psychiatric disorders. Pervasive hyperactivity or pervasive misery refer to problems that are present in a range of different settings. In the

---

Box 2.2   A do-it-yourself cluster analysis.

Look at the next list of different animals and divide them into groups:

- Tortoise
- Duck-billed platypus
- Cat
- Snail

- Dolphin
- Crocodile
- Mouse
- Giant squid.

You will probably have identified some of the key features and limitations of a cluster analysis. Firstly, you may have noticed that how you grouped the animals depended on what features you concentrated on. If you had focused on measures of size and habitat, you might have grouped dolphins, crocodiles and giant squid together as large aquatic animals, and snails and mice together as small terrestrial animals. If, however, you concentrated on morphological and physiological measures, you would have generated a more typically zoological taxonomy, e.g. generating a mollusc grouping comprising snails and giant squid. A second notable feature of cluster analysis is that the method does not tell you how many groups to identify. For instance, you could have gone for a 'two group' solution (e.g. mollusc v. vertebrate) or a 'three group' solution (e.g. mollusc v. reptile v. mammal). You have to decide for yourself what degree of lumping or splitting is most appropriate (which depends on what use you plan to make of the classification). Finally, the case of the duck-billed platypus with its mixture of reptilian and mammalian features is a reminder that some individuals fall midway between neighbouring categories. It is somewhat arbitrary whether they are assigned to either of the neighbouring categories or to a category of their own.

---

term 'pervasive developmental disorder', however, 'pervasive' refers primarily to the fact that multiple domains of development are affected by autistic disorders (in contrast to the specific developmental disorders affecting just one domain of development, e.g. reading or speech). This is confusing since both sorts of developmental disorder – pervasive and specific – are pervasive in the sense of being present in a range of different settings.

Classifying disordered individuals or disordered families?

Diagnosis of the 'identified patient' might be focusing attention on the wrong organisational level, e.g. on one family member rather than on the family system as a whole. Conversely, family therapists might be making the opposite error in their formulations. Multiaxial diagnostic systems potentially provide the best of both worlds since they can record abnormalities at both the individual and the family level. Unfortunately, there is no widely accepted and well validated system for classifying disordered families.

DIAGNOSTIC GROUPINGS: CURRENT PRACTICE

ICD–10 and DSM–IV

There are two main classifications in current use: the International Classification of Diseases (ICD) of the World Health Organization, and the Diagnostic and Statistical Manual (DSM) of the American Psychiatric Association. There used to be many differences between the two schemes but the latest versions (ICD–10 and DSM–IV) have converged on very similar classifications. It is worth noting that ICD–10 comes as a clinical version that provides clinical descriptions and somewhat impressionistic diagnostic *guidelines* for each disorder, and as a research version that provides more clearly defined diagnostic *criteria* – often identical to those used by DSM–IV. This agreement owes at least as much to improved international collaboration as to increased scientific knowledge. Fashion continues to be important in classification and there are likely to be minor and major revisions of the schemes for many years yet. Our current ideas are like early maps of largely unexplored territory – better than nothing provided you do not take the details too seriously.

Operationalised diagnoses: pluses and minuses

DSM–IV and the research version of ICD–10 both provide operationalised diagnostic criteria for many disorders. For each of these disorders, there are clear criteria that must be fulfilled if the diagnosis is to be made. The main advantage of this approach is that different clinicians and researchers are more likely to be referring to similar conditions when they use a particular diagnostic label. There are disadvantages, however. The DSM and ICD criteria can come to seem like Holy Writ, making it easy to forget that the criteria are often built on very shaky foundations. They have become a straightjacket as well as an aid for clinicians and researchers. Furthermore, many children who clearly do have psychiatric disorders – since they have symptoms that result in substantial distress, disruption or social impairment – fail to meet the full criteria for an operationalised diagnosis and have to be given one of the 'not otherwise specified' labels. Most of these children have partial or undifferentiated syndromes. Children with partial syndromes have some of the features of operationalised disorders but not enough to reach the diagnostic threshold. For example, many children have pronounced autistic features but fall short of the full criteria for autism. Children with undifferentiated syndromes have a mixture of symptoms from different operationalised disorders but do not reach the diagnostic threshold for any one of them. This may apply, for instance, to children with a mixture of worries, fears, misery and somatic complaints. Yet other children fall between the cracks of the current schemes, having constellations of problems that have not yet been recognised; the mapping of child psychiatry still has a long way to go.

The main diagnostic groupings

Three broad diagnostic groupings are particularly relevant to child psychiatrists (Table 2.1). The emotional disorders are also sometimes described as internalising disorders, dating back to the notion that 'stresses' could be turned

Table 2.1 The three main diagnostic groupings.

Emotional disorders	Disruptive behaviour disorders	Developmental disorders
• Anxiety disorders • Phobias • Depression • Obsessive–compulsive disorder • Some somatisation	• Conduct disorder • Oppositional defiant disorder • Hyperactivity	• Speech/language delay • Reading delay • Autistic disorders • Mental retardation • Enuresis and encopresis

inwards (internalised), leading to worries, fears, misery, stomach-aches etc. Similarly, the disruptive behaviour disorders are sometimes described as externalising disorders, with the notion that 'stresses' can also be turned outwards (externalised), resulting in disruptive, defiant, aggressive or antisocial behaviours that impinge on others.

The developmental disorders are a heterogeneous group characterised by delays or abnormalities in the development of functions that normally unfold in a predictable sequence as a result of biological maturation. The partition of developmental disorders between different disciplines has largely been determined by history and convenience. Conventionally, some developmental disorders, most notably the autistic disorders, are considered primary psychiatric disorders. Enuresis is sometimes considered a child psychiatric problem, though there is little justification for this practice. Most developmental disorders are not considered psychiatric disorders themselves but are covered in this book because they are important risk factors for child psychiatric disorders.

The three main groupings overlap. Hyperactivity, for example, is usually grouped in the disruptive behaviour disorders, though it could equally be considered a disorder in the development of attention and activity control. There is also an overlap between emotional disorders and disruptive behavioural disorders. For instance, many children present with a mixture of disruptive and depressive symptoms.

Opinions differ on the extent to which it is helpful to subdivide the main groupings. Until relatively recently, for example, few clinicians saw much merit in subdividing the emotional disorders into different subgroups, and ICD–9 offered little opportunity to do so. Of late, however, the pendulum has swung from lumping to splitting, and both ICD–10 and DSM–IV offer a multitude of possible subtypes of emotional disorder. The pendulum may swing again since splitting has probably gone too far; it is distinctly unusual to find any child with a 'pure' version of any of the new diagnoses.

The swing of the pendulum has also been evident in the extent to which children are regarded as being 'little adults' as far as diagnosis is concerned. There are two polar views of childhood: one view holds that children are radically different from adults, rather like tadpoles and frogs; the other view holds that children and adults are fundamentally similar. As far as psychiatric classification goes, the 'tadpole and frog' view used to dominate, but this is being eroded. For the emotional disorders, adult-type diagnoses such as dysthymia or generalised anxiety disorder are used where possible, though there are still a few childhood-specific disorders such as separation anxiety disorder. The developmental disorders and disruptive behavioural disorders remain childhood-specific.

Finally, it is important to remember that child mental health problems are not limited to the three main groupings. There are inevitably disorders that do not fit into this neat tripartite classification: early-onset schizophrenia, anorexia nervosa, disinhibited attachment disorder, Tourette's syndrome, and many others. In addition, many child mental health professionals currently spend much of their time on tasks that do not necessarily involve a child with a formal psychiatric disorder. This is often the case, for example, when assessing dysfunctional families, juvenile offenders, or the victims of abuse.

Multiaxial diagnosis

Diagnostic labels are a useful aid to clinical and research work, allowing similar cases to be grouped together. Sometimes, however, being forced to settle on just one label is too restricting. Should this patient be labelled as having autism or mental retardation? Often it will be essential to record both. This idea has been taken further in the multiaxial assessment that is an optional part of DSM–IV, and by the multiaxial version of ICD–10. In these multiaxial schemes, each axis reflects one important aspect of the child's presentation (Table 2.2).

Table 2.2   The multiaxial schemes of ICD–10 and DSM–IV.

ICD–10 axis	DSM–IV axis	Aspect of the child
1	I	*Psychiatric disorder* e.g. separation anxiety disorder
2	I	*Specific delays in development* e.g. reading disorder
3	II	*Intellectual level* e.g. mild mental retardation
4	III	*Medical conditions* e.g. epilepsy
5	IV	*Psychosocial adversity* e.g. institutional upbringing
6	V	*Adaptive functioning* e.g. serious social disability

Though many people would regard five or six axes as rather too much of a good thing, the scheme does have advantages. It is not necessary to decide whether the child has conduct disorder, specific reading disorder or mental retardation; if the child has all three, each can be coded. Equally, it is not necessary to decide if one or more of these problems is due to the child's epilepsy or institutional upbringing: these are coded whether or not they seem to be causes (thereby capturing data that can eventually be used to explore the association statistically). The final axis provides a means for recording how far the child's psychiatric and developmental problems interfere with his or her everyday life. The five axes of DSM–IV do the same job as the six axes of ICD–

10 because DSM–IV allows multiple diagnoses on its axis I, an axis that encompasses both psychiatric disorders and specific developmental disorders.

Subject reviews

Cantwell, D.P. and Rutter, M. (1994) Classification: conceptual issues and substantive findings. In *Child and Adolescent Psychiatry: Modern Approaches*, 3rd edn (M. Rutter, E. Taylor & L. Hersov, eds) Blackwell Science, Oxford, pp. 3–21.
Volkmar, F.R. and Schwab-Stone, M. (1996) Childhood disorders in DSM–IV. *Journal of Child Psychology and Psychiatry*, 37, 779–784.

Further reading

American Psychiatric Association (1994) *Diagnostic and Statistical Manual of Mental Disorders, 4th ed; DSM–IV*. American Psychiatric Association, Washington DC.
Taylor, E. *et al.* (1986) Conduct disorder and hyperactivity: I & II. *British Journal of Psychiatry*, 149, 760–777. (This elegant study used factor and cluster analyses to identify dimensions and categories respectively, and then validated the findings by examining associated features, developmental history and treatment response.)
World Health Organization (1993) *The ICD–10 Classification of Mental and Behavioural Disorders: Diagnostic Criteria for Research*. World Health Organization, Geneva.

3 Epidemiology

Epidemiology can be defined as the study of the distribution of disorders and associated factors in defined populations. The defined population may be a representative community sample, but it might also be a high-risk or particularly informative sample, e.g. all children with hemiplegic cerebral palsy in London, or all children living in an area with high lead pollution.

ADVANTAGES OF AN EPIDEMIOLOGICAL APPROACH

(1) Essential to estimate incidence and prevalence – relevant to service needs.

(2) Being free (or freer) of referral bias, epidemiological studies are better than clinic-based studies as sources of accurate information about demographic characteristics, associated problems, and natural history. All these benefits are important for studies aiming to improve classification. They are also relevant to aetiology, with causal relationships being suggested, but not proven, by epidemiological associations that are strong, dose-related, and persistent despite controlling for 'confounders' such as socioeconomic status. The power of epidemiological studies to distinguish between causal and non-causal associations is increased when the study is longitudinal or capitalises on a 'natural experiment' such as adoption, twin birth or migration.

(3) Epidemiological studies (e.g. of individuals exposed to some particular risk) are useful for examining protective factors. For example, why do some children remain well adjusted despite exposure to acrimonious marital conflict? Clinic-based studies are almost bound to miss the children who have benefited most from exposure to protective factors.

EPIDEMIOLOGICAL STUDIES ARE NOT ALWAYS THE BEST APPROACH

(1) A detailed study of a few (unrepresentative) cases may be more instructive than a superficial study of a large and representative population. Understanding phenylketonuria or general paresis of the insane did not require an epidemiological approach.

(2)   Epidemiological studies rarely address pathogenesis – different approaches are needed to clarify the processes involved.

(3)   In practice, epidemiological studies rarely include the evaluation of an intervention.

STAGES IN AN EPIDEMIOLOGICAL STUDY

(1)   *Define* the population to be studied: catchment area; inclusion criteria; everyone *v.* random sample *v.* stratified random sample. Examples include a random 1 in 4 sample of three-year-olds living in a London borough, and all children with new-onset severe head injuries in South East England.

(2)   *Identify* individuals who meet the criteria. For community samples, identification is often via some sort of population register (e.g. for schools or immunisations). For rare disorders or risks, identification is often via agencies who are particularly likely to be in contact with relevant individuals, e.g. doctors, special schools, voluntary organizations. Use of multiple sources (known as 'multiple ascertainment') is likely to identify more relevant individuals than use of any one source. Even with multiple ascertainment, there is still the risk of missing some affected individuals who have never been diagnosed or sent to a special school. There is no straightforward way of estimating the size of this problem.

(3)   *Recruit* identified individuals. It is far easier to spot problems with recruitment than problems with identification – problems with recruitment show up as low participation rates. Ideally, all studies should compare participants and non-participants on any available information.

(4)   *Assess* subjects. There are two main possibilities: full assessment of all subjects, or use a two-stage procedure:
  (a)   Use single or multiple screening tests (e.g. parent, teacher, or self-report questionnaires) to divide the sample up into 'screen positive' and 'screen negative' subjects.
  (b)   Fully assess a mixture of 'screen positive' and 'screen negative' subjects, sampling disproportionately more of the former (e.g. 100% of 'screen positive' and a randomly chosen 50% of 'screen negative' subjects). Inclusion of a random sample of 'screen negative' subjects makes it possible to determine how often the screening procedure generates *false* negatives.

EPIDEMIOLOGICAL FINDINGS IN CHILD PSYCHIATRY

The first major epidemiological study of psychiatric disorders in childhood was carried out by Michael Rutter and his colleagues on the Isle of Wight over 30 years ago. The methods and findings of this first Isle of Wight study are summarised in Box 3.1. It is hardly an exaggeration to say that this was the beginning of scientific child psychiatry. By and large, the Isle of Wight findings have withstood the test of time remarkably well, with subsequent epidemiological studies confirming the main findings and extending them in various directions.

Comparable epidemiological surveys have since been carried out all over the world – each is of local interest, but some have attracted international attention because of their wide implications for service provision and aetiology. Particularly notable studies have been carried out in Ontario (Canada), Dunedin (New Zealand), Christchurch (New Zealand), the Great Smoky Mountains (USA) and Puerto Rico.

While the first Isle of Wight study focused on middle childhood, other studies have examined different age groups. Examples include the Preschool to School study of problems in early childhood and their consequences (Box 20.1) and the Isle of Wight study of adolescence (Box 21.1). Whereas the Isle of Wight studies covered a broad range of psychiatric disorders, some subsequent studies have focused on specific disorders, such as depression, anxiety, hyperactivity, obsessive–compulsive disorder, tic disorders, autistic disorders, and eating disorders. Yet other epidemiological studies have focused on particular risk factors such as head injury, marital discord or divorce, low-level lead, disasters, or school influences. Finally, epidemiological studies of twins and adoptees have increasingly been used to investigate the relative aetiological importance of genetic and environmental factors. The main conclusions that have emerged from epidemiological studies are as follows:

Overall prevalence

The 7% rate of psychiatric disorder reported by the first Isle of Wight study was on the low side. Most subsequent studies have reported that psychiatric disorders are present in roughly 10–25% of children, with some estimates being as high as 50%. These alarmingly high rates are probably a great overestimate, reflecting the inadequacy of DSM–III and DSM–III–R diagnostic criteria. Until the most recent revision, DSM criteria were met when children had a particular set of symptoms irrespective of whether those symptoms had a significant impact (in terms of social impairment, distress, or disruption for others). As a result, many of the children who met DSM–III and DSM–III–R symptom checklists were not in need of treatment and did not correspond to what clinicians recognised as 'cases'. Thus many of the children identified as psychiatrically disordered in epidemiological studies using unmodified DSM–III or DSM–III–R criteria were probably not 'real' cases in any meaningful sense. Since DSM–IV and ICD–10 now use impact as well as symptom criteria,

Box 3.1   The Isle of Wight Study (Rutter *et al.*, 1970)

Method

There were 2193 10- and 11-year-olds whose homes were on the Island and who attended state schools (or schools for which the local authority paid the fees). Teacher questionnaires were completed on 99.8%. Parent questionnaires were completed on 88.5%. In a second stage, more detailed assessments were carried out on all children who scored above the cut-off on either questionnaire or who were known to have had recent contact with child guidance or the probation service. (There was no random sample of 'screen negative' subjects). Complete parent interviews were obtained on 94% of selected children. There was satisfactory inter-rater reliability on presence and type of psychiatric disorder.

Main findings

Overall prevalence
Correcting for the 'best guess' rate of false negatives, the estimated prevalence of psychiatric disorder was 6.8%, largely comprising conduct and mixed disorders (4% combined) and emotional disorders (2.5%).

Specific disorders
(a)   *Conduct disorders:* male:female = 4:1 Over-representation of children from large families. Associated with parental discord.
(b)   *Emotional disorders:* male:female = 0.7:1 Specific animal phobias only in females. Overt depressive disorder rare – 0.2%.
(c)   *Mixed disorders of conduct and emotion:* The emotional symptoms were usually misery rather than anxiety. In most respects, mixed disorders were closer to 'pure' conduct disorders than to 'pure' emotional disorders, e.g. in sex ratio, link with large families, link with reading problems. Consequently, mixed disorders are usually counted in with conduct disorders.
(d)   *Hyperactivity:* Restlessness and inattentiveness were common in all psychiatric disorders. Hyperkinesis was only diagnosed in 0.1%, but subsequent reanalysis of questionnaire data suggested that about 2% of children had pervasive hyperactivity – a clinically distinctive behaviour pattern associated with marked cognitive impairment, general behavioural disturbance, and chronicity.

Risk factors
(a)   *Link with specific reading disorder (SRD):* SRD and conduct disorder (CD) overlapped to a considerable extent – one-third of children with SRD had CD, and one-third of children with CD had SRD. Mixed SRD/CD was more similar to 'pure' SRD than to 'pure' CD. SRD was not particularly associated with emotional disorders.
(b)   *Link with low IQ:* Across the entire normal range of IQ, lower IQ was associated with more psychiatric symptoms – most markedly for poor concentration and speech problems, less markedly for conduct symptoms, and least markedly for emotional symptoms.
(c)   *Little link with socioeconomic status:* After allowing for IQ, there was no link between socioeconomic status and psychiatric symptoms. There was a non-significant trend for conduct disorder to be commoner in children of low socioeconomic status.

Parental concern and service use

Even when the research team thought that children had a psychiatric disorder, only half of the parents thought that their children had definite problems that were more serious than shown by most children. 10% of children with psychiatric disorders were under psychiatric care. Another 10% were seeing a GP or probation officer, or attending a special school for maladjusted children. Of the remaining children with psychiatric disorders, only 18% of parents wanted help.

future prevalence estimates of child psychiatric disorders may drop to more realistic levels (provided the problems involved in measuring impact reliably and validly can be solved).

What is common?

Disruptive behaviour disorders – oppositional–defiant disorder and conduct disorder – are common. So too are anxiety and depressive disorders, though the exact frequency of these emotional disorders is somewhat uncertain because of the problems described in the previous paragraph. Thus although some studies have reported that anxiety disorders are more common than any other disorders, many of the children with supposed anxiety disorders have worries or fears that do not result in much distress or social impairment. Opinion has been divided in the past on whether or not hyperactivity disorders are common, with most British researchers and clinicians regarding hyperkinesis as a rare disorder affecting less than 0.1% of children, and with most North American researchers and clinicians regarding attention–deficit/hyperactivity disorder (ADHD) as a very common disorder affecting some 5% of children. The empirical evidence supports an intermediate position: now that the ICD–10 criteria for hyperkinesis have been made more lenient and the DSM–IV criteria for ADHD have been made stricter, prevalence studies using either scheme should converge rather better, probably generating prevalence estimates in the region of 1–3%.

Comorbidity

Many children with psychiatric disorders meet the criteria for more than one psychiatric diagnosis. For example, children who meet the criteria for generalised anxiety disorder commonly also meet the criteria for other anxiety disorders too, including specific phobias, social phobia, and separation anxiety disorder. Similarly, children who meet the criteria for ADHD commonly also meet the criteria for oppositional–defiant or conduct disorders. For some disorders, comorbidity is the rule rather than the exception. Depression, for instance, is usually accompanied by anxiety or a disruptive behavioural disorder. There are several possible explanations for comorbidity. Firstly, the current psychiatric classification may have erred too far in the direction of splitting rather than lumping. If we labelled 'sore throat' and 'runny nose' as separate disorders, many people would be comorbid for the two. Secondly, one disorder may be a risk factor for another. For example, conduct disorder may be a risk factor for depression, perhaps because conduct problems result in the child being isolated and criticised. Finally, the same biological and psychosocial factors that predispose a child to one disorder may simultaneously predispose the child to other disorders.

Most disorders go untreated

Even when children do have psychiatric symptoms that result in significant social impairment or distress, only a minority of these children are in contact with specialist mental health services. Children are most likely to be referred for specialist help when their problems are a substantial burden to their parents. Conversely, children whose parents do not feel burdened are unlikely to receive specialist mental health care. Although some of the children with psychiatric problems who are not being seen by specialist mental health services do get help from elsewhere in the health sector, or from education or social services, the majority get no professional help at all.

Persistence

When an individual has a disorder at two different ages, the continuity is said to be *homotypic* if the disorders are similar at both ages, and *heterotypic* when the type of disorder has changed with age. For example, when children with conduct disorders are followed up into adult life, some continue to have disruptive and antisocial problems (homotypic continuity) while others become depressed adults (heterotypic continuity). In this instance, homotypic continuity is more likely in males, heterotypic in females.

Many studies have shown that conduct problems are somewhat more persistent than emotional problems. For example, when children from the Isle of Wight with psychiatric disorders at the age of 10 or 11 were followed up, only a quarter of those with conduct disorder were free from psychiatric disorder four years later, as compared with half of those who had originally had an emotional disorder. The continuity from childhood to adulthood can be substantial. In the Dunedin longitudinal study, for example, three-quarters of all 21-year-olds with psychiatric diagnoses had previously had a mental disorder when studied between the ages of 11 and 18.

Sex ratio and age of onset

While child mental health services tend to see more boys than girls, epidemiological studies do not show marked gender differences in the overall rate of psychiatric disorder – boys are more likely than girls to have a disorder before puberty, but the reverse is true after puberty. The sex ratio varies markedly with the type of problem (see Box 3.2). The usual age of onset also varies markedly from problem to problem, with some problems characteristically beginning early in childhood, and with other adult-type problems being much commoner in the teenage years than in earlier childhood (see Box 3.3). It is tempting to suppose that these striking differences in sex ratio and age of onset are important clues to the underlying aetiology or pathogenesis, but sadly the clues remain largely undeciphered.

Box 3.2   Sex ratio.

Marked male excess	Male ≈ female	Marked female excess
Autistic disorders	Depression (prepubertal)	Specific phobias,
Hyperactivity disorders	Selective mutism	e.g. insects
Conduct/oppositional	School refusal.	Diurnal enuresis
disorders		Deliberate self-harm
Juvenile delinquency		(postpubertal)
Completed suicide		Depression (postpubertal)
Tic disorders (e.g. Tourette's)		Anorexia and bulimia
Nocturnal enuresis in older		nervosa.
children		
Specific developmental		
disorders, e.g. language		
and reading disorders.		

Box 3.3   Age at onset.

Characteristic early onset	Mostly teenage onset
Autistic disorders	Depression
Hyperactivity disorders	Mania
Attachment disorders	Psychosis
Selective mutism	Suicide and deliberate self-harm
Oppositional-defiant disorder	Anorexia and bulimia nervosa
Separation anxiety	Panic attacks and agoraphobia
Specific phobias, e.g. insects	Substance abuse
Enuresis	Juvenile delinquency.
Mental retardation	
Specific developmental disorders,	
e.g. language and reading disorders.	

Aetiology

Epidemiological studies have provided evidence for the aetiological importance of psychosocial, genetic and neurological factors. A particularly influential study of psychosocial factors involved a direct comparison of children from a run-down area of inner London with children from the small towns and countryside of the Isle of Wight. The same two-stage measures were applied to representative samples of 10-year-olds from both areas. By comparison with the Isle of Wight children, the inner city children had roughly double the rate of conduct, emotional and reading disorders. These differences seemed to be attributable primarily to higher rates of the following psychosocial problems in the inner city: marital breakdown, parental illness and criminality, social disadvantage, and schools with high turnovers of pupils and teachers.

Epidemiological twin and adoption studies have pointed to substantial genetic contributions to many child psychiatric disorders. In the case of autism, for example, epidemiological twin studies have demonstrated a very high heritability for a 'broad phenotype' that includes autism and lesser variants. Genetic factors also seem to play a prominent role in bipolar affective disorders, schizophrenia, tic disorders, and hyperactivity – and somewhat lesser roles in the common conduct and emotional disorders of childhood.

Child psychiatric disorders are often associated with lower intelligence or specific learning disorders. Though these links are well established, the underlying causal mechanisms are still in doubt. In some instances, psychiatric problems such as hyperactivity may interfere with learning. In other instances, the frustration and stress caused by learning problems may lead to psychiatric problems. In yet other instances, both learning and behavioural problems may reflect the operation of some 'third factor', whether psychosocial, genetic or neurological.

Epidemiological studies of children with congenital and acquired brain disorders have found particularly high rates of associated psychiatric disorders – much higher rates than those found among children with chronic non-cerebral disorders that result in comparable disability and stigmatisation. This persuasive evidence for direct brain–behaviour links will come as no surprise to anyone who believes that the brain is the organ of the mind.

Cross-cultural differences

In a multicultural society there is obvious interest and importance in epide-miological studies examining whether different communities have different child psychiatric profiles. How else could one determine whether minority groups were being appropriately served? In addition, our current knowledge of child psychiatry is almost entirely based on studies of white children; cross-cultural studies are needed to show whether our current ideas on classification, aetiology, prognosis, treatment and prevention apply equally to children from all backgrounds. It is important to remember that cross-cultural differences in child mental health could arise from many factors, including cultural differ-ences in child rearing practices; physical and social consequences of migration; different experiences of racism or poverty; or biological differences. Epide-miological studies have generated some interesting findings in this field. In one London study, for example, children whose parents were born on the Indian subcontinent were less hyperactive than comparison children as judged by objective measures of activity and attention, but were equally or more hyper-active as judged by teacher ratings, raising the possibility of inter-ethnic bias. Another London study showed that by comparison with white children, Afro-Caribbean children were more likely to have conduct disorders at school, but were no more likely to have conduct disorders at home. One possible expla-nation is that the disruptive behaviour of the black children at school was commonly a response to their experience of racism in the school environment. Several studies from different countries have reported higher rates of autism in the children of immigrants. One possible but unproven explanation is that this excess of autism is due to prenatal infections with viruses that immigrant mothers had not previously been exposed to in their countries of origin. Even from these few examples, it is evident that many possible explanations need to be considered when cross-cultural differences are found.

Time trends

A growing body of empirical evidence supports the pessimists' view that things are getting worse as the years go by. Since diagnostic criteria and research tools have changed over time, it is obviously hard to establish whether some particular problem has really become more common, or whether we are setting our threshold lower nowadays, or getting better at recognising that sort of problem. Taking account of these methodological issues, it still seems likely that there has been a real rise over the last 50 years in psychosocial disorders of youth. The increase is clearest for crime, substance abuse, depression and suicide. For eating disorders, the evidence is suggestive but not conclusive.

Subject review

Rutter, M. (1989) Isle of Wight revisited: 25 years of epidemiological research in child psychiatry. *Journal of the American Academy of Child and Adolescent Psychiatry*, **28**, 633–653.

Further reading

Bird, H.R. (1996) Epidemiology of childhood disorders in a cross-cultural context. *Journal of Child Psychology and Psychiatry*, **37**, 35–49.
Rutter, M., Tizard, J. and Whitmore, K. eds (1970) *Education, Health and Behaviour*. Longman, London. (This is the original description of the first Isle of Wight study.)
Rutter, M. (1976) Isle of Wight studies, 1964–1974. *Psychological Medicine*, **6**, 313–332.
Rutter, M. and Smith, D.J. eds (1995) *Psychosocial Disorders in Young People: Time Trends and Their Causes*. Wiley, Chichester. (This extensive review documents the rising tide of psychosocial problems affecting young people.)
Verhulst, F.C. and Koot, H.M., eds (1995) *The Epidemiology of Child and Adolescent Psychopathology*. Oxford University Press, Oxford. (A mixture of methodological and substantive chapters by distinguished researchers.)

Part II
Specific Disorders and Presentations

4 Autistic Disorders

Autistic disorders are also known as *pervasive developmental disorders*. They used to be known as *infantile psychoses* – a term best avoided since it misleads people into thinking that autistic disorders are akin to adult psychoses. Childhood (or infantile) autism is the best known and best researched of the autistic disorders. The other autistic disorders can be thought of as less extreme variations on the same theme – meeting some but not all of the diagnostic criteria for childhood autism. Though autistic disorders always begin in childhood, they often persist into adulthood too.

Epidemiology

Roughly two children per 1000 have a pervasive developmental disorder, of whom some 10–50% have childhood autism, depending on how narrowly or broadly the disorder is defined. Current estimates of the prevalence of autism are around 0.5 per 1000. The male:female ratio is approximately 3:1. There is no clear relation to socioeconomic status; the links with high socioeconomic status reported by early studies were probably due to ascertainment bias.

Characteristic features

Infantile autism is defined by the combination of four sets of features.

- Social impairment
- Communication impairment
- Restricted and repetitive activities and interests
- Early onset.

Social impairment

These concern the quality of reciprocal interactions with others. The young autistic child is aloof with poor eye contact, shows a lack of interest in people as people (though they may be of interest as tickling machines, biscuit dispensers, etc.), and fails to seek comfort when hurt. If social interest subsequently develops, as it does in just over 50% of autistic children, problems persist in social responsiveness, reciprocity and the capacity for empathy. The child has difficulty adjusting his or her behaviour according to the social context, and is poor at recognising other people's emotions and responding appropriately. Attachment to parents is *not* unusual, and the child may be affectionate (or even over-affectionate), although he or she is more likely to initiate cuddles than to accept cuddles initiated by his or her parents. Social interactions are on the child's terms – adults and much younger children typically adjust better to this than children of the same age. Interactions with peers are generally very restricted. Even among older high-functioning autistic individuals, a limited ability to form close friendships (involving mutual sharing of interests, activities, and emotions) is probably the most sensitive index of residual social impairments.

Communication impairment

This affects comprehension as well as expression, and gesture as well as spoken language. Babble may be reduced. Roughly 50% of autistic individuals never acquire useful speech. In the remainder, speech development is typically markedly delayed (though a minority acquire single words and even phrases at the normal time before losing these skills again). Speech, if it emerges, is typically deviant as well as delayed. Possible abnormalities include: immediate or delayed parroting of words or phrases (echolalia); pronominal reversal (e.g. 'you' for 'I'); idiosyncratic use of words or phrases; invented words (neologisms); and reliance on stock phrases or repetitive questioning. Instead of chatting in a to-and-fro way *with* other people, the autistic individual primarily talks *at* other people. For example, some autistic individuals use speech mainly for demanding things. Others talk at length about one of their current preoccupations, oblivious of the social cues indicating that their listener has long since lost interest in the topic. Speech is often abnormal in intonation or pitch, e.g. sing-song or a monotonous drone. Gestures are similarly reduced and poorly integrated (e.g. abnormal pointing).

Restricted and repetitive activities and interests

These include: resistance to change; insistence on routines and rituals; hand-flapping, twirling, or other stereotypies; ordering play (e.g. lining things up); attachment to unusual objects (e.g. a dustbin); fascination with unusual aspects of the world (e.g. the feel of zips or people's hair); and consuming preoccupations with restricted subjects (e.g. train timetables, car prices). Make-believe play is typically lacking, except in older higher-functioning individuals. When present, pretend play is often limited to simple repetitive enactments of just one or two incidents from a favourite story or TV programme.

Early onset

Though the disorder is rarely recognised in the first year of life, it is usually clear retrospectively that development was never entirely normal, even though the parents may not have been seriously concerned about early signs of a lack of social interest, e.g. not liking being cuddled, or not reaching out to be picked up. In a substantial minority of cases, however, there is a clear 'setback' in the second or third year of life; after a period of normal or near normal development, these children go through a phase of regression when they lose previously acquired skills in social interaction, communication, and play. Both ICD–10 and DSM–IV define early onset in terms of developmental abnormalities that were evident by 36 months, but this is an arbitrary cut-off and other schemes have set earlier or later cut-offs.

While some children meet all four criteria and warrant a diagnosis of infantile autism, others meet only some of the criteria and so may warrant a diagnosis of *atypical autism* (ICD–10) or *pervasive developmental disorder, not otherwise specified* (DSM–IV).

Associated features

Mental retardation

This is present in the majority. A useful mnemonic is that 50% have an IQ under 50, 70% have an IQ under 70, and almost 100% (95%) have an IQ under 100. In autism, the IQ should be judged by non-verbal tests. Verbal IQ is almost always lower than non-verbal IQ because of the associated language problems.

Seizures

These affect about a third of mentally retarded autistic individuals, and about 5% of autistic individuals with normal IQ. These seizures often begin in adolescence, whereas the seizures of non-autistic individuals with mental retardation usually begin in early childhood.

Other psychiatric problems

In addition to the characteristic features already described, many autistic children have additional behavioural and emotional problems. Hyperactivity is common. Severe and frequent temper tantrums are common and may be triggered by the child's inability to communicate his or her needs, or by someone interfering with their rituals and routines. Interference by others may also unleash aggressive outbursts. Children with an autistic disorder and mental retardation are particularly prone to self-injurious behaviours, such as head banging, eye poking or hand biting. Extreme food fads represent one particular form of ritualistic behaviour. Intense fears may lead to phobic avoidance. Some of these phobias are exaggerations of common childhood fears (e.g. of large dogs) while others are idiosyncratic (e.g. fear of petrol pumps). Hallucinations and delusions are *not* associated with autism.

Differential diagnosis

Developmental or acquired language disorders

The desire to communicate by gesture, and the capacity for social interaction are intact in children with 'pure' phonological-syntactic language disorders (see Chapter 25). However, there are 'overlap' cases involving a mixture of severe phonological-syntactic language problems and mild autistic features. In addition, there is continuing controversy as to whether semantic-pragmatic language disorder (see Chapter 25) is a distinctive condition or describes the linguistic component of mild autism.

Asperger's syndrome

This is regarded by some as a mild version of autism. It differs from classical autism in several respects:

Firstly, there is little or no delay in the development of vocabulary and grammar, though other aspects of language are abnormal as in autism. Thus speech is often stilted and pedantic, with abnormal intonation; gesturing may be restricted or exaggerated; and monologues on favourite topics are easily triggered and hard to stop.

Secondly, early aloofness is less likely than in autism. The child with Asperger's syndrome is often interested in other people, although his or her social interactions are gauche, reflecting impaired empathy and social responsiveness. In these respects, the individual with Asperger's syndrome resembles higher-functioning autistic individuals who have grown out of their aloofness.

Thirdly, restricted and repetitive behaviours are mostly evident in preoccupations or circumscribed interests (such as plane spotting or geographical maps) rather than in motor stereotypies.

Finally, marked clumsiness is probably commoner in Asperger's syndrome than in autism.

Mental retardation without autistic features

Language and pretend play will be absent if mental age is under 12 months. Simple stereotypies are common. These children are socially responsive in line with their mental age.

Mental retardation with autistic features

Many mentally retarded children have a 'triad' of impairments affecting (1) social interaction, (2) communication and (3) play – plus varying degrees of repetitive and restricted behaviours. Only some of these children meet the full diagnostic criteria for infantile autism, but many more can be diagnosed as having atypical autism (though not all clinicians think it is useful to do so).

Rett's syndrome

This occurs only in girls and may be confused with autism. There is regression at about 12 months accompanied by: deceleration of head growth; characteristic 'hand washing' stereotypies and restricted hand use; episodic over-breathing and unprovoked laughter; and progressively impaired mobility. Most girls with Rett's syndrome are appropriately socially responsive once allowance is made for their low mental age and physical disabilities. The disease is progressive and most are in wheelchairs by their late teens and die before 30.

Neurodegenerative disorders with progressive dementia

These need to be considered when regression and the emergence of autistic features occur after a period of normal or nearly normal development. With time, frank neurological impairments emerge and the child eventually dies.

Disintegrative disorder

Also known as disintegrative psychosis or Heller's syndrome, it involves entirely normal development for two to six years, followed first by a phase of regression (often accompanied by marked anxiety and loss of bladder and bowel control), leading to lifelong severe mental retardation with pronounced autistic features.

Intense early deprivation

This is sometimes followed by autistic features. This has been evident from studies of transnationally adopted children who have been deprived in their first year or two of life of adequate nutrition, physical care, cognitive and linguistic stimulation, and ordinary social interaction. Though most such children do remarkably well within a few years of being adopted, a small minority continue to have social and communicative impairments associated with intense circumscribed interests, and preoccupations with specific sensations. In many instances, these autistic features subsequently resolve surprisingly well.

The fragile X syndrome

This is commonly associated with behaviours that bear a superficial resemblance to autism. Social avoidance and poor eye contact are common, but they seem to result from social anxiety rather than social indifference. Setting aside these superficially autistic behaviours, it remains controversial whether the fragile X syndrome is any more likely than other mental retardation syndromes to result in classical autism.

Deafness

This is often suspected when young autistic children pay no heed to people speaking to them. A careful history usually establishes that they have no difficulty hearing sounds that interest them, e.g. the rustle of a crisp packet! Unlike autistic children, deaf children are typically sociable and keen to communicate, e.g. by gesture.

Aetiology and pathogenesis

Most estimates suggest that roughly 10% of autistic children have known medical conditions, though some estimates put the proportion considerably higher. The likelihood of finding an underlying medical cause is probably higher when the child is severely or profoundly mentally retarded, or when the autism is atypical rather than classical. A wide variety of medical disorders have been reported; some may be chance associations and others may reflect a non-specific increase in the rate of autistic disorders in any condition that results in mental retardation. It is unlikely that the link with mental retardation is entirely non-specific, however, since autistic disorders are over-represented in some mentally retarding conditions, such as tuberous sclerosis with seizures, but much less commonly seen in others, such as severe cerebral palsy.

For the majority of classically autistic children without a known medical disorder, genetic factors seem of primary importance, with twin studies suggesting a heritability of over 90%, and with an adverse combination of genes seeming more likely than a single major gene. The heritable phenotype seems to be broad, stretching from classical autism at the one extreme to mild partial variants at the other extreme. The recurrence rate in siblings is roughly 3% for narrowly defined autism, but is about 10–20% for milder variants. Genetic factors may be less important in the aetiology of the autistic features associated with severe and profound mental retardation; these may be primarily determined by widespread brain damage (phenocopies). Obstetric adversity is of dubious aetiological significance.

Though extreme and prolonged early deprivation in grossly inadequate institutions may result in autistic features, there is no evidence that 'ordinary' psychosocial adversities play any part in the aetiology of autism. There is no evidence for the theory that autism is caused by an early traumatic event, parental insensitivity or lack of responsiveness to their child.

Many researchers have hypothesised that autism results from a primary fault in just one neurological system or just one psychological function. It is equally plausible that autism reflects a distinctive combination of structural or functional abnormalities. Neurobiological studies have not identified a characteristic focal deficit: almost every portion of the brain has been implicated by some neuroimaging or neuropathology study and no localisation has been consistently replicated. Since a substantial minority of autistic individuals have abnormally large brains and head circumferences, widespread neurodevelopmental abnormalities may turn out to be more important than focal abnormalities.

Attempts to identify a primary psychological deficit in autism have fared slightly better. Though no one theory has won universal acceptance, two rival theories are both supported by a large and growing body of empirical evidence. One theory suggests that the primary deficit in autism is in 'Theory of Mind', i.e. the capacity to attribute independent mental states to self and others in order to predict and explain actions (see Box 4.1). This sort of 'mentalising' deficit would disrupt abilities that depended on the capacity to see another person's point of view but would not interfere with abilities that simply required a mechanical or behavioural understanding of objects and people. The main alternative theory is that the primary deficit in autism is in executive function, with the sorts of problems in planning and organisational skills that result in poor performance on 'frontal lobe' tests. Other suggestions for the primary psychological deficit in autism include an innate impairment in the ability to become emotionally engaged with others and an impaired ability to extract high-level meaning by synthesising diverse sorts of information. However none of these theories accounts satisfactorily for the repetitive and stereotyped behaviours seen in autism, nor for the low IQ seen in the majority.

Box 4.1   The Sally-Anne story – a test of first-order 'Theory of Mind'.

The following story is enacted with puppets and props: Sally has a marble. She puts it in a basket and then goes out. While Sally is out, Anne decides to play a trick on Sally. Anne takes the marble out from the basket and puts it in a box instead. Then Anne leaves. When Sally comes home, she wants her marble. Where will Sally look for the marble?

Normal three-year-olds fail the test, saying that Sally will look in the box; they know the marble is there and they find it hard to see that Sally does not.

Normal four-year-olds pass the test, predicting that Sally will act on her false belief and look in the basket.

Children with Down's syndrome usually pass the Sally-Anne test if they have a mental age of four or more (on verbal tests).

Autistic children, by contrast, usually fail the Sally-Anne test even when they do have a verbal mental age of four or more. The minority of high-functioning autistic individuals who do pass the Sally-Anne test nearly always fail more complex tests of mentalising ability.

Treatment

The mainstays of treatment are appropriate school placement and the provision of adequate support for parents. Autistic children generally do best in a well-structured educational setting where the teachers have special experience of autism. Home- and school-based behavioural programmes can reduce tantrums, aggressive outbursts, fears and rituals, as well as fostering more normal development. Many families welcome respite care.

Standard anticonvulsants are used to manage any associated epilepsy.

Psychotropic medication does not improve the core symptoms of autism but may sometimes improve associated symptoms. Stimulants may reduce associated hyperactivity, though often at the cost of an unacceptable increase in repetitive behaviours. Low doses of a neuroleptic may reduce agitation and repetitive behaviours and make the children more manageable; higher doses may reduce hyperactivity, withdrawal and emotional lability. These potential advantages have to be set against the hazards of neuroleptic medication (see Chapter 31). Fenfluramine, a serotonergic stimulant, also has its advocates but possible benefits in terms of reduced hyperactivity have to be weighed against the risk of serious complications such as pulmonary hypertension. Contrary to early claims, the effect of fenfluramine on any given individual does not seem to be related to whether or not that individual has reduced blood serotonin levels.

Prognosis

For children with the full autistic syndrome approximately half acquire useful speech. Children who have not done so by the age of five years are unlikely to do so subsequently. Autistic aloofness improves in just over half of all cases, being replaced by an 'active but odd' social interest.

Adolescence is associated with several changes:

- The peak age for onset of seizures is 11–14 years.
- Earlier hyperactivity may be replaced by marked underactivity and inertia.
- About 10% of autistic individuals go through a phase in adolescence when they lose language skills, sometimes with intellectual deterioration as well; this decline is not progressive, but the lost skills are not generally regained.
- Agitation seems more common, sometimes leading to serious aggressive outbursts.
- Inappropriate sexual behaviour can become troublesome.

In adult life, roughly 10% of autistic individuals are working and able to look after themselves. Fewer still have good friends, marry, or become parents. The child's IQ and the presence or absence of speech by five years of age are the best predictors of long-term social independence. Children with a non-verbal IQ of under 60 will almost certainly be severely handicapped in adult life and unable to live independently. Children with higher IQs are more likely to become independent, particularly if they have acquired useful speech by the age of five. Even with IQ and speech on their side, however, autistic individuals only have a 50% chance of a good social outcome. Autistic individuals are not at an increased risk of developing schizophrenia in adult life.

Subject review

Lord, C. and Rutter, M. (1994) Autism and pervasive developmental disorders. In *Child and Adolescent Psychiatry: Modern Approaches*, 3rd edn (M. Rutter, E. Taylor & L. Hersov, eds) Blackwell Science, Oxford. pp. 569–593.

Further reading

Bailey, A. *et al.* (1996) Autism: towards an integration of clinical, genetic, neuropsychological, and neurobiological perspectives. *Journal of Child Psychology and Psychiatry*, **37**, 89–126.

Cohen, D.J. and Volkmar, F.R. (1997) *Handbook of Autism and Pervasive Developmental Disorders*, 2nd edn. Wiley, New York. (This is the encyclopedia of autism.)

Happé, F.G.E. (1994) Current psychological theories of autism: the 'Theory of Mind' account and rival theories. *Journal of Child Psychology and Psychiatry*, **35**, 215–229.

Le Couteur, A. *et al.* (1996) A broader phenotype of autism: the clinical spectrum in twins. *Journal of Child Psychology and Psychiatry*, **37**, 785–801.

Wing, L. (1981) Asperger's syndrome: a clinical account. *Psychological Medicine*, **11**, 115–129.

Wing, L. and Gould, J. (1979) Severe impairments of social interaction and associated abnormalities in children: epidemiology and classification. *Journal of Autism and Developmental Disorders*, **9**, 11–30. (This is the classical account of the high rate of the autistic 'triad' in mentally retarded children.)

5 Hyperactivity

Parents may use hyperactivity as a label for all manner of behaviours, including frequent night wakenings, naughtiness, exuberance, and extraversion. Child psychiatrists use hyperactivity in a more restricted sense, defining it in terms of restlessness and inattentiveness (and sometimes impulsiveness as well). There is a continuum of attention and activity in the general population. Hyperactivity is sometimes used in a dimensional sense to refer to the continuum as a whole, and sometimes used in a categorical sense to refer to individuals who have extreme values. Even when used in a categorical sense to make a diagnosis, the dividing line between normality and hyperactivity has been drawn in very different places by different diagnostic schemes. The British have traditionally used very stringent criteria for 'hyperkinesis', making it a severe disorder affecting around 0.1% of children. Under DSM–III, by contrast, North Americans used far broader criteria for 'attention deficit disorder with hyperactivity' (ADDH), making it a milder disorder affecting around 10% of children. More recently, empirical approaches to classification have supported the validity of a category that lies somewhere between these extremes. These findings have guided the ICD–10 and DSM–IV definitions, which are now very similar, although the terms used are hyperkinesis and attention-deficit/hyperactivity disorder (ADHD) respectively.

Epidemiology

Prevalence is 1–3% for the new ICD–10 and DSM–IV categories. Male:female ratio is 3:1. It is more common in younger children. Hyperactivity is linked with deprivation. It is more common in inner cities, very poor rural areas, in families of low socioeconomic status and among children reared in institutions.

Characteristic features

Marked restlessness, inattentiveness and impulsiveness

These features must allow for the child's chronological and mental age. Hyperactive children wriggle and squirm in their seats, fiddle with objects or clothing, repeatedly get up and wander about when they should be seated, have difficulty persisting with any one task, change activity frequently, and are easily distracted. The most obvious abnormality is not in the amount but in the control of activity. In the playground, the hyperactive child may be no more active than anyone else. However, what stands out is the child's inability to suppress activity when stillness is required, e.g. in the classroom or at the meal table. Hyperactive children are also likely to be impulsive: acting without due reflection, engaging in rash and sometimes dangerous behaviours, blurting out answers in class, interrupting adults and children, and not waiting their turn in games. However, impulsiveness is also a common feature of conduct disorder (see Box 6.3), so it is not useful when trying to distinguish between hyperactivity and conduct disorder.

Pervasiveness

Pervasiveness across situations is a key requirement of the new ICD–10 and DSM–IV definitions. Severe hyperactivity in just one setting is not enough for a diagnosis of hyperkinesis or attention-deficit/hyperactivity disorder. The hyperactivity must be evident across different settings, e.g. at home *and* at school. It is important to note, however, that pervasive hyperactivity may not be evident during a brief clinic visit since the child may be intimidated by unfamiliar professionals, or may be happy to settle to interesting tasks when given plenty of adult attention. Pervasiveness was not a requirement in earlier versions of the DSM diagnosis, and DSM–IV still allows situational hyperactivity (e.g. hyperactivity that is noted at school but not at home, or *vice versa*) to be coded under the clumsy rubric of 'Attention-deficit/hyperactivity disorder not otherwise specified'.

Chronicity and early onset

Both ICD–10 and DSM–IV require chronicity (at least 6 months of symptoms) and early onset (by seven years of age). Though hyperactivity generally dates back to the preschool years, referral is often delayed until the primary school years. This is the period when the child's inattentiveness, learning problems, and disruptiveness become increasingly troublesome.

Exclusion criteria

In both ICD–10 and DSM–IV, autistic disorders (pervasive developmental disorders) take precedence over hyperactivity disorders. Though many children with autistic disorders are restless and inattentive, these children are not given a second diagnosis of hyperkinesis or ADHD. A hyperactivity diagnosis is not made when restlessness and poor concentration are due to a mood disorder, an anxiety disorder, or schizophrenia.

Assessment of symptoms

(1) *Attention* is primarily assessed from the child's persistence (in minutes) when engaged in a range of tasks including playing alone, reading, drawing, or playing with a friend. Some children who are reported to persist for fairly long periods when playing alone or with others turn out, on more searching enquiry, to have a brief attention span, switching frequently from one play activity to another. Since all but the most hyperactive of children are able to watch TV or play computer games for long periods, this is not a very discriminating measure of attention.

(2) *Motor activity* is assessed from: (a) how long the child can stay seated during the aforementioned tasks; (b) what proportion of the time they are fidgeting; and (c) how often they run off on family outings or at the supermarket.

Common associated features

(1) *Defiant, aggressive, and antisocial behaviours* are often sufficiently marked to warrant a diagnosis of conduct disorder. Child psychiatrists using DSM–IV will give dual diagnoses of ADHD and conduct disorder (or oppositional defiant disorder); child psychiatrists using ICD–10 will use the specific combined diagnosis of hyperkinetic conduct disorder.

(2) *Problems with social relationships.* Hyperactive children are often socially disinhibited with adults, being overfamiliar and cheeky. Peer rejection is common, partly in response to hyperactive children's disruptiveness and impulsive disregard for rules and turns. Hyperactive children are easily led or dared into all manner of mischief.

(3) *IQ under 100* in many but not all children.

(4) *Specific learning problems* (e.g. with reading or spelling), even when IQ is taken into account.

(5) *Clumsiness* and neurodevelopmental immaturities ('soft neurological signs').

(6) A history of specific *developmental delay*, e.g. in language acquisition.

Differential diagnosis

(1) *Normality.* Parents may complain of minor degrees of restlessness and inattention that are well within the normal range. Simple exuberance can be wearing for parents and teachers; this requires sympathy rather than a diagnostic label!

(2) *Situational hyperactivity.* Some children seem hyperactive at school but

not at home, or *vice versa*. These children cannot be diagnosed as hyperkinetic (ICD–10) or ADHD (DSM–IV) under current guidelines since cross-situational pervasiveness is required. However, they can be diagnosed as 'ADHD, not otherwise specified' under DSM–IV. The nature of situational hyperactivity is still unclear. One possibility is that situational hyperactivity is a milder variant of pervasive hyperactivity. Alternatively, hyperactivity limited to school may be particularly linked to (unrecognised) specific learning difficulties, while hyperactivity limited to the home may be an aspect of home-based relationship difficulties or conduct disorder.

(3) *Conduct disorder*. This is often mixed with true hyperactivity, but even 'pure' conduct disorder may mimic hyperactivity. Impulsiveness is a feature of both disorders (see Box 6.3). In addition, children with conduct problems at school may not want to settle to school work and may wander about the classroom creating trouble. Similarly, children with conduct problems at home may not settle to their chores or their homework. The key question is: do restlessness and inattentiveness persist during chosen activities, such as drawing, reading comics, building models, or playing with friends? If 'no', this is unlikely to be hyperactivity; if 'yes', this may be a mixed hyperactivity/conduct disorder (depending on pervasiveness, age of onset, etc.)

(4) *Emotional disorder*. Severe anxiety, depression or mania can all result in restlessness and inattentiveness (in which case a diagnosis of hyperactivity is ruled out). If a child presents with a mixture of hyperactivity and emotional symptoms, it is essential to take a careful history to establish which began first. If the emotional symptoms came first, this should be diagnosed simply as an emotional disorder. However if the hyperactivity symptoms came first, this may be an acute emotional disorder on top of a chronic hyperactivity problem.

(5) *Tics, chorea, and other dyskinesias*. These may be mistaken for fidgetiness. Observe the movements carefully. Children with tic disorders may also be hyperactive and the hyperactivity may have been evident long before the first tic.

(6) *Pervasive developmental disorders*. These are suggested if the restlessness and inattentiveness are accompanied by autistic types of social impairment, communication deviance, rigid and repetitive behaviours, or lack of spontaneous pretend play.

(7) *Mental retardation*. The child's attention and activity control may be impaired relative to chronological age but appropriate for mental age. However, even allowing for mental age, many children with mental retardation are also hyperactive. Hyperactivity is some 10–30 times more common among children with mental retardation.

Causation

Family, adoption and twin studies suggest that genetic factors make a major contribution. Though children with epilepsy or other brain disorders are particularly prone to hyperactivity (and other psychiatric problems), most children with hyperactivity have no neurological symptoms or signs: hyperactivity is not synonymous with overt brain damage. Do hyperactive children have 'minimal brain damage'? This sort of catch-all term has proved a barrier rather than an aid to thought. If neurobiological explanations are to be helpful, they need to be as specific and testable as possible. There is limited evidence from neuroimaging and neuropsychological studies that hyperactivity may result from a reduction in the normal inhibitory function of the frontal lobes. Since barbiturates, benzodiazepines and other anticonvulsants sometimes precipitate severe hyperactivity, and since stimulants and other medications are useful in the treatment of hyperactivity (see below), it seems plausible that hyperactivity reflects a neurochemical imbalance. Unfortunately, it has not proved possible to take this notion much further, partly because hyperactivity is influenced by a very wide range of drugs, affecting many different neurotransmitters and receptors. Despite popular stereotypes to the contrary, perinatal complications and exposure to low-level lead are not common causes of hyperactivity. However, there is rather more evidence for the widely held view that hyperactivity can be triggered by adverse reactions to specific foods or drinks.

Psychosocial as well as biological factors influence hyperactivity, as indicated by the link with deprivation and institutional rearing. The responses of parents, teachers and peers to a child's hyperactivity may influence the prognosis. There is some evidence to suggest that parents who respond to hyperactivity with criticism, coldness, and lack of involvement can increase the chance of their child becoming defiant, aggressive, and antisocial.

Treatment

Education

The nature of the disorder needs to be explained to the child, the family and the school. Hyperactivity is neither the parents' fault nor the child's fault. Since hyperactive children can be extremely exasperating, they often come in for much criticism and little praise. The balance may improve, however, once adults accept that the child's problems are not just wilful naughtiness. Rules about unacceptable behaviours should be clear, consistently and calmly enforced, and backed up by immediate (but not harsh) sanctions. A key objective of treatment is to maximise the chances of normal development, thus reducing the probability of conduct disorder emerging. Special learning problems may need remedial help, and all teaching will need to take account of the child's limited attention span.

Cognitive and behavioural approaches

Behavioural management is often useful, and may be the only treatment needed for the mildest cases. For example, praise or other rewards may help a child who normally only remains on a task for two minutes to persist for three minutes instead, with the target being increased slowly and progressively as time goes by. For maximum effect, the reinforcement of desirable behaviour needs to be clear and immediate. Other suitable targets for behavioural programmes include associated conduct problems. Even when a child responds to medication, behavioural approaches often continue to provide additional benefit. The value of cognitive approaches – such as 'stop and think' self-commands – is less well established. An initial phase of enthusiasm for cognitive therapy was followed by widespread disillusionment when it became clear that the benefits seen in training sessions often failed to generalise to everyday life. As the pendulum settles down, it should become clearer whether cognitive approaches are beneficial for a particular subset of hyperactive children – perhaps older and brighter children who are highly motivated and psychologically minded.

Medication

Stimulant medication is a well-tested treatment for hyperactivity that tends to be under-used in the UK and over-used in the USA. The most commonly used stimulant is methylphenidate (Ritalin), but dexamphetamine has very similar properties. Pemoline has been used but there is currently considerable concern about its hepatotoxicity. A good response to stimulant medication is predicted by severe and pervasive hyperactivity, and by the absence of emotional symptoms. Many parents are understandably reluctant to consider medication, but the benefits can be so striking that it is often worth trying to persuade parents to accept a brief trial of medication if the child seems likely to respond. When medication does improve attention and activity level, there are often parallel improvements in compliance, peer relationships, family relationships and learning ability. Methylphenidate and dexamphetamine are not addictive for children, do not make them 'high', and do not cause sedation. Side-effects are rarely troublesome. Appetite suppression or difficulty getting to sleep can usually be overcome by adjusting the dosage or timing. If stimulants lead to a severe dysphoric reaction, with marked misery and tearfulness lasting more than a few days, the trial should usually be abandoned. Repetitive activities or stereotypies can be provoked by over-medication which disappear when the dose is reduced. Stimulants can exacerbate tics, and so are not usually the first choice in children with tics or a strong family history of tics. If the initial trial is successful parents are usually keen to continue; stimulants can be administered for months or years. Long-term use of stimulants is remarkably safe – the only known complication of long-term use is a very slight reduction in adult height, and even this is controversial. Other drugs that are sometimes used for hyperactivity include imipramine, other antidepressants and clonidine (second-line treatments) and neuroleptics (third-line treatments). Medication should always be part of an integrated treatment package. A good response to stimulants is the beginning rather than the end of treatment – increasing the chance of successful work with the family and the school to get the child back on to as normal a developmental trajectory as possible. Though medication can be a useful symptomatic treatment, it remains unclear whether the long-term prognosis is altered. Even if there were no long-term benefit, this would not be a reason for withholding treatment – children would deserve symptomatic relief anyway. After all, most adults use medication to obtain symptomatic relief from colds or aches that would go away anyway.

Diet

Dietary treatment is popular with parents, and often needs to be explored before the family are willing to try anything else. Recent evidence suggests that some children are substantially better when specific foods are excluded from their diets – though it is still uncertain whether diet-responsive children are rare or common. It is not possible to predict on the basis of blood or skin tests which children will respond, or which foods are responsible. Additives are rarely the only culprits; one or more natural foods, such as milk or wheat products or oranges, are usually involved as well. As described in Chapter 31, a proper trial of dietary treatment is very hard work for all concerned.

Prognosis

Hyperactivity typically wanes in adolescence, though many affected individuals have residual problems with restlessness and inattentiveness even in adult life. Educational attainments are likely to be poor. Children who are both hyperactive and conduct disordered are at high risk of antisocial personality disorder and substance abuse in adult life; children with 'pure' hyperactivity are at less risk, though they are still vulnerable.

Subject reviews

Hinshaw, S.P. (1994) *Attention Deficits and Hyperactivity in Children*. Sage, Thousand Oaks, CA.
Taylor, E. (1994) Syndromes of attention deficit and overactivity. In *Child and Adolescent Psychiatry: Modern Approaches*, 3rd edn (M. Rutter, E. Taylor and L. Hersov, eds) Blackwell Science, Oxford, pp. 285–307.

Further reading

Schachar, R. *et al.* (1987) Changes in family function and relationships in children who respond to methylphenidate. *Journal of the American Academy of Child and Adolescent Psychiatry*, **26**, 728–732.

Taylor, E. *et al.* (1996) Hyperactivity and conduct problems as risk factors for adolescent development. *Journal of the American Academy of Child and Adolescent Psychiatry*, 35, 1213–1226.

6   Conduct Disorder

Conduct disorder (CD) is a term used to denote a syndrome of core symptoms characterised by the *persistent failure to control behaviour appropriately within socially defined rules*. According to most epidemiological studies, it is the commonest child psychiatric problem. It is often persistent, has a heavy cost for society, and yet has proved to be largely untreatable. Conduct problems involve three overlapping domains of behaviour: *defiance* of the will of someone in authority, *aggressiveness*, and *antisocial behaviour* that violates other people's rights, property, or person. None of these is in itself abnormal or pathological and indeed there are occasions when one tries to promote some of these behaviours in overdependent children. Disobedient and destructive behaviour is a part of normal development that usually diminishes with maturity, and a diagnosis should only be made when the behaviours are both extreme and persistent.

Psychiatric labelling and social control

But should children be given a psychiatric label simply because their behaviour is unacceptable to people in authority? Totalitarian regimes have used similar rationales in order to justify the incarceration of dissidents in psychiatric hospitals. Partly for this reason, many psychiatrists will only make a diagnosis of CD if a further criterion is met, namely that the conduct problems result in impairment in everyday functioning (e.g. in interpersonal relations or school work). This impairment criterion is included in DSM–IV but not in ICD–10.

Dimension or category?

It is arguably more appropriate to think of conduct problems as a dimension (like blood pressure) than as an all-or-nothing category (normal *v.* hypertensive). In medicine, cut-offs are often imposed on continuous variables in order to distinguish between normality and abnormality. In psychology, the thinking is much more likely to be in dimensional terms, retaining the continuous variable and investigating the extent to which increasingly abnormal scores have increasingly maladaptive outcomes. In the case of conduct problems, the dimensional approach has much to recommend it. Thus as the variety and severity of conduct problems increases, so the prognosis progressively worsens.

There is not a relatively sudden transition from a good prognosis for children just below the CD threshold to a bad prognosis for children above the threshold (although it does seem to be the case that children with conduct problems confined to just one area – such as aggression – do have a good prognosis). In addition, there is the risk that an all-or-nothing classification that divides children into those with and without CD might create an us-and-them attitude that adds to the marginalisation of troubled families. Nevertheless, the categorical approach is not only simpler but has the advantage of focusing on the most severely affected individuals; they are particularly relevant clinically and most studies of causation and treatment have been based on this group.

Is conduct disorder a psychiatric problem?

Whether conduct problems should be assessed or treated by child mental health professionals is debatable. Certainly, the difficulty is one of behaviour that is beyond the normal range and is causing impairment or burden to others. However, so is smoking 40 cigarettes a day as a teenager or driving motorcycles at 100 mph, yet these are more likely to be seen as social or moral problems than health problems.

Perhaps those cases of conduct disorder that are clearly socially determined and where management is solely a matter of discipline or behaviour management could be seen as the province of social services, education, or voluntary agencies. To be maximally effective, these other agencies would need to acquire a wide range of assessment and management skills, many of which were originally developed within mental health disciplines. They would need to be able to recognise the minority of conduct-disordered children with problems such as hyperactivity or depression that could benefit from referral to mental health professionals. They would also need to be able to recognise learning problems that could benefit from referral to specialist educational services. Given the high prevalence of conduct problems, and the relatively small number of child mental health professionals, the practicalities of effective service provision demand some such spread of expertise and responsibility.

Symptoms and signs

The manifestations change with age. Younger children are more likely to show the signs of *oppositional–defiant disorder* (ODD) which is a subtype of CD in ICD–10 but a separate condition in DSM–IV. The criterion behaviours for ODD (Box 6.1) should occur 'considerably more frequently than in other children of the same mental age'. The DSM–IV criteria for CD (Box 6.2) are more likely to be met by older children, and are closer to those for adult antisocial personality disorder. This definition is less likely to include girls than previous definitions since early sexual experience, early substance abuse and chronic violation of rules have been dropped:

Box 6.1　DSM–IV criteria for oppositional–defiant disorder.

Six months involving at least four of the following:

(1) Often loses temper
(2) Often argues with adults
(3) Often defies adult requests or rules
(4) Often deliberately annoys others

(5) Often shifts blame to others
(6) Often touchy or easily annoyed
(7) Often angry and resentful
(8) Often spiteful or vindictive.

Box 6.2　DSM–IV criteria for conduct disorder.

Disturbance for 12 months involving at least three of the following:

(1) Often bullies, threatens or intimidates
(2) Often starts fights
(3) Has used serious weapons in fights
(4) Physically cruel to people
(5) Physically cruel to animals
(6) Stealing with force
(7) Has forced someone into sexual acts
(8) Fire-setting to cause damage

(9) Has destroyed other's property
(10) Has broken into car or house
(11) Cons others
(12) Stealing without force
(13) Often out at night without permission
(14) Ran away from home overnight twice
(15) Often truants, beginning under 13 years.

Associated features

Psychiatric symptoms

- *Hyperactivity* Restlessness, inattentiveness, impulsiveness and general overactivity often co-exist but tend to be underplayed in the UK. The combination makes the outcome worse.
- *'Depression'*. About a third show significant emotional symptoms, most commonly unhappiness and misery. Whether this should be seen as a separate co-morbid condition, or is a part of the general underlying distress is debated; it does not seem to lead to a better or worse outcome in terms of CD, and neither is it clearly a risk factor for adult depression.

Educational failure

Many have poor achievements in terms of grades and level of work, and often have specific learning deficits. On testing, a third of children with CD have specific reading disorder (SRD), defined as being more than two standard deviations below the reading level expected for their age and intelligence (see Chapter 26). Conversely, a third of children with SRD have CD. The association between CD and SRD could be due to any of three possibilities. Firstly, disruptive behaviour may interfere with classroom learning. Secondly, children who do not have the ability to understand and participate in class may become frustrated and disruptive as a result. Thirdly, both disruptiveness and reading problems may stem from a third factor such as hyperactivity. Lower IQ is associated with CD but probably not as strongly as poor achievement.

Poor interpersonal relations

Disruptive children often become unpopular with their peers and frequently have no enduring friends. They commonly show poor social skills with both peers and adults, e.g. they have difficulty sustaining a game or promoting positive social interchanges. Poor peer relationships predict an unfavourable outcome. ICD–10 divides CD into 'unsocialised' and 'socialised' types according to whether the young person has normal peer relationships or not; DSM–IV has no comparable categories. In clinical practice, the great majority of children with CD do have impaired peer relationships. Nevertheless, there is limited evidence from cluster analytic studies for a relatively small group of conduct-disordered youngsters who do make enduring friendships, display altruistic behaviour, feel guilt or remorse, refrain from blaming others, and show concern for others. These individuals with socialised CD tend to be older and to engage in less aggressive antisocial acts such as stealing, truanting and drinking alcohol. They could be considered 'well-adjusted criminals' who are not regarded as deviant within their own subculture.

Differential diagnosis

There is usually not much doubt about the diagnosis if detailed information is obtained from more than one source. Multiple informants are vital since conduct problems may only occur in one setting, e.g. just at home or just at school. Epidemiological studies have shown that there is fairly low correlation between teacher and parent ratings of conduct problems.

Differential diagnoses to consider include:

(1) *Adjustment disorder* This can be diagnosed when onset occurs soon after exposure to an identifiable psychosocial stressor such as divorce, bereavement, adoption, trauma, and abuse – within one month according to ICD–10 and within three months according to DSM–IV – and when symptoms do not persist for more than six months after the cessation of the stress or its consequences.

(2) *Hyperactivity* Conduct disorder can be mistaken for hyperactivity and *vice versa*. This is partly due to overlap in symptoms, as shown in Box 6.3. Defiance, aggression and intentionally antisocial behaviour are not part of pure hyperactivity. In clinically referred populations, CD and hyperactivity often co-exist, when there is a danger of missing the hyperactivity.

(3) *Normal child* The child's behaviour is within the normal range, but parents or teachers have unrealistically high expectations.

(4) *Subcultural deviance* Some youngsters are antisocial but not particularly aggressive or defiant, and they are well adjusted within a deviant peer culture that approves of drug use, shoplifting, etc. They could be assigned

an ICD–10 diagnosis of socialised CD, but it is arguably a mistake to pathologise what can be seen as a cultural variant.

(5) *Autistic disorders* These are often accompanied by marked tantrums or destructiveness, and these conduct problems are occasionally the principal cause for referral.

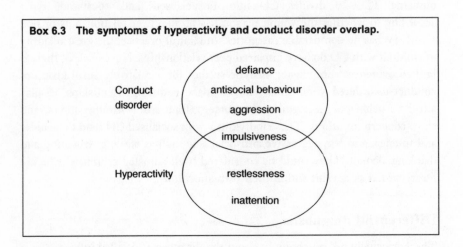

Box 6.3   The symptoms of hyperactivity and conduct disorder overlap.

Epidemiology

CD was diagnosed in 4% of children on the Isle of Wight, and many subsequent studies have reported even higher rates. The prevalence is particularly high in deprived inner-city areas. Boys are conduct disordered around three times more commonly than girls. The age of onset can vary considerably. CD is associated with lower socioeconomic status (this covers a multitude of variables), and large family size.

Causes

Genes or environment?

Though CD commonly clusters in families, shared environment may be more important than shared genes. Thus although twin studies have shown a high concordance for monozygotic pairs, the concordance for dizygotic pairs is also high. Adoption studies have shown the influence of the biological parents to be less than that of the adoptive ones. Genetic influences seem to play a stronger role in the development of adult antisocial personality and criminality. Cytogenetic and molecular genetic studies have added little so far. Epidemiological studies do not support the notion that individuals with the XYY karyotype are particularly prone to severe aggression.

Child-based mechanisms

Constitutional characteristics proposed include neurotransmitter imbalance, hormonal excess (notably testosterone), and metabolic variations such as low cholesterol. There are also abnormal arousal patterns with failure to calm down after frustration. None of these show replicable findings of any generality. However, infants with temperaments classified as 'difficult' are more likely to be referred for aggressive problems later on.

Psychological processes. Significant cognitive attributional bias has been shown in aggressive children whereby they are more likely to perceive neutral acts by others as hostile. As the child gets more disliked and rejected by his or her peers, the opportunity for seeing things this way increases. Social skills are lacking. Emotional processes in CD children have been little studied, although self-esteem is often low and co-existent misery common. The role of academic achievement is discussed above.

Immediate environment

(1) *Parental psychiatric disorder.* This is an important influence but is mainly mediated through marital discord and child-rearing practices and is not specific to any particular psychiatric condition in the parents.

(2) *Parental criminality.* Similar environmental considerations apply.

(3) *Child-rearing practices.* CD is strongly associated with discord between parents, hostility directed at the child, and lack of warmth. While these factors may partly be a reaction to the child's behaviour, follow-up and intervention studies suggest that they do also have a causal role in initiating and maintaining the child's disorder. Lack of supervision and inconsistent discipline are also clearly associated with CD, perhaps because the child is not given the opportunity to experience and learn predictable social rules. Overly harsh discipline is also associated with CD.

(4) *Parent-child interaction patterns.* Fine-grained analysis by Patterson (1994) has shown that children's disruptive behaviour escalates if this enables them to get more attention, avoid unpleasant demands or get their own way more often. By responding in ways that reward disruptive behaviour, and by failing to encourage socially acceptable behaviour, parents are training their children to behave antisocially. Interventions to break this cycle have been shown to be effective.

(5) *Sexual abuse* can lead to the emergence of conduct problems in girls or boys who were previously free of such problems.

Wider environment

(1) *School factors* have been shown to affect CD rates independently of home background: poorly-organised, unfriendly schools with low staff morale,

high staff turnover, and poor contact with parents have higher CD rates even when catchment area characteristics have been allowed for.

(2) *Wider social influences*. Though conduct problems are associated with overcrowding, poor housing, and poor neighbourhoods, it is still unclear if these factors are causal or simply markers for other family or socio-economic variables.

Assessment

The severity and frequency of defiant, aggressive and antisocial acts in the last month or so should be established in detail. Some parents are prone to catalogue all 'bad' things done over the last year or even since birth. Attention and activity should be enquired about in the same detailed way (see Chapter 5) since hyperactivity is a common and easily overlooked accompaniment (or differential diagnosis) of conduct problems. Though it is worth enquiring about impulsiveness, this could be part of either hyperactivity or conduct problems. Do not forget to enquire about emotional symptoms, particularly unhappiness and misery. Part of the problem may derive from things that are upsetting the child, e.g. a father who often fails to turn up for his access visits, or a mother who never seems to appreciate them however hard they try. The strength of these concerns may only come out in an individual interview with the child, and could easily be missed if the family are only ever seen together.

Parenting practices should be enquired about in detail, with a blow-by-blow account of what happens before, during and after a recent episode of troublesome behaviour. Who 'won' the encounter? What was said? How long did it take for relations to return to normal? More generally, ask how much praise and encouragement is given for constructive behaviour, and how much time is spent in joint activities. Try to gauge the parents' sensitivity to the child's moods and needs, and how much they take these into account when negotiating conflicts and planning the child's life.

Consider the parents' emotional tone and attitude towards the child. Asking about the child's good qualities can be helpful. Is there some warmth and approval despite the child's difficulties, or is the tone entirely negative? Powerful beliefs may be discovered which will need to be addressed if treatment is to progress, e.g. 'There's something wrong in his head', or 'He's just like his father. He was rotten too'.

Direct observation of parents and children is invaluable in getting a picture of their interactions, albeit in atypical circumstances. Are clear boundaries set, or is the child allowed to get away with almost anything? For example, how do the parents react when the child tries to leave the room? Is good behaviour praised or ignored? Is the child handled sensitively?

A school report is essential, covering antisocial behaviour, ability to concentrate and sit still, peer relations, and scholastic attainments, including test results. There are occasions when troublesome behaviour in class can take up so much of the teacher's time that significant reading difficulties can be overlooked or simply regarded as a consequence of the bad behaviour.

Treatment

Child-focused

(1) *Behaviour modification* can be very effective in modifying one or two specific antisocial behaviours, but does not usually generalise.

(2) *Problem-solving skills training and social skills training.* Both of these have been shown to have definite although so far modest effects.

(3) *Individual psychotherapy* is usually unfruitful as these children have little insight into why they behave the way they do. Furthermore, when they can identify what is upsetting them, they are not usually in a position to modify it or find another way of coping.

(4) *Medication and diet.* When children are hyperactive as well as conduct disordered, it may be appropriate to treat their restlessness and inattention with medication or diet (see Chapters 5 and 31). When stimulant medication reduces restlessness and inattention, it may well reduce defiance, aggression and antisocial behaviour too. There is no evidence that stimulants reduce conduct problems in children who are not also hyperactive. There is some evidence that lithium may be of value for children who have explosive outbursts in response to minimal provocation, and who have not responded to appropriate psychological management, but it is very rarely prescribed for this purpose. When diet helps hyperactivity, it often reduces irritability too.

Family-focused

(5) *Family counselling and social work* is essential to address the more gross disruptive influences to provide a setting for more specific therapeutic work.

(6) *Family therapy* is frequently used but has hardly been evaluated. Judging from clinical experience, it is often useful in fairly well-functioning families where after only a few sessions parents may collaborate in setting clear boundaries for their child and improve the emotional atmosphere; it is less useful for chaotic, disorganised families who lack coping skills.

(7) *Parent management training* is probably the most promising approach, being of well-replicated effectiveness. It gets parents to pay attention to desired behaviour rather than get caught up in lengthy slanging matches;

positive aspects of parent-child relationships are promoted, and parents are also taught effective techniques for handling undesired behaviour.

Community-focused

(8) *Prevention programmes* are currently under evaluation.

Continuity and outcome

- Forwards continuity: 40% of children with CD become delinquent young adults with ongoing behaviour problems and disrupted relationships.
- Backwards continuity: 90% of young adult delinquents had CD as children.

Factors predicting outcome

In child: A poor outcome is predicted by early onset, a wide range and high total number of symptoms, greater severity and frequency of individual symptoms, pervasiveness across situations (home, school and other), and associated hyperactivity. Conversely, having only one area of problem behaviour, such as aggressiveness alone, has a good prognosis provided there are no problems in other areas, including peer relationships and educational achievements. The presence or absence of a *constellation* of problems is what is important.

In family: A poor outcome is predicted by parental psychiatric disorder, parental criminality, high hostility, and high discord focused on the child.

Type of adult outcome

- *Homotypic* continuity seen more in males (i.e. the symptoms remain much the same): aggressiveness and violence, antisocial personality, alcohol, drugs; crime.
- *Heterotypic* continuity seen more in females (i.e. different types of symptoms come to predominate): wide range of emotional and personality disorders, less aggressiveness and criminality.

In addition to being at greater psychiatric and forensic risk, individuals with a history of CD are also more likely to be socially impaired in adulthood, being more likely to have few if any educational qualifications, a poor job history, and impaired social relations, e.g. more marital breakup.

Subject review

Earls, F. (1994) Oppositional-defiant and conduct disorders. In *Child and Adolescent Psychiatry: Modern Approaches*, 3rd edn (M. Rutter, E. Taylor and L. Hersov, eds) Blackwell Science, Oxford. pp. 308–329.

Kazdin, A.E. (1995) *Conduct Disorders in Childhood and Adolescence*, 2nd edn. Sage, Beverly Hills, CA.

Further reading

Loeber, R. & Hay, D.F. (1994) Developmental approaches to aggression and conduct problems. In *Development Through Life: A Handbook For Clinicians* (M. Rutter and D.F. Hay, eds) Blackwell Science, Oxford. pp. 488–516.

Quay, H.C. (1993) The psychobiology of undersocialised aggressive conduct disorder: a theoretical perspective. *Development and Psychopathology*, 5, 165–180.

Patterson, G.R. (1994) Some alternatives to seven myths about treating families of antisocial children. In *Crime and the Family* (C. Henricson, ed.) Family Policy Studies Centre, London. pp. 26–49. (This is an accessible introduction to the thinking of one of the most influential figures in the field.)

Webster-Stratton, C. *et al.* (1989) The long-term effectiveness and clinical significance of three cost-effective training programs for families with conduct-problem children. *Journal of Consulting and Clinical Psychology*, 57, 550–553.

7 Juvenile Delinquency

In the UK, this is defined as a person between the ages of 10 and 17 who has been found guilty of an offence which would be criminal in an adult. Thus the definition is legal and is not directly related to mental health. Contrary to popular belief, more than 90% of the offences are against property rather than persons: thieving, driving away cars, breaking in, and destructive vandalism. Personal violence, drug offences and sex offences comprise less than 10%. Comparisons of official records with delinquents' self-reports and the results of victim surveys suggest that official records only cover about one tenth of all offences committed. This discrepancy between actual and reported offences applies mainly to smaller crimes; more serious ones are reported in the majority of cases. For relatively minor offences, the chance of being caught decreases if the perpetrator is white, attends a high-achieving school, is from an orderly home, and is of normal intelligence. This is not true for more serious offences – personal and demographic characteristics are closely similar whether judged from self-reports or from official records. Once caught, the chances of being charged are increased if there is a previous criminal record, if the type of offence is considered serious, and if the individual is older or black.

Epidemiology

Age. There is an overall peak in law-breaking in the late teens, when theft and property offences are at a maximum; violence peaks in the early twenties and there is a rapid decrease overall by the mid-twenties. One half to three-quarters of people convicted will never be convicted again, leaving a 'hard core' of around a quarter who repeat. The characteristics which predict repeaters are similar in kind to those which predict delinquency overall, but are more marked. Starting young is a major predictor of persistence. Thus in the influential 'Cambridge' Longitudinal Study carried out in inner London by West and Farrington, three-quarters of those with more than three convictions as a juvenile went on to repeated offending as a young adult.

Sex. Both in Europe and North America, male delinquents are 3 to 10 times commoner than female delinquents, irrespective of whether this is judged from official records or self-reports. The male preponderance is most marked for aggressive offences. Some offences, most notably shoplifting, are commoner in females. There are many possible explanations for the gender differences, ranging from the biological, supported by the cross-cultural invariance and parallel gender differences in non-human primates, to the cultural, looking at which behaviours are differentially encouraged and sanctioned in boys and girls. Current evidence suggests that both biological predisposition and psychosocial factors are relevant. Thus, boys are more liable to biologically based syndromes such as hyperkinesis that increase the risk of delinquency; and boys are also more likely to be accepted and praised when they display aggression.

Socioeconomic status (SES). There are substantial effects, although many authors like to play this down as it covaries with many other factors. The magnitude of the SES gradient is evident from UK surveys showing that the rates of juvenile delinquency were around 5% for professional and managerial families, as opposed to around 25% for unskilled manual workers' families. Self-reports confirm this trend for the more serious offences, but the ratio comes down to 2:1 for less serious ones. By comparison, conduct disorder shows less SES gradient.

Race. In the UK, both official records and victim reports suggest that Afro-Caribbean youths are between five and ten times more likely than their white counterparts to be involved in assault, robbery, violence and theft. This was not true for first-generation Afro-Caribbean immigrants 30 years ago. For other juvenile offences, the current Afro-Caribbean rates are around double the white rates. These black-white differences are partly but not totally explained by socioeconomic factors and family characteristics; decades of prejudice and harassment may also have much to answer for. At present, delinquency rates for 'Asian' youths are lower than, or equal to, white rates.

Epoch. Historical accounts seem to indicate that violent crime was very prevalent in the middle of the 18th century, but then declined, reaching a trough in the late 19th and early 20th century, before rising again. The last 50 years have probably seen a fairly steady rise in juvenile offending. Internationally, officially reported crime rates have mostly increased by a factor of between two and six in most countries over this period, though this is partly attributable to better recording. Changes in officially recorded juvenile delinquency rates are more inconsistent, at least partly because these official rates are very sensitive to changes in policy. For example, the official delinquency rates can dramatically increase or decrease if the police switch from unrecorded warnings to recorded cautions, or *vice versa*. Over recent decades, the proportion of offences involving violence has stayed fairly constant at well under 10%, but the proportion of women perpetrators involved has increased from around one-tenth to around one-fifth.

Locality. There are clear neighbourhood differences in delinquency rates that cannot be entirely explained by social class or other socioeconomic factors. The architectural design of buildings on estates has been shown to have some effect; the ability to keep an eye on people and the feeling of responsibility for what has been termed 'defensible space' seems important. At a broader level, the Isle of Wight/Inner London comparison found more than double the rate of conduct disorders in the inner city area compared with a rural area, and this was all accounted for by psychosocial family factors such as parental psychiatric disorder, parental criminality, and family discord. It has been suggested that where there are stable cohesive neighbourhoods without too much change in those living there, the social network inhibits crime. The 'Cambridge' study found that convicted juveniles who then moved out of a deprived area of inner London had a lower reconviction rate than those who stayed, even when other risk factors were controlled for.

Associated factors

Family

- *Size*. Particularly in lower socioeconomic groups, there is a strong association with large family size, especially having a number of brothers rather than sisters. Conversely, the delinquency rate is considerably lower among only children.

- *Income*. Low income is strongly associated with greater delinquency.

- *Criminality*. Serious juvenile offences are particularly strongly associated with a history of criminality in parents or siblings. Is this due to shared genes, shared deprivation, or social learning? Twin and adoption studies of adult recidivist criminals do suggest a modest genetic influence. Studies of juvenile delinquency also suggest a small genetic influence, but shared environmental effects generally seem more important.

- *Child rearing experiences*. Juvenile delinquency, like conduct disorder, is strongly associated with lack of caring supervision and broken homes. The emotional tone is frequently one of hostility and discord. There is often a lack of house rules, and a low level of monitoring of the child's behaviour and feelings; parents respond infrequently to either desired or deviant behaviour, so that any punishments are inconsistent and such praising as there is, is irregular. A lack of techniques for dealing with family crises and problems means that conflict leads to ongoing tension and disputes.

Individual factors

- *Behaviour*. Around 90% of recidivist delinquents were antisocial enough to meet criteria for conduct disorder in middle childhood. Thus the notion that the majority of this persistently delinquent group were fine initially but then 'fell in with a bad crowd' in adolescence is a myth. On the other hand, the majority of one-time offenders have unremarkable earlier histories – it is indeed often part of 'a phase teenagers commonly go through'.

- *Intelligence*. There is a fairly strong association between lower IQ and greater delinquency. Thus in one study 20% of youths with an IQ of less than 90 were recidivist, as opposed to 2% of youths with an IQ of 110 or more. Self-report figures show the association between delinquency and low IQ is not simply due to brighter delinquents escaping detection. Perhaps the link between low IQ and delinquency is mediated by educational failure, poor self-esteem and frustration. Alternatively, low IQ may simply be a marker for other biological or social disadvantages. It is interesting that the link between low IQ and conduct problems has been found at as young an age as three years old.

- *Biology*. The genetic contribution to adult criminality has already been mentioned. By comparison with controls, adult criminals have been shown to have less autonomic reactivity to stress, impaired passive avoidance learning, greater aggression, poorer attention skills and a greater tendency to seek thrills. Whether these characteristics are acquired or inherited is unclear. Offending is only rarely attributable to specific organic syndromes. Though EEG studies of delinquents do not show any consistent abnormalities, seriously aggressive outbursts are sometimes attributed to an 'episodic dyscontrol syndrome', perhaps linked to temporal lobe pathology and complex partial seizures. The XYY chromosome anomaly is not associated with an increase in violent crime, but does seem to be associated with an excess of petty criminality, perhaps mediated by the link with low intelligence.

- *Relationships*. Juvenile delinquents are more likely than non-delinquents to have impaired and disharmonious relationships with same-sex peers and with members of the opposite sex.

- *Attitudes*. Do delinquents have a consistently anti-establishment set of values? Most studies suggest not. When asked why they commit offences, young delinquents commonly mention the thrill, the relief from boredom, and the satisfaction of demonstrating their prowess to peers; material gain is often not the main objective. Studies of young offenders' moral reasoning shows more egoism and less altruism; they are less able to take another person's point of view or think about the consequences of actions.

- *Personality*. There have been no consistent differences in personality using Eysenck's or others' measures.

Management

Most effort is directed at the quarter of offenders who repeatedly break the law. There is little evidence for the effectiveness of punishments such as prison or other judicial approaches, and beliefs in 'short, sharp shocks' at one extreme and prolonged individual therapy at the other owe more to fashion and political ideology than empirical evidence.

Two treatment approaches have been well evaluated and shown to be effective. Functional family therapy and the more broadly-based multisystemic therapy (MST) have been shown in replicated studies to reduce re-offending rates (usually by around one half) and increase sociable behaviour. MST has six elements which are flexibly applied according to the needs of the young person (Box 7.1). Parent-training has also been shown to reduce offending rates, but at considerable emotional cost to staff involved.

Box 7.1   Elements of multisystemic therapy (MST).

(1) Family therapy which focuses on effective communication, systematic reward and punishment systems, and taking a problem-solving approach to day-to-day conflicts.
(2) Encouragement to spend more time with peers who do not have problems, and to stop seeing other delinquents.
(3) Liaison with school to improve learning and homework performance, and restructure after-school hours.
(4) Individual development, including assertiveness training against negative peer influences.
(5) Empowerment of youths and their parents to cope with family, school, peer and neighbourhood problems. The emphasis is on promoting the family's own problem-solving abilities, not providing ready-made answers.
(6) Coordination with other agencies, e.g. juvenile justice, social work, mental health, education.

Preventative programmes are theoretically attractive as they operate before antisocial behaviour is thoroughly ingrained. These programmes are targeted at early or middle childhood and can be at one of three levels: *universal* interventions for all children; interventions for children at *high risk* of becoming offenders; and interventions aiming for the *secondary prevention* of offending behaviour in referred populations who already have established conduct problems. Few universal programmes have yet been evaluated, but there are promising high-risk programmes that involve the following three components: parent-management training, reading remediation, and teacher-training in classroom management techniques. Secondary prevention may well be feasible since parent-management training has been shown to reduce conduct problems in middle childhood, though it has yet to be established that this does reduce subsequent delinquency. One problem with all prevention approaches is the difficulty of enrolling those families whose children are most likely to need this help.

Subject reviews

Rutter, M.L., Giller, H. and Hagell, A. (1997) *Juvenile Delinquency*, in press.
Sheldrick, C. (1994) Treatment of delinquents. In *Child and Adolescent Psychiatry:*

Modern Approaches, 3rd edn (M. Rutter, E. Taylor and L. Hersov, eds) Blackwell Science, Oxford, pp. 968–982.

Further reading

Borduin, C.M. *et al.* (1995) Multisystemic treatment of serious juvenile offenders: Long-term prevention of criminality and violence. *Journal of Consulting and Clinical Psychology*, **63**, 569–578.

Farrington, D.P. (1995) The development of offending and antisocial behaviour from childhood: key findings from the Cambridge study in delinquent development. *Journal of Child Psychology and Psychiatry*, **36**, 929–964. (This summarises a particularly influential longitudinal study of delinquency and its predictors.)

Henggeler, S.W. and Schoenwald, S.K. (1994) Boot camps for juvenile offenders: Just say no. *Journal of Child and Family Studies*, **3**, 243–248.

Robins, L. (1978) Sturdy childhood predictors of adult antisocial behaviour: replications from longitudinal studies. *Psychological Medicine*, **8**, 611–622.

8   School Refusal

Roughly 5% of child psychiatric referrals present with refusal to attend school associated with anxiety or misery. This presentation is labelled 'school refusal'. The term 'school phobia' is probably best avoided since refusal to go to school is more often due to reluctance to leave home than to fear of school itself. It is important to remember that school refusal is not a diagnosis – it is a presenting complaint that can reflect a variety of problems in the child, family or school system as a whole. It is also worth noting that school refusal is salient because we live in a society that particularly values schooling and makes it compulsory. There is no administrative or psychiatric category for 'shopping refusal' or 'weeding refusal', though there probably would be if children were expected and obliged to spend much of their time shopping or weeding the garden.

Epidemiology

School refusal peaks at three ages: at five to six on starting school; around 11 after transfer to secondary school; and in the early teens. Though many primary school children express reluctance to go to school, their parents are generally able to get them to school despite that reluctance. 'Successful' school refusal is commoner among secondary than primary school children, partly because it is harder to compel older children to attend school against their will. In the Isle of Wight survey, no cases of school refusal were found among over 2000 children assessed in their last two years of primary school. When the same children were assessed at 14 and 15 years of age, there were 15 cases of school refusal (representing a prevalence of 0.7%).

School refusal is equally common in boys and girls. No one socioeconomic group is particularly vulnerable.

Characteristic features

The child either refuses to go to school or sets out for school but returns home before or shortly after arriving at school. In some cases the child is explicit that he or she is frightened to leave home or attend school. In other cases school refusal assumes a 'somatic disguise' without overtly expressed fears, e.g. there are complaints of headache, stomach-ache, malaise or tachycardia before leaving for school or once at school. The absence of complaints at weekends or during school holidays is a helpful clue.

Attempts to force the reluctant child to attend school are met with tears, pleading, tantrums or physical resistance. In contrast to truancy, the children do not make a secret of their non-attendance – the parents know where their child is, generally for the good reason that the child is in or near the home.

The onset of school refusal may be abrupt, or may be gradual with the child expressing increasing reluctance to attend school and staying away for more and more days each week. Precipitating factors can often be identified, e.g. a change of teacher, a move to a new school, the loss of a friend, or an illness. The onset is more likely to be insidious in adolescence, with a progressive withdrawal from peer group activities that were previously enjoyed. Onset or relapse of school refusal is particularly common after a period off school due to holiday or illness.

School refusal usually results from a combination of the child's unwillingness to attend and parental inability or unwillingness to make them go. It can be a manifestation of a variety of underlying psychiatric disorders. These disorders commonly result in symptoms other than the school refusal itself, and these additional symptoms provide useful clues to the nature of the school refusal. For example, a child who refuses to go to school because of separation anxiety may also refuse to go to Scouts or birthday parties, whereas a child who refuses to go to school because of fear of being bullied may be happy to go to Scouts or parties. Symptoms of misery and hopelessness even when the child is not under pressure to attend school suggest an underlying depressive disorder.

Associated features

Family factors

As well as the child's unwillingness to attend, there is often a lack of effective pressure from the parents to get the child to school and keep them there. In some cases this may seem justified by the marked distress experienced by the child. Often, however, it reflects some combination of three family processes:

(1) Ineffectual home organisation and discipline. This may be seen in a general lack of enforced house rules, and is more likely to come about if the father is absent or ineffectual.

(2) Emotional over-involvement with the child. For example, the mother may be anxious not to upset the child and incur his or her disapproval by being firm; she may also feel the better for having the child around her during the day. The child may be perceived as particularly precious or vulnerable, e.g. having survived a very premature birth contrary to the doctors' expectations.

(3) Difficulty negotiating with outside agencies, e.g. liaising with the school to address bullying or academic stress, or getting help for emotional difficulties.

Intelligence and attainments

As a group, school refusers are of average intelligence and academic ability. Problems with school work may be present but are not usually the main factors leading to school refusal. Objective measures of the child's attainment level – from school tests or psychometric tests – are frequently useful, if only to reassure the child.

Child's personality

The child may always have been a rather quiet conformist who has relatively few friends and who is easily 'thrown' by minor mishaps. On the other hand, the child's previous personality may have been unremarkable or outgoing. There is commonly a history of previous separation difficulties when first attending nursery or school.

Family composition

Family size is irrelevant, i.e. there is no over-representation of only children or children from large families. Youngest (rather than middle or eldest) children are probably at greatest risk.

Differential diagnosis

Truants stay away from school to engage in alternative activities without parental permission. In many schools, this is the commonest cause of non-attendance in the last year or so before teenagers are officially allowed to leave school. In most cases truants spend the day in groups, and their parents are unaware of their whereabouts. Whereas school refusal is often secondary to an emotional disorder, truancy is often linked to conduct disorder. Unlike school refusal, therefore, truancy is associated with the predictors of conduct disorder: male sex, social disadvantage, large family, parental criminality, marital discord, poor school attainment, inconsistent discipline, and lax supervision.

Some parents deliberately *withhold* their children from school, either because they think school is useless or because they need their child's help. An ill mother, for example, may choose to keep one of her children home for company or to do the housework. The distinction between withholding and school refusal is not always clear since the parents of school refusers are often anxious themselves and may collude with their child's decision to stay at home.

Physical illness is by far the commonest reason for non-attendance at school, except during the last year or so of compulsory education when truancy rates are often high. It is not always easy to distinguish between this and school refusal in a 'somatic disguise'. Being better at weekends is not an infallible guide: genuine illnesses may be aggravated by school-related stresses, and most children are capable of exaggerating genuine symptoms when it suits them.

Underlying psychiatric conditions in the child

School refusal can be the presenting complaint for children with a variety of underlying disorders, with *separation anxiety* being the commonest diagnosis, particularly among younger children. In many cases, school refusal results when a child who does not want to separate has parents who do not insist very forcefully on school attendance, either because they are poor at imposing limits in general or because they share their child's anxieties about separation.

In a minority of cases, school refusal arises not from anxiety about leaving home but from a *specific phobia* related to school or to the journey to and from school. There may be a specific travel phobia, a fear of bullies, of one particular teacher, or of one particular subject. Children's complaints about school may be a smoke-screen for separation anxiety, but they should not be dismissed without investigation.

Depression is particularly important as a cause of school refusal in teenagers, though different studies have generated very different prevalence estimates.

Psychosis is a rare cause of adolescent school refusal.

Treatment

A behavioural 'back to school' approach is particularly likely to be successful when refusal to attend school began recently and relatively suddenly. A rapid return to full-time school is often possible once parents are persuaded that consistent firmness is in the child's best interests. With motivated parents and supportive teachers, this approach can be very effective. When the anxiety level in the child or parents is particularly high, or when the child has been out of school for a long time, a gradual desensitisation approach may be more appropriate, e.g. visiting the school out of hours first and then spending progressively longer periods at school every day.

Informing parents about the detrimental effects on social development of being out of school may help them see the need for a return to school. They are usually already well aware of the academic disadvantages. Family therapy approaches can empower parents to set firm boundaries and exert control over the child while reducing over-involvement.

Once school refusal has become chronic, there are a variety of additional obstacles that need to be overcome in order to get the child back to school. As time goes on, the child gets increasingly far behind with school work, former friends find new people to play with, and the prospect of explaining the prolonged absence to classmates becomes ever more daunting. At the same time, extra parental attention while at home all day may be very rewarding. If the child is to return to school, the obstacles need to be overcome (e.g. coaching the child in an acceptable explanation of his or her absence) and the balance of rewards and disincentives needs to be altered to favour school attendance rather than non-attendance.

Liaison with education is essential. Teachers need to be as well prepared as possible to support the child's return to school, often backed up by educational social workers and educational psychologists. Providing home tuition during the period when the child is out of school is often inappropriate since it reduces the pressure on all concerned to achieve a more definitive solution and legitimises the child spending all day at home. If return to school is delayed, attending a tutorial unit with other children is a more satisfactory interim solution. Though parents and children often maintain that a change in school would solve the problem, this is rarely the case. Instead, the slow process of arranging a school transfer delays the implementation of a more appropriate solution. Even when school factors (such as bullying) are important, the school should generally be given a reasonable chance to overcome the problems rather than opting at once for a school transfer.

The evidence does not favour the use of medication for school refusal due to separation anxiety disorder (see Chapter 9). One possible indication for medication is the use of tricyclics for adolescents whose school refusal is associated with panic attacks. The value of medication is also uncertain when school refusal is due to depression. As discussed in Chapter 10, conventional antidepressants often seem ineffective in the treatment of childhood or teenage depression.

In-patient treatment is sometimes appropriate when the child's problems are so severe or entrenched that there is no response to other forms of treatment, and when the family environment actively maintains the disorder and blocks effective treatment.

Prognosis

Even though many reported series include a disproportionate number of severe cases, the success rate for return to school is generally 70% or better. This success rate is higher when the child is younger, when the symptoms are less severe, and when intervention is soon after the onset. Even when return to school is successful, emotional symptoms and relationship problems commonly persist. Though most school refusers become normal adults, social relationships may be somewhat limited and around a third have persisting emotional disorders. Only a small minority develop agoraphobia or become unable to face going to work.

Subject review

Berg, I. (1992) Absence from school and mental health. *British Journal of Psychiatry*, **161**, 154–166.

Further reading

Bernstein, G.A. and Garfinkel, B.D. (1986) School phobia: the overlap of affective and anxiety disorders. *Journal of the American Academy of Child Psychiatry*, **25**, 235–241.

Flakierska, N. *et al.* (1988) School refusal: a 15–20 year follow-up of 35 Swedish urban children. *British Journal of Psychiatry*, **152**, 834–837.

9 Anxiety Disorders

Worries, fears and misery often cluster together, along with somatic complaints in many cases. Given the considerable overlap, children with socially incapacitating fears, worries or misery were traditionally 'lumped' into a relatively broad-band category of *emotional disorders of childhood*. Of late, the 'splitters' have been more influential, delineating the large number of specific anxiety and depressive disorders included in ICD–10 and DSM–IV. This attempt to increase diagnostic precision has its drawbacks. Some children do not quite match any set of operationalised diagnostic criteria, while other children with broad-band symptomatology qualify for several labels simultaneously.

Epidemiology

The Isle of Wight study diagnosed clinically significant anxiety disorders in 2% of 10- and 11-year-olds, whereas more recent surveys of children and adolescents suggest a prevalence of roughly 5–10%. Prevalence estimates depend on assessment methods, e.g. studies that ask both children and parents find higher rates of anxiety disorders than studies that rely entirely on parent reports. The definition of a disorder also influences the apparent prevalence – the highest estimates generally derive from studies that do not stipulate that the child should be socially impaired by the worries or fears. Does a child have a disorder if he or she has a variety of worries or fears but is not incapacitated by them? There is no definite answer at present, but follow-up or treatment studies of youngsters who have symptoms without social incapacity may help provide an answer. The effects of gender, age and socioeconomic status on prevalence vary from one anxiety disorder to another.

Causation

Anxiety disorders run in families: affected parents are more likely to have affected children, and *vice versa*. The twin and adoption studies needed to distinguish between cultural and genetic transmission have yet to be carried out.

Catastrophic life events are clearly relevant to post-traumatic stress disorder. Other anxiety disorders may also be related to adverse life events, including the cumulative impact of a series of relatively minor life events.

Many theories suggest that anxiety is due to experiencing threat (while depression is due to experiencing loss). According to Bowlby's influential formulation based on attachment theory (see Chapter 27), anxiety – and particularly separation anxiety – often arises from threatened or actual separations from key attachment figures (e.g. when parents punish their children by threatening to send them away). Psychodynamic theories formulate the threat in terms of intrapsychic conflicts.

Classical conditioning can potentially explain the way in which previously neutral stimuli can, by association with a frightening experience, become fear-evoking in themselves. Operant conditioning theory predicts subsequent avoidance of these stimuli (thereby blocking the opportunity for natural exposure and the extinction of the fear).

VARIETIES OF ANXIETY DISORDER

The three most common anxiety disorders are separation anxiety disorder, generalised anxiety disorder, and specific phobias. Avoidant disorder and panic disorder are less common, as is post-traumatic stress disorder (PTSD – covered in Chapter 12).

Separation anxiety disorder

Anxiety about separation from parents and other major attachment figures usually emerges around six months and remains prominent during the pre-school years, subsequently waning as the child acquires the ability to keep attachment figures, and the security they provide, 'in mind' even when they are not physically present. Separation anxiety disorder is diagnosed when the intensity of separation anxiety is developmentally inappropriate and leads to substantial social incapacity, e.g. refusal to go to school.

Characteristic features

Affected children worry unrealistically that their parents will come to harm or leave and not return. They also worry about themselves, fearing that they will get lost, be kidnapped, be admitted to hospital, or be separated from their parents by some other calamity. These worries may also emerge as themes of recurrent nightmares. The children are commonly clingy even in their own home, e.g. following a parent from room to room. There may be reluctance or refusal to attend school, or to sleep alone, or to sleep away from home. Separations, or the anticipation of separations, may result in pleading, tantrums and tears, or may result in purely physical complaints e.g. headaches, stomach-aches, nausea.

Epidemiology

Several surveys have reported separation anxiety disorder in about 2–4% of children. It is the commonest anxiety disorder in prepubertal children. The disorder is less common in adolescence. The disorder may be commoner in females and in children from lower socioeconomic groups.

Treatment

Operant techniques (e.g. star charts or contingency management) may be used to alter the balance of rewards and disincentives that favour clinging rather than separation. Graded exposure to increasingly more demanding separations can be useful. Cognitive therapy may have a place, teaching coping self-statements to the child. Sometimes the child's clinginess is increased by the parents' own need to stay close to the child, by the parents' own anxieties, or by the parents' underestimation of their child's capacity for independence – issues that can be the focus of work with the parents or with the family as a whole. Parents can be encouraged to take practical steps to make their child feel more secure, e.g. providing adequate warning and explanation before leaving the child with a baby-sitter. Though one controlled trial suggested that tricyclic antidepressants reduced separation anxiety and thereby facilitated a return to school, subsequent studies have not replicated this finding. The only controlled trial of a benzodiazepine for school refusal due to separation anxiety was also negative. Overall, therefore, there is no convincing evidence that tricyclics or benzodiazepines have a useful role.

Course

Some children experience a chronic low level of separation anxiety punctuated by episodes of exacerbated anxiety, e.g. precipitated by a change of school or by illness in a parent. Over the years, anxieties about separations may be replaced by a wider range of anxieties more typical of generalized anxiety disorder. It is uncertain if there is any continuity with agoraphobia or panic disorder.

Generalised anxiety disorder

This is a category used for both children and adults in DSM–IV and ICD–10 (incorporating what used to be the child-specific 'overanxious disorder' of DSM–III–R).

Characteristic features

Children and adolescents with generalised anxiety disorder are marked and persistent worriers whose anxieties are not consistently focused on any one object or situation. Typical worries focus on the future, on past behaviour, and on personal competence. These worries are commonly accompanied by tension, inability to relax, self-consciousness, need for frequent reassurance, and somatic complaints, such as headaches and stomach-aches. DSM–IV criteria stipulate that the symptoms must have caused clinically significant distress or social impairment. ICD–10 does not have comparable impact criteria, increasing the likelihood that children who are 'worriers' by temperament will be given a disorder label even if their quality of life is hardly affected by their anxieties.

Epidemiology

Roughly 3% of children are affected, with higher rates in adolescents. The sex ratio may be equal, or there may be a slight female preponderance. Children of high socioeconomic status are over-represented. Many children with generalized anxiety disorder also fulfil the criteria for other DSM–IV and ICD–10 diagnoses, particularly relating to separation anxiety, depression and specific phobias.

Treatment

Relaxation and cognitive therapy may be helpful. There is no good evidence for drug treatment.

Course

The disorder often persists for years, and may continue into adult life.

Specific phobias

Characteristic features

Specific persistent fears of circumscribed stimuli are very common in childhood, with different fears peaking at different ages, e.g. fear of animals peaks at age two to four years, fear of the dark or of imaginary creatures peaks at age four to six, and fear of death or war is particularly common during adolescence. To be classified as a specific phobia, both ICD–10 and DSM–IV stipulate that the feared object or event must be avoided, or endured with intense anxiety. DSM–IV also stipulates that the avoidance, anxious anticipation, or distress in the feared situation results in significant social incapacity (e.g. preventing the child from engaging in age-appropriate leisure activities), or there is marked distress about having the phobia. Children may lack the cognitive maturity to recognise the irrational nature of their fear.

Epidemiology

Specific phobias probably affect 2–4% of children and adolescents, though the great majority of these phobias are relatively mild. Girls report more fears than boys at all ages, and phobias are correspondingly commoner in girls too.

Though younger children report more fears than adolescents, there are no clear age trends in clinically significant phobias.

Treatment

Desensitisation, contingency management and cognitive techniques may all be helpful.

Course

Though mild fears are often transient, true phobias – particularly if they are severe – are more likely to be persistent and may continue into adulthood.

Social anxiety disorder of childhood

This ICD–10 diagnosis corresponds to DSM–III–R's category of avoidant disorder but has no counterpart in DSM–IV. The condition can be thought of as an exaggeration and undue persistence of the normal phase of stranger anxiety (which is commonly prominent up to the age of 30 months in ordinary children). Affected children have good social relationships with family members and other familiar individuals but show marked avoidance of contact with unfamiliar people, resulting in social incapacity (e.g. in peer relationships). They may remain unassertive and socially impaired into adolescence, or they may improve spontaneously. It is not clear how useful it is to think of these children as having an anxiety disorder as opposed to extremely shy personalities. In practice, many affected children meet the criteria for other anxiety disorders, most commonly generalised anxiety disorder. Though social anxiety disorder is clearly not exactly the same condition as social phobia (with the latter typically starting in the mid-teens and involving fear of public scrutiny and humiliation), social phobia can arise from a background of long-standing childhood shyness and inhibition. This suggests that social anxiety disorder may sometimes evolve into more typical social phobia. The relationship with avoidant personality disorder in adulthood is unknown.

Panic disorder

The key feature of panic disorder, which may or may not be accompanied by agoraphobia, is the presence of discrete panic attacks, at least some of which occur unexpectedly without any obvious precipitant. The peak age of onset is 15–19 years. Panic attacks are rare in prepubertal children, and when they do occur the affected individuals are particularly likely to have a positive family history. Treatment options include tricyclic antidepressants and cognitive therapy.

Subject reviews

Bernstein, G.A. *et al.* (1996) Anxiety disorders in children and adolescents: a review of the past 10 years. *Journal of the American Academy of Child Psychology and Psychiatry*, 35, 1110–1119.

Klein, R.G. (1994) Anxiety disorders. In *Child and Adolescent Psychiatry: Modern Approaches*, 3rd edn (M. Rutter, E. Taylor and L. Hersov, eds) Blackwell Science, Oxford, pp. 351–374.

Further reading

Biederman, J. *et al.* (1993) A 3-year follow-up of children with and without behavioral inhibition. *Journal of the American Academy of Child Psychology and Psychiatry*, 32, 814–821. (This examines the extent to which childhood anxiety disorders are in continuity with one of the most widely studied traits of early childhood.)

Engel, N.A. *et al.* (1994) Parent–child agreement on ratings of anxiety in children. *Psychological Reports*, 75, 1251–1260. (It is sobering to see how poorly parents and children agree on anxiety symptoms.)

10 Depression and Mania

DEPRESSION

The term depression can refer to a single symptom, a symptom cluster, or a disorder.

Depression as a single symptom

Epidemiological studies show that many children are miserable. In the Isle of Wight studies, about 10% of 10-year-olds were miserable according to their parents, and over 40% of 14-year-olds were miserable by their own account (with almost 15% being observably sad at interview). Among children with psychiatric disorders, the symptom of misery is commoner still (being common among conduct-disordered children as well as among emotionally disordered children). It is uncertain whether the symptom of depression differs from ordinary sadness in kind or just in degree. Possible distinguishing features between normal sadness and abnormal depression include severity, persistence, and quality of mood, i.e. the child describes the mood as qualitatively different from ordinary sadness.

Depression as a symptom cluster

In children as in adults, the symptom of depression is sometimes part of a wider constellation of affective, cognitive and behavioural symptoms. Associated symptoms include: reduction or loss of ability to experience pleasure (anhedonia); low self-esteem; self-blame; guilt; helplessness; hopelessness; suicidal thoughts and acts; loss of energy; poor concentration; restlessness; and changes in appetite, weight and sleep. The symptom cluster of depression is not necessarily abnormal – it is a part of normal grief, for example.

Depression as a disorder

When should a child with the symptom cluster of depression be described as suffering from a depressive disorder? There is no consensus yet, but the criteria have certainly become more inclusive over the last decade, so that rates of diagnosed depression have risen dramatically. DSM–IV and the research version of ICD–10 both specify that symptoms must persist for at least two weeks to constitute a depressive episode, and core symptoms have to be present for most of the day for the majority of these days. Some definitions state that a disorder is only present if the depressive symptoms result in social incapacity as well as distress: an additional criterion that has the advantage of sharpening the distinction between normality and abnormality, but the disadvantage of excluding children who manage to continue with their everyday lives even though their depressive symptoms cause them much suffering. Some children who do not meet the full diagnostic criteria for a depressive disorder do have depressive symptoms as part of a relatively undifferentiated emotional disorder that also involves symptoms of anxiety, fearfulness or obsessionality – such children are common but are not well handled by the current diagnostic systems. By convention, depressive disorders are not diagnosed if the child also meets criteria for schizophrenia.

Features of depression at different ages

Children under five who are separated from their attachment figures will often go through a phase of despair, but it is unclear whether this despair is equivalent to depression. From roughly the age of eight, however, some children do experience depressive disorders that are phenomenologically very similar to adult depressive disorders. This similarity enables childhood depressive disorders to be diagnosed using unmodified (or only slightly modified) adult criteria. Sleep and appetite disturbance seem less common than in adults. Guilt and hopelessness are probably less common in depressed children than in depressed adolescents and adults (perhaps reflecting the cognitive sophistication needed to experience guilt or hopelessness). The suicidal plans of depressed children are typically less lethal than the plans of depressed adolescents or adults, e.g. trying to drown by putting their head under water in the bath. In childhood, the constellation of depressive symptoms may include refusal or reluctance to attend school, irritability, abdominal pain and headache. Indeed, somatic complaints are probably the rule rather than the exception, are not simply due to coexisting anxiety, and should always be asked about.

Depressive equivalents

It has been suggested that many child psychiatric disorders, ranging from enuresis to conduct disorder, are the childhood equivalents of adult depression even if the children do not appear miserable in childhood. There is no good evidence for this view, and children should not be diagnosed as depressed in the absence of clear affective symptoms.

Epidemiology

The Isle of Wight study found that 0.2% of 10-year-olds and 2% of 14-year-olds were depressed. More recent studies, using broader diagnostic criteria, have found higher rates, with major depressive disorder being present in roughly 1–2% of prepubertal children and roughly 2–5% of adolescents. The rise in adolescence seems to be more closely linked to pubertal status than to chronological age. Studies that rely primarily on informants (parents and teachers) report lower rates of depression than studies that rely primarily on the children and adolescents' self-reports. The long-term significance of inner misery that is not apparent to parents and teachers is still uncertain. The female preponderance seen in adult depression is evident from middle or late adolescence – the sex ratio is 1:1 prepubertally, or there may even be a male preponderance. A link with social disadvantage has been suggested but the evidence is contradictory. Over recent decades, the evidence suggests that the prevalence of childhood depression has risen and the average age of onset has fallen. These trends are probably real and not just a reflection of improving recognition or less stringent diagnostic criteria.

Classification

Children and adolescents who have enough persistent depressive symptoms to meet the criteria for a depressive episode can be assigned one of several diagnoses, depending on how many episodes they have had and whether they have also had any manic, hypomanic or mixed episodes. Thus children with two or more major depressive episodes but no manic, hypomanic or mixed episodes can be classified under DSM–IV as having major depressive disorder, recurrent. Children with lesser symptomatology may meet the diagnostic criteria for dysthymia or adjustment disorder with depressed mood. Dysthymia involves chronic mild symptoms for at least one year (as opposed to the two years stipulated for adults). An adjustment disorder can be diagnosed if the symptoms occur shortly after an identifiable stressor – within one month according to ICD–10 and within three months according to DSM–IV – and do not outlast the stressor by more than six months.

Associated features

(1) *Comorbidity* Roughly 50% of depressed children in epidemiological samples have at least one other psychiatric disorder as well (typically a conduct or anxiety disorder), and the rate of comorbidity is often even higher in clinic samples. Mixed depressive disorders may behave quite differently from pure depressive disorders. Judging from adult outcome, for example, mixed depression and conduct disorder seems more akin to pure conduct disorder than to pure depression.

(2) *Friendship difficulties* are common during depressed episodes, and may precede (and possibly precipitate) these episodes.

(3) *Biological features*   Sleep and cortisol studies do not consistently show the sorts of abnormalities described in adults (but these are less marked in young adults too). Prepubertally depressed children hyposecrete growth hormone in response to a hypoglycaemic challenge. Nocturnal growth hormone secretion is increased in depressed adolescents.

Differential diagnosis

(1) Normal sadness, including that of a normal bereavement reaction (though DSM–IV allows a depressive episode to be diagnosed if a depressive symptom cluster persists for more than two months after a major bereavement or is particularly severe, e.g. with suicidal ideation, psychotic symptoms or marked functional impairment).

(2) Misery as just one feature of another psychiatric disorder, without the additional affective, cognitive and behavioural features needed to diagnose a true depressive disorder (but beware of the reverse danger of under-diagnosing comorbid depression in children with other disorders).

Causation

Depression runs in families. Depressed children are more likely than children with other psychiatric disorders to have parents or siblings who are themselves depressed. Parents with depression are more likely to have depressed children. The relative importance of genetic and environmental transmission has yet to be established. Family dysfunction and life events are associated with higher rates of childhood depression (and other child psychiatric disorders as well).

Treatment

Family therapy, school liaison, and supportive therapy with the child or teenager are commonly used to change factors thought to be contributing to high stress levels. These 'common sense' measures are equally relevant for children with broad-band emotional disorders with depressive components. There is increasing interest in cognitive-behavioural therapy (CBT) and interpersonal therapy (IPT), discussed in Chapter 33. The cognitive component of CBT is designed to alter negative cognitions, improve self-esteem, and enhance coping skills. The behavioural component, which seems just as important as the cognitive component, is designed to increase the young person's involvement in normal and rewarding activities. Social skills training and remedial help with specific learning problems may also be offered. Sensible though they seem, these sorts of psychosocial interventions are only just beginning to be evaluated by properly conducted trials to distinguish between natural remission, non-specific 'placebo' effects, and specific treatment effects. Initial results do suggest some specific effects. For example, a recent comparison of brief CBT and relaxation therapy showed a significant post-treatment advantage for those depressed children and adolescents who had been randomised to CBT. This advantage had largely worn off by the time of the six-month follow-up.

The role of medication is controversial. Although open trials of various tricyclic antidepressants have reported successes with children and teenagers, meta-analyses of controlled double-blind trials suggest that tricyclic antidepressants are little or no better than placebos for this age range, though dosage and duration of treatment may not have been optimal. While two controlled trials suggest that selective serotonin reuptake inhibitors (SSRIs) may be more effective than placebos, further confirmation is needed. Despite the generally negative trial evidence, many clinicians are convinced that conventional antidepressants are effective treatments for some severely depressed children and teenagers. These may include those with adult-type endogenous features, similarly affected adult relatives, or 'out of the blue' depressive disorders that were not preceded by conduct disorder or separation anxiety disorder. It is possible that the current definition of childhood depression is too inclusive, with the value of medication for the minority of children with 'true depression' being masked by its inefficacy for the majority of children who are understandably miserable but not truly depressed. This is pure supposition, however, and does not justify the widespread use of antidepressants outside of expert centres. If medication is used, SSRIs seem to be the most appropriate first-line treatment. If tricyclics are used, they may need to be administered in high doses to achieve the blood levels recommended for the treatment of adult depression; in these doses, particularly with desipramine, there is a risk of precipitating potentially fatal cardiac arrhythmias and ECG monitoring is essential (see Chapter 31). For bipolar disorders, lithium is probably as effective in young people as in adults (and carbamazepine can also be considered). Resistant depression is sometimes treated with combinations of different medications or with ECT, techniques that should probably only be used in specialist centres.

Prognosis

An adjustment disorder with depressed mood usually lasts a few months and does not recur. Major depressive episodes often last six to nine months and commonly recur. Dysthymia typically persists for several years; dysthymic children are at a high risk of major depressive episodes. Children with 'double depression' (i.e. major depressive episodes superimposed on dysthymia) are particularly likely to experience recurrent major episodes. Coexistent conduct disorder may affect outcome – with mixed depression and conduct disorder increasing the adult risk of criminality but not depression, and with pure childhood depression increasing the adult risk for depression but not criminality. Prepubertal onset carries a better prognosis.

MANIA

Classical mania and hypomania do occur in childhood but are very rare. Neurochemical immaturity may account for this since prepubertal children do not have a euphoric response to amphetamines or related stimulants. Irritability may be a more common presentation than euphoria. Chronic mania in childhood has been described, but may simply represent misdiagnosed hyperkinesis. This is an understandable error since hyperkinetic children can display a variety of 'manic features' including social disinhibition, fatuous cheerfulness, high energy level, and a tendency to tell fantastic and sometimes grandiose stories. Mania can only safely be diagnosed in childhood when the symptoms have a definite onset and are clearly out of keeping with the child's prior characteristics. In adolescence, mania and depression are probably equally common as first episodes of bipolar disorders, with mania being more commonr thereafter. Mania in adolescence is commonly misdiagnosed as schizophrenia because the mood changes are often accompanied by prominent disturbances in perception and thinking, including the sorts of 'first rank' delusions and hallucinations characteristic of schizophrenia. Neuroleptics (or lithium) are commonly used to control acute episodes, with lithium (or carbamazepine) being used to reduce the risk of recurrence (see Chapter 31).

Subject review

Harrington, R. (1994) Affective disorders. In *Child and Adolescent Psychiatry: Modern Approaches*, 3rd edn (M. Rutter, E. Taylor and L. Hersov, eds) Blackwell Science, Oxford, pp. 330–350.

Further reading

Harrington, R. *et al.* (1990) Adult outcomes of childhood and adolescent depression – I. Psychiatric status. *Archives of General Psychiatry*, **47**, 465–473.
Harrington, R. *et al.* (1991) Adult outcomes of childhood and adolescent depression – II. Links with antisocial disorders. *Journal of the American Academy of Child and Adolescent Psychiatry*, **30**, 434–439.
Hazell, P. *et al.* (1995) Efficacy of tricyclic drugs in treating child and adolescent depression: a meta-analysis. *British Medical Journal*, **310**, 897–901.
Wood, A. *et al.* (1996) Controlled trial of a brief cognitive–behavioural intervention in adolescent patients with depressive disorders. *Journal of Child Psychology and Psychiatry*, **37**, 737–746.

11 Suicide and Deliberate Self-harm

COMPLETED SUICIDE

Epidemiology

Completed suicide is very rare under the age of 12 and becomes progressively more common thereafter, with peak rates in the elderly. In Britain, there are roughly five suicides per million children aged 10–14 per year (including definite suicides and the more common 'undetermined deaths', which are very often suicides). The rate rises to roughly 30 suicides per million for 15–19 year olds, which is still substantially lower than adult rates. There is a male excess at all ages, partly reflecting the male predilection for violent and more lethal methods (hanging, shooting, electrocution), as opposed to the female predilection for poisoning (mostly with analgesics and antidepressants). Rates vary by country and ethnicity, e.g. being higher in the USA, where the rate in whites is roughly twice that in blacks. Between the early 1950s and the early 1980s, teenage suicide rates increased in Europe and the USA, particularly in males. Over the last decade, suicide rates in young females have generally remained fairly stable, while rates for males have continued to rise in some countries.

What protects younger children?

Though children commonly believe that death is reversible, it seems implausible that this belief inhibits suicidal ideas or acts. More plausible protective factors include: the relative rarity of severe depressive disorders before puberty; the lack of sufficient cognitive maturity to experience profound hopelessness or plan a successful suicide; restricted access to lethal methods; and the presence of a supportive network of relationships at home or school.

Background factors

(1) *Disrupted home circumstances*, e.g. broken home, marital discord, deaths.

(2) *Family members with a psychiatric disorder* – mainly (a) alcohol and drug abuse, (b) depression and other emotional disorders, and (c) suicide and self-harm.

(3) *Psychiatric disorder in the young person.* Among older teenagers, ret-
rospective assessments by means of 'psychological autopsies' suggest that
over 90% had some psychiatric disorder, with affective disorders being
especially common in both sexes; conduct disorder and substance abuse
are also common, particularly in males. About half had been in contact
with professionals for their mental health problems. The proportion with
a psychiatric disorder is probably somewhat lower in young teenagers,
who are correspondingly more likely to be responding to an impending
threat, e.g. the imminent arrival of a bad school report.

(4) *Models of successful or attempted suicide.* These include family, friends,
media, books.

(5) *Previous suicidal threats or behaviour* in roughly half of all cases, often
occurring in the 24 hours prior to the young person's death.

(6) *Availability of highly lethal means*, e.g. firearms, coal gas.

Precipitating factors and motivation

There is often a precipitant. For younger teenagers, the most common
precipitant is a disciplinary crisis, with the young person having got into trouble
with the school or the police, and with the parents being about to find out.
Other precipitants include problems with a psychotic parent or rows with
parents, friends, or boy/girlfriend. Young people who are out of school at the
time may be at particular risk because of lack of support. Judging from suicide
notes, the desire to escape from a recent crisis is a common motivation, with
hostility being more often directed outwards to others or external circumstances
than inwards.

DELIBERATE SELF-HARM (DSH)

DSH (attempted suicide, parasuicide) is roughly 100 times more common than
completed suicide in childhood or adolescence; many episodes never come to
the attention of professionals. The rate of DSH is relatively low in childhood,
rises to a peak in adolescence and early adulthood, and then falls again. Among
community samples of adolescents, as many as 10–20% may have had relatively
serious suicidal ideation at some time over the previous year – although it is
only a minority who act on these ideas. Thoughts and threats of suicide are
fairly common among child psychiatric patients and do sometimes lead to
attempted suicide (even among preschool children). Under the age of 12, DSH
is commoner among boys than girls. The ratio reverses dramatically during the
teenage years, with females predominating by roughly 5:1. Self-poisoning is by
far the most common form of DSH, particularly among females. Rates have

increased dramatically since the early 1950s, but have shown some signs of stabilising over recent years.

Background factors

(1) Lack of supportive family relationships. Associated with 'broken homes', placement in a children's home, and disharmonious family environments with low affection. Girls are particularly likely to be in conflict with their fathers and unable to discuss problems with them. For boys, conflict with their mother seems particularly likely when there is no father at home and they are under pressure to be the 'man about the house'.

(2) Family members with a psychiatric disorder. Alcohol abuse is common in parents, particularly fathers.

(3) A minority have a definite psychiatric disorder, which may be a conduct or an emotional disorder. The great majority of deliberate self-harmers are not severely depressed. The likelihood of associated substance abuse varies greatly from place to place.

(4) A history of physical or sexual abuse. Children from abusing backgrounds may be particularly liable to hate themselves.

(5) School or work problems are common. Academic attainments are typically below average, and there have commonly been problems relating to teachers and peers. Unemployment is common among older teenagers.

(6) Family members, friends, or media reports may have provided models for imitation. Contagion within adolescent units is well described.

(7) Roughly 20% have made a previous attempt.

(8) Since most DSH is on the spur of the moment, impulses are more likely to be acted on when there is immediate access to prescribed or over-the-counter medication.

Precipitating factors

A clear precipitant in the two days before DSH can be identified in about two-thirds of cases. (Psychiatric disorder is more likely when there is no identifiable precipitant.) In many cases, a relatively minor additional stress seems to be the 'last straw' for an individual who has been rendered vulnerable by a multiplicity of prior and concurrent adversities. Acute precipitants sometimes trigger DSH in young people who are otherwise well-adjusted. The commonest precipitants are rows with family, friends, or boy/girlfriend. An episode of physical or sexual abuse may also precipitate DSH.

Motivation

At the time they harm themselves, young people commonly feel angry with someone, or feel lonely and unwanted. Worry about the future is more prominent in older teenagers. Hopelessness is prominent only in the depressed minority. DSH typically reflects a desire for temporary respite from distressing circumstances (functioning rather like getting drunk), or a wish to influence family and friends. It is rarely a 'cry for help' directed at professionals (which is one reason why offers of help from professionals are commonly rejected). The circumstances of the DSH do not usually suggest a serious intent to die or advanced planning. DSH is usually impulsive: roughly half of the young people have contemplated it for less than 15 minutes before carrying it out.

Assessment

All children and adolescents who harm themselves should have a mental health and psychosocial assessment. This may involve a child psychiatrist but could equally involve a suitably trained nurse, social worker, etc. Informants can be interviewed at once, but assessment of the young person may need to wait until toxic effects of the overdose have worn off. The assessment should cover the following areas:

(1) The circumstances of the self-harm and the degree of suicidal intent (Box 11.1).
(2) Possible precipitating factors in the preceding days.
(3) Predisposing factors – previous and current life circumstances, family history, models for suicidal behaviour.
(4) History and mental state examination to evaluate current psychiatric state and suicide risk. Have suicidal talk or behaviour been escalating progressively?
(5) Was the episode of self-harm typical of a long-standing difficulty in coping with stress or obtaining support in a more adaptive way?
(6) Attitude of individual and family to professional help.

Box 11.1   Characteristics suggesting serious suicidal intent.

(1) Carried out in isolation
(2) Timed so that intervention unlikely
(3) Precautions taken to avoid discovery
(4) Preparations made in anticipation of death
(5) Other people informed beforehand of the individual's intention
(6) Extensive premeditation
(7) Suicide note left
(8) Failure to alert other people following the episode.

Management

When DSH is an out-of-character response to acute stress in an otherwise well-adjusted young person, referral back to the GP is usually all that is necessary. At the other extreme, psychiatric admission is occasionally necessary for further assessment, for treatment of a major psychiatric disorder, or because of continuing high suicide risk. Most self-harmers should be offered outpatient treatment (though many will never turn up). A family approach often seems indicated, though the families are usually difficult to engage or change. Some families dismiss the episode as trivial; they should be encouraged to regard the episode as a serious challenge to solve problems or reduce stresses. Brief individual therapy may be helpful, particularly if it is focused on improving the young person's capacity to solve problems and handle stresses in a more adaptive way. Occasionally this sort of crisis intervention will lead on to longer-term psychotherapy. Individuals and families are more likely to accept treatment when there is continuity of care between the assessment and treatment phases.

Prognosis

There are few good follow-up studies of young people who have harmed themselves because of the difficulties involved in tracing and recruiting subjects. One month later, the overall adjustment is generally better than at the time of DSH, but a substantial minority are still experiencing considerable difficulties a year later. Continuing difficulties are predicted by coexistent antisocial traits. Individuals who harm themselves during an acute crisis but who were previously well-adjusted have a particularly good prognosis. Roughly 10% of young people who harm themselves do so again within the next year. Predictors of repetition include male sex, more than one previous episode of DSH, extensive family psychopathology, poor social adjustment, and a psychiatric disorder (including substance abuse). Subsequent episodes may be fatal, either by design or because the individual underestimates the lethality of what was intended to be a non-fatal overdose or injury. Roughly 1% of young people who harm themselves do subsequently kill themselves, usually within the next two years. Factors that increase the risk of eventual suicide are male sex, being an older adolescent, the presence of a psychiatric disorder, and use of active rather than passive means (e.g. hanging rather than an overdose) in the initial episode.

Subject review

Shaffer, D. and Piacentini, J. (1994) Suicide and attempted suicide. In *Child and Adolescent Psychiatry: Modern Approaches*, 3rd edn (M. Rutter, E. Taylor and L. Hersov, eds) Blackwell Science, Oxford. pp. 407–424.

Hawton, K. (1986) *Suicide and Attempted Suicide Among Children and Adolescents*. Sage, Beverly Hills.

Further reading

Hawton, K. and Fagg, J. (1992) Deliberate self-poisoning and self-injury in adolescents. A study of characteristics and trends in Oxford, 1976–89. *British Journal of Psychiatry*, **161**, 816–823.

Kerfoot, M. *et al.* (1995) Brief home-based intervention with young suicide attempters and their families. *Journal of Adolescence*, **18**, 557–568. (A description of the sort of programme that is currently being evaluated.)

Shaffer, D. (1974) Suicide in childhood and early adolescence. *Journal of Child Psychology and Psychiatry*, **15**, 275–291. (This is an excellent descriptive study of completed suicide in 12–14 year olds; most other studies focus on older teenagers.)

Shaffer, D. *et al.* (1996) Psychiatric diagnosis in child and adolescent suicide. *Archives of General Psychiatry*, **53**, 339–348.

12 Acute Reactions to Stress

This chapter is concerned with discrete major shocks, rather than major longer-term stresses such as parental fighting, chronic psychosocial adversity, disabling illness, obesity, psychiatric illness of a parent, problems with school, and repeated disruption of the immediate world of the child. The short-term reaction to bereavement will be considered but not longer-term effects.

Until recently researchers have judged the severity of the *reaction* primarily from parent or teacher reports, without paying much attention to the children themselves. The picture has changed dramatically as a result of a careful appraisal of the stressed children's emotions, cognitions and behaviour. Thus it is now recognised to be important to consider specific circumscribed fears and not just general fearfulness, to enquire about intrusive thoughts or images, and to ask about avoidance. It is also important to consider any effect on psychosocial functioning as seen in friendships and schoolwork.

BEREAVEMENT

Three main stages of grief in children were observed by analytic writers such as Anna Freud and John Bowlby; empirical observations have broadly confirmed these. Firstly there is an *initial crisis response* with shock, denial and disbelief, emotional numbness and feelings of detachment; thoughts and behaviour are mainly directed towards the lost one. *Emotional disorganisation* follows, with sadness and crying, anger and resentment, feelings of despair, disappointment, hopelessness and worthlessness, poor sleep and appetite, and sometimes guilt or self-blame. *Adjustment* to the loss is eventually evident in reduced anxiety, increased enjoyment of life, greater engagement in everyday activities and the formation of new attachments. These stages merge into each other and may coexist. The rate of progress from one stage to another is very variable, and transitions are not irreversible – the child may temporarily go back a stage when stressed again.

POST-TRAUMATIC STRESS DISORDER (PTSD)

It is now increasingly recognised that PTSD occurs in children in a similar form to that recognised in adults. As well as occurring after experiencing or witnessing disasters and gross violence, it can also occur after sexual or physical abuse, life-threatening illnesses and medical procedures. While disasters are uncommon, physical and sexual abuse are not. Children also commonly witness serious domestic violence; it has been estimated, for example, that 10–20% of murders are witnessed by children (the majority of murders arise out of domestic disputes). Children in hospital with serious injuries or illnesses are also at higher risk, as are refugees from war-torn countries. At one extreme, one study using DSM criteria found 100% of sexually molested children had PTSD, as did 70% of those who were physically abused and 60% of those involved in disasters. In many such cases, the PTSD goes unrecognised and untreated. While it is important to recognise and treat PTSD symptoms, this often needs to be done as one part of a broad management plan that takes adequate account of the child and family's wide-ranging problems, a plan in which education and social services may play larger roles than health services.

Diagnostic criteria for PTSD

In the aftermath of an event that would have distressed almost anyone, the child experiences for at least a month some symptoms from each of the following three groups:

(1)   The traumatic event is *persistently re-experienced*, e.g. intrusive images, traumatic dreams, repetitive re-enactment in play, distress at reminders.

(2)   There is continued *avoidance* of stimuli associated with the trauma or *numbing* of responsiveness: avoidance of thoughts, feelings, locations, situations; feelings of being alone or detached, reduced interests and restricted emotional range; poor memory for important aspects of the trauma; loss of belief in the future.

(3)   There are new symptoms of *increased arousal*, including sleep disturbance, irritability, poor concentration, hypervigilance and alertness, exaggerated startle response.

Ordinary psychiatric scales completed by teachers or parents may not detect any problems in affected children; indeed, preoccupied and numbed children may seem particularly well behaved to adults. Self-report questionnaires for the children may also miss PTSD since general screening questions are not good at tapping PTSD symptoms. With specific enquiries, however, affected children are generally able to give a clear account from as young as three years of age. Many affected children report not telling their parents in order not to upset them.

The degree of exposure to the trauma influences the extent of symptoms, with those directly experiencing pain or coming very close to death tending to be the worst affected. There is typically marked fear and avoidance of objects or events directly connected to the trauma, and lesser fear and avoidance of tangentially related stimuli. For example, children who have been on a sinking ship are subsequently likely to have marked fears related to boats, and may also have lesser fears relating to travel by train or plane; they are no more likely than other children to fear objects or events unrelated to the disaster. While general anxiety and depression tends to wane over time, specific fears and avoidance can be remarkably persistent.

Moderating variables

Both in childhood and adulthood, apparently similar traumas can have extremely different effects on different individuals. In part, this may reflect differences in temperament, personality or genetic liability to specific disorders. Some cognitive attributes, such as good problem-solving skills, may also be relevant. It also seems likely from the literature on resilience that children will be better able to buffer stress if they have a good relationship with one parent, a cohesive and harmonious family, and support from a wider social network of peers and teachers. Conversely, family dysfunction, peer problems and severe social disadvantage are all likely to impair resilience.

Treatment

Many traumatised children have never had the opportunity to talk freely about their experiences to a sympathetic and informed adult. They may have feared that they were going mad when they began to experience intrusive thoughts, and may have been very frightened by what have seemed inexplicable panic attacks. Hearing that these are normal responses to abnormal experiences can help such children to make sense of their world and so begin to be reassured.

Parents and teachers may also need to be helped to acknowledge what has happened. When adults feel that the trauma and its aftermath should not be talked about, or feel frightened about what might be said, children often read the signs and keep obligingly quiet. Early experience suggests that group discussions with fellow victims and their parents can be helpful.

A number of cognitive approaches that have proved successful with adults can also be used with children. Triggers for anxiety attacks can be identified and then addressed by teaching relaxation and other anxiety-reducing techniques. These can then be followed by graded exposure to the distressing scene; exposure generally needs to be vivid and long to overcome avoidance. Other cognitive techniques include challenging maladaptive thoughts and using guided imagery to gain mastery over distressing feelings.

Difficulty getting to sleep may be helped by simple techniques such as listening to a music or story tape when in bed to help banish unpleasant intrusive thoughts. Bad dreams can be retold during the day with the child giving them a happy ending.

In addition to treating the specific symptoms of PTSD, it may be necessary to address wider issues. For example, when children have been orphaned by the disaster, it may be vital to help the children and their new caregivers adjust to one another's needs.

Subject reviews

Udwin, O. (1993) Children's reactions to traumatic events. *Journal of Child Psychology and Psychiatry*, **34**, 115–127.

Yule, W. (1994) Post-traumatic stress disorder. In *Child and Adolescent Psychiatry: Modern Approaches*, 3rd edn (M. Rutter, E. Taylor and L. Hersov, eds) Blackwell Science, Oxford, pp. 392–406.

Further reading

Deblinger, E. *et al.* (1990) Cognitive behavioral treatment for sexually abused children suffering post-traumatic stress: preliminary findings. *Journal of the American Academy of Child and Adolescent Psychiatry*, **29**, 747–752. (This paper presents an appealing treatment package that targets PTSD symptoms and much, much more!)

Sack, W. *et al.* (1996) Multiple forms of stress in Cambodian adolescent refugees. *Child Development*, **67**, 107–116.

13 Obsessive-Compulsive Disorder

Child psychiatrists have long been aware that children sometimes develop troublesome and distressing rituals and ruminations, but until recently these were generally considered relatively non-specific symptoms of broad-band emotional disorders. Recent studies have emphasised the value of subclassifying the emotional disorders, with obsessive–compulsive disorder (OCD) being a particularly distinctive subgroup in terms of symptomatology, aetiology, treatment and prognosis.

Epidemiology

Roughly a third to a half of adults with OCD have their first symptoms before the age of 15. Epidemiological studies suggest a prevalence of roughly 0.5% in adolescents, with symptoms sometimes dating back to the preschool years. Males and females are equally commonly affected from adolescence onwards, but males predominate in prepubertal OCD.

Characteristic features

There are surprisingly few differences between the presentation of a five-year-old and a 25-year-old. The most common compulsions involve washing, cleaning, repeating, checking, and touching. The most common obsessions focus on contamination, disasters, and symmetry. Resistance to the obsessions and compulsions is not always present.

Associated features

Secondary anxiety and depression are common and may be the cause of psychiatric referral (and children may fail to disclose the underlying obsessive-compulsive symptoms unless specific inquiry is made). Parents and siblings may be drawn into rituals and demands for reassurance. About 20% have premorbid obsessive personality. There is no premorbid excess of bedtime rituals, and children with OCD can generally distinguish clearly between their obsessive–compulsive symptoms and their ordinary rituals and superstitions.

Differential diagnosis

(1) *Normal childhood rituals.* Bedtime rituals often peak at two to three years and rarely persist much beyond eight years. Rule-bound play increases from five years. Collecting often begins around seven. Adolescent 'obsessions' with an activity or an idol are culturally sanctioned and aid peer integration. OCD has some resemblance to normal rituals, with a bedtime peak and some common themes, e.g. counting, order. OCD also differs from normal rituals: there is no age trend in OCD rituals, and symptoms interfere with, rather than enhance, socialisation and the growth of independence.

(2) *Primary depressive disorders* can result in secondary obsessive-compulsive symptoms. It is important to take a careful history to determine whether the depressive or obsessive-compulsive symptoms started first.

(3) *Undifferentiated emotional disorders.* Like adults, children may present with relatively undifferentiated emotional disorders in which mild obsessive–compulsive symptoms are mixed with fears, worries and misery, with no one element predominating.

(4) *Autistic disorders.* The ritualistic and repetitive behaviours characteristic of autistic disorders are accompanied by other autistic impairments in communication and social interaction, are often simpler than OCD rituals, and are not ego-dystonic. It is important to remember, though, that children and teenagers with autistic disorders do sometimes develop an additional OCD which may respond well to behavioural therapy or medication.

(5) *Schizophrenia* can be accompanied by obsessions and compulsions. It is important to clarify if an 'obsession' is actually a voice, and if a 'compulsion' is actually a response to a command.

(6) *Anorexia nervosa* has obsessive-compulsive qualities relating to food and exercise, and may be accompanied by washing, checking and counting rituals. OCD involving avoidance of 'contaminated' food, or compulsive exercising, may resemble anorexia nervosa except for a normal body image.

(7) *Tourette's syndrome* is commonly accompanied by obsessive-compulsive features (see Chapter 14). Complex tics preceded by an 'urge' are arguably compulsions by a different name.

Causation

Despite an earlier enthusiasm for psychodynamic explanations, current theories emphasise biological and behavioural explanations. Neurological and neuro-imaging studies point to structural or functional abnormalities of the basal ganglia. There is also growing interest in the ethological suggestion that compulsions are fixed action patterns related to grooming and cleaning that have escaped suppression by 'higher centres' and taken on a life of their own. Once initiated, rituals may persist because of their anxiety-reducing effects. A positive family history of OCD is fairly common. Tic disorders and OCD may cluster in the same families, suggesting that these disorders may sometimes reflect the same underlying gene or genes (see Chapter 14). There may be other genes that predispose to OCD but not to tic disorders, perhaps associated with elevated levels of oxytocin in cerebrospinal fluid. Yet other cases seem to be phenocopies, following streptococcal infections that initiate an immune response that also damages the individual's own basal ganglia.

Treatment

Both behaviour therapy and medication seem effective in children, though medication has been better evaluated. The behavioural management of compulsions often begins with an initial period of diary keeping. The child then helps to draw up a hierarchy of compulsions, ranging from the easiest to tackle to the hardest (most anxiety provoking). Starting with the easiest, the child is encouraged and helped to avoid carrying out the compulsion. When all goes well, this 'response prevention' only leads to a temporary surge of anxiety, followed by a more lasting reduction in the compulsive drive. Obsessions that have no behavioural accompaniment (ruminations) are harder to tackle using behavioural approaches. Family work can be particularly helpful when family members are being drawn into the rituals. Medication has an important role in many cases, whether as an adjunct or an alternative to behavioural approaches. Serotonin reuptake inhibitors such as clomipramine and selective serotonin reuptake inhibitors (SSRIs) such as fluoxetine are particularly effective, and are generally well tolerated even by children as young as six years old. Immunological approaches, including plasmapheresis, have been used to treat acute-onset OCD after a streptococcal infection; some dramatic responses have been reported from open trials and the results of controlled trials are awaited.

Prognosis

Unlike many other emotional disorders of childhood, OCD seems to be remarkably persistent, with only a small minority fully recovering two to five years later.

Subject review

Rapoport, J.L. *et al.* (1994) Obsessive-compulsive disorder. In *Child and Adolescent Psychiatry: Modern Approaches*, 3rd edn (M. Rutter, E. Taylor and L. Hersov, eds) Blackwell Science, Oxford, pp. 441–454.

Further reading

Allen, A.J. *et al.* (1995) Case study: a new infection–triggered, autoimmune subtype of pediatric OCD and Tourette's syndrome. *Journal of the American Academy of Child and Adolescent Psychiatry*, **34**, 307–311.

Leckman, J.F. *et al.* (1994) Elevated cerebrospinal fluid level of oxytocin in obsessive–compulsive disorder. *Archives of General Psychiatry*, **51**, 782–792.

Thomsen, P.H. (1996) Treatment of obsessive–compulsive disorder in children and adolescents: a review of the literature. *European Child and Adolescent Psychiatry*, **5**, 55–66.

14 Tourette's Syndrome and Other Tic Disorders

Tics are sudden, repetitive, stereotyped motor movements or phonic productions. They are either involuntary or partly voluntary in response to a premonitory 'urge'. Simple motor tics (such as blinks, grimaces or shrugs) and simple phonic tics (such as grunts, sniffs or barks) are clearly purposeless. Complex motor tics (such as brushing hair back, gyrating, touching) and complex phonic tics (such as words or phrases) may seem more purposeful but are out of context. Tics characteristically vary in intensity from hour to hour and from day to day. They can briefly be suppressed, are often better during sleep or an absorbing activity, and usually worsen with stress or relaxation.

Classification

Tourette's Syndrome (TS) involves chronic motor *and* vocal tics: more than one type of motor tic plus at least one type of phonic tic, lasting for over a year and starting before 21 years of age. Other disorders recognised by DSM–IV and ICD–10 are 'chronic motor or vocal tic disorder' and 'transient tic disorder'.

Epidemiology

TS affects roughly 3–5 per 10 000 children. Male:female = 3–9:1. Chronic motor tics are probably at least three times more common. Transient tics are much more common still, affecting up to 4–16% of children at some stage.

Characteristic features

The average age of onset of motor tics is seven, with onset being rare before two or after 15. The motor tics are usually simple, primarily involving eyes, face, head or neck. Vocal tics usually start later, between eight and 15 years. Complex phonic tics involving obscene speech (coprolalia) only occur in a minority, starting about four to eight years after onset. It is a mistake, therefore, to rule out the diagnosis of TS on the basis that coprolalia is absent. Echoed speech (echolalia), echoed actions (echopraxia), and obscene actions or gestures (copropraxia) may also occur.

Associated features

(1) Obsessive–compulsive symptoms (sometimes amounting to OCD) occur in a third to two-thirds, particularly among older subjects. 'Evening up', counting, and ritualistic touching are particularly common, though the checking and contamination concerns of 'ordinary' OCD may also occur.

(2) Inattention/hyperactivity problems occur in 25–50%, typically preceding the onset of tics. It is probably this comorbid hyperactivity rather than the presence of tics *per se* that best predicts associated learning difficulties.

(3) Other reported associations include self-injury, failure to inhibit aggression, sleep problems, affective disorders, schizotypal personality, pervasive developmental disorders – in fact, almost anything!

Differential diagnosis

(1) Other dyskinesias may resemble simple tics, but they all differ from tics in some respects (e.g. not increased by relaxation).

(2) The stereotypies that are commonly seen in severe mental retardation and the autistic disorders may look like complex motor tics, but it is very rare to have complex tics without some simple tics too.

(3) Compulsions cannot clearly be distinguished from complex tics preceded by 'urges', but the latter are nearly always accompanied by simple tics too.

Causation

TS, chronic tics and OCD often run together in families. This may reflect an autosomal dominant gene present in about 1% of the population with very variable expression and penetrance, resulting in TS in a minority (mainly male), chronic tics in a larger proportion, and OCD in some (particularly females). The notion of a single major gene is undermined, however, by the fact that it has not yet been found in searches that have now covered practically the whole genome. Whatever the genetic basis for the familial clustering of tic disorders, it seems likely that a minority of cases are sporadic. It is unclear whether the gene or genes that load for TS are also 'hyperactivity genes', or whether TS simply exacerbates any coexistent tendency to hyperactivity.

Treatment

It is essential to explain to the child, family and school that TS is a medical disorder that is beyond the child's control. It is not cheekiness or possession by evil spirits. Mild tics may need no specific treatment. Psychological treatments such as relaxation training and habit reversal may help but the evidence is not yet strong. These may be the appropriate first line of treatment for children with relatively mild tic disorders. They may also be appropriate for children with more severe tic disorders, who are strongly motivated to try psychological approaches before considering medication.

Neuroleptics can generally reduce tic severity by about two-thirds, although sometimes at the price of cognitive dulling or extrapyramidal symptoms. Complete abolition of tics is often not possible without pushing neuroleptics to levels that result in unacceptable side-effects. Historically, haloperidol and pimozide have been the most widely used neuroleptics, but concerns about side-effects (including the risk of potentially fatal cardiac arrhythmias with pimozide) have prompted trials of other neuroleptics such as sulpiride and risperidone. It is not yet clear if these newer neuroleptics are as effective as haloperidol or pimozide. Since tic disorders characteristically wax and wane, it will sometimes be necessary to push up the dose of medication to cover acute exacerbations. It is important to remember to bring the dose down again subsequently. The dosage needs to be titrated against clinical need in order to ensure that the child is always treated with the lowest possible dose compatible with adequate (rather than total) tic control.

Clonidine can be used instead of neuroleptics: the advantage is fewer side effects, but the corresponding disadvantage is lower efficacy – tic severity is generally reduced by about one third instead of two-thirds. Associated obsessions and compulsions may be helped by behaviour therapy or medication: usually clomipramine or a selective serotonin reuptake inhibitor (SSRI) such as fluoxetine. When a child with a tic disorder also has a significant problem with inattention and restlessness, these hyperactivity symptoms may be reduced by clonidine or by a tricyclic such as imipramine. Since stimulants can aggravate tics, they are best reserved for severe hyperactivity that has failed to respond to other drugs.

Prognosis of TS

Complete or partial resolution is common in late teens or early twenties. TS may persist throughout adulthood, but if it does the severity gradually wanes.

Subject review

Leckham, J.F. and Cohen, D.J. (1994) Tic disorders. In *Child and Adolescent Psychiatry: Modern Approaches*, 3rd edn (M. Rutter, E. Taylor and L. Hersov, eds) Blackwell Science, Oxford, pp. 455–466.

Further reading

Pauls, D.L. *et al.* (1991) A family study of Gilles de la Tourette syndrome. *American Journal of Human Genetics*, **48**, 154–163. (This study provides evidence for a genetic link between some tic and obsessive–compulsive disorders.)

Sandor, P. (1995) Clinical management of Tourette's syndrome and associated disorders. *Canadian Journal of Psychiatry*, **40**, 577–583.

15 Selective Mutism

Children with selective mutism speak only to a small group of intimates in specific circumstances. Typically, the child talks freely to parents and siblings at home, but does not speak to classmates or teachers at school, though comprehension is normal. Much more rarely, the child speaks at school but not at home. Mutism usually develops at about three to five years of age. However, it does not usually lead to specialist referral while the child is at playgroup; referral is more often after the start of formal schooling. Many clinicians only make the diagnosis if the period of mutism exceeds six months, though DSM–IV and ICD–10 only stipulate a period of one month.

Epidemiology

Refusal to speak at school is relatively common during the first few months after school entry, affecting almost 1% of children in one study (with higher rates among the children of immigrants). These problems are nearly all short-lived. By the age of six or seven, the rate has fallen to about 2–5 per 10 000 (almost identical to the rate of narrowly defined autism). Whereas boys are more prone than girls to developmental language disorders, selective mutism is as common, or even more common, in girls. There is no clear association with socio-economic status, family size, or birth order.

Associated features

(1) *Other psychiatric problems*. Increased rates of anxiety, depression, enuresis, encopresis, hyperactivity and tics have all been described. Recent studies have particularly emphasised the high rate of social anxiety, with most children meeting diagnostic criteria for social phobia (DSM–IV) or social anxiety disorder of childhood (ICD–10). Indeed, some argue that selective mutism should be seen simply as a symptom of a social anxiety disorder rather than as a distinct diagnostic syndrome.

(2) *Language problems*. By definition, the child must be able to chat fairly normally in some situations, but there is often a history of somewhat delayed speech milestones, or continuing minor problems with articula-

tion. Since selectively mute children are unlikely to talk to you, it is important to assess the child's articulation and language level in some other way, e.g. by listening to a tape recording of the child chatting at home, and asking to see written work. A formal assessment of language level by a psychologist or speech therapist can sometimes be very helpful. Picture vocabulary tests that require the child to point to the picture illustrating a particular word are helpful screening tests for receptive language problems.

(3) *Intelligence*. This obviously needs to be assessed using tests that do not require the child to speak, e.g. visuospatial subtests from wide-ranging intelligence tests. The average non-verbal IQ in selective mutism was 85 in one study, but ranged from above 100 to under 70. Selective mutism can occur in children with mild or severe mental retardation.

(4) *Relationships*. Most children have been noted to be markedly shy from the preschool years onwards, and are withdrawn both with children and adults.

(5) *Personality*. An unshakeable determination not to speak in some settings is often accompanied by other evidence of a strong will. Some children are sulky with strangers and aggressive at home; other children are shy with strangers and submissive at home; and yet other children are sensitive and easily distressed both at home and elsewhere. Mixtures of these personality styles are common.

(6) *Family factors*. There is often a history of social anxiety or selective mutism in a parent or sibling. Maternal over-protectiveness is commonly described, as is an association with marital discord (but not marital breakdown), parental mental illness (neurotic and depressive disorders), and parental personality problems (marked aggression or shyness).

(7) *Traumatic experiences*. Although studies of selective mutism have generally emphasised personality factors rather than specific traumas, one recent study reported that selectively mute children were more likely than classroom controls or children with developmental speech or language problems to have suffered definite or probable abuse, usually sexual abuse. The role of abuse and other traumatic experiences needs further exploration.

Differential diagnosis

(1) *Normality*. Young children vary markedly in how forthcoming they are in unfamiliar situations. Is transient mutism at school entry an exaggeration of normal shyness? Is persistent mutism also on the same continuum, or is it qualitatively distinct?

(2) Serious *developmental or acquired language disorders* can only be ruled out when there is convincing evidence that the child's language is fairly normal in some settings.

(3) *Autistic disorders* are ruled out by the same sort of evidence, combined with direct observations of normal play and social interactions with family members.

(4) *Hysterical muteness* generally involves loss of speech in all settings. It is usually sudden in onset (sometimes following a definite stress), and is not typically preceded by marked lifelong shyness.

Causation

This rare disorder may result from a combination of constitutional and environmental factors. Perhaps marked constitutional shyness is exacerbated by stress at home, by immigrant status, or by self-consciousness about relatively minor articulation difficulties or cognitive problems. The mutism may be rewarded by extra attention and affection at home and at school. Without twin or adoption studies, it is impossible to determine whether family clustering points to genetic transmission or social modelling. Do anxious and over-protective parents fill their children with social anxieties? Or do the same genes that predispose parents to be anxious and over-protective also predispose their children to be anxious and selectively mute?

Treatment

Behavioural techniques may be helpful, e.g. desensitising the child to speaking in large groups by starting with just one familiar person and gradually increasing the size of the group. It is obviously essential to ensure that the rewards for speaking are greater than the rewards for not speaking (in terms of attention, for example). Since selective mutism is usually a school-based problem, teachers and classroom assistants are often the most appropriate 'front line' behaviour therapists, advised by clinicians or educational psychologists. Speech therapy can be used to tackle articulation problems and thereby reduce the children's embarrassment about speaking in front of others. Social skills training and family therapy can be included in the therapeutic package to tackle associated problems with social relationships.

There has recently been a flurry of interest in the possible role of selective serotonin reuptake inhibitors (SSRIs) such as fluoxetine in the treatment of social phobia and elective mutism. However, a small double-blind placebo-controlled study of fluoxetine for selective mutism showed only a small advantage for the active medication. The advantage might have been greater if medication had been administered for longer and if dosage had been adjusted individually.

Prognosis

Although mutism at school entry is usually transient, the likelihood of resolution drops dramatically once the mutism has persisted for at least 6–12 months. One study of established cases found that half showed little or no improvement five to ten years later. Improvement is most likely to occur in the primary school years, but may occur at a later stage. Resolution of the mutism is usually but not always accompanied by improved relationships too.

Subject review

Dow, S.P. *et al.* (1995) Practical guidelines for the assessment and treatment of selective mutism. *Journal of the American Academy of Child and Adolescent Psychiatry*, **34**, 836–846.

Further reading

Black, B. and Uhde, T.W. (1995) Psychiatric characteristics of children with selective mutism: a pilot study. *Journal of the American Academy of Child and Adolescent Psychiatry*, **34**, 847–856.

MacGregor, R. *et al.* (1994) Silent at school – elective mutism and abuse. *Archives of Disease in Childhood*, **70**, 540–541.

16   Attachment Disorders

Children's attachment to their parents and other caregivers is of great developmental importance, with the quality of these selective attachments being predictive of their subsequent development. As discussed in Chapter 27, insecurely attached children tend to fare worse than securely attached children in many aspects of their psychological and social development. Nevertheless, insecure attachment is best seen as a risk factor for psychosocial maladjustment rather than as a disorder in itself; many insecurely attached children are well-adapted to their environment and do not develop any psychiatric problems. There are, however, some children who are markedly distressed or socially impaired as a result of an extremely abnormal pattern of attachment; these are the children who can be thought of as having an attachment disorder.

Varieties of attachment disorder

Both ICD–10 and DSM–IV recognise two varieties of attachment disorder: *non-attachment with emotional withdrawal*, typically resulting from abuse; and *non-attachment with indiscriminate sociability*. These typically result from repeated changes in caregiver (from frequent changes in foster placement, or rearing in a group home with a high turnover of staff).

Non-attachment with emotional withdrawal is called 'reactive attachment disorder' by ICD–10 and 'reactive attachment disorder, inhibited type' by DSM–IV. Social interactions are inhibited, ambivalent or hypervigilant. Thus the child may respond to caregivers with a mixture of approach, avoidance, and resistance to comforting, or may exhibit frozen watchfulness. These children tend to be miserable and lacking in emotional responsiveness, and may act aggressively in response to their own or another person's distress.

Non-attachment with indiscriminate sociability is called 'disinhibited attachment disorder' by ICD–10 and 'reactive attachment disorder, disinhibited type' by DSM–IV. The child does seek comfort when distressed but lacks the normal degree of selectivity in the people from whom comfort is sought. Social interactions with unfamiliar people are poorly modulated with generally clinging behaviour in infancy, or attention-seeking and indiscriminately friendly behaviour in early or middle childhood.

Diagnosis

Although both ICD–10 and DSM–IV include attachment disorders because of their 'obvious clinical importance', there is almost no research evidence for the validity of the current definitions. For the present, the following diagnostic criteria are relevant:

(1) *Severity*. The children are not attached in any meaningful sense. They do not have enduring relationships with people who provide them with a 'secure base' and a 'safe haven'.

(2) *Pervasiveness*. A seriously troubled relationship with one particular parent or other caregiver is insufficient. The attachment problems must be evident across a number of different caregivers.

(3) *Distress or Disability*. Attachment disorders cause the child persistent distress or social disability, partly as a consequence of the lack of normal attachment relationships, and partly as a consequence of a wider range of associated social difficulties (e.g. with poor peer relationships).

(4) *Onset before the age of five years*. Along with autism, it is one of the few psychiatric disorders that can be diagnosed in a child of three or under.

(5) *Not autistic*. The child's impaired social relationships are not attributable to autism or some other pervasive developmental disorder (see Chapter 4). Relevant evidence is the lack of other autistic impairments, such as ritualistic and repetitive behaviours, or communication difficulties. In addition, some capacity for social reciprocity and responsiveness is usually evident in interactions with normal adults. In extreme cases, though, the child's social potential may not be apparent for as long as he or she lives in adverse social circumstances. The response to a more favourable caregiving environment is then of diagnostic value. For example, the rapid emergence of social responsiveness and reciprocity in a foster placement points to an attachment disorder rather than an autistic disorder.

(6) *Mental age over 10–12 months*. Severely retarded children may lack selective attachments simply because they have not yet reached a mental age when these would normally emerge. This does not warrant an additional diagnosis of an attachment disorder.

(7) *Pathogenic care*. DSM–IV insists on an abnormal caregiving context, involving either repeated changes of primary caregiver preventing the formation of stable attachments, or persistent disregard of the child's basic emotional or physical needs. ICD–10 also makes it clear that an attachment disorder is usually associated with pathogenic care but does not make this a diagnostic requirement. This makes sense, if only because some transnationally adopted children may meet all the other criteria without much being known of their care history.

Attachment disorders *v.* insecure attachment

Attachment has been one of the key themes in developmental research for decades, with much being written about secure and insecure attachment (see Chapter 27). How do attachment disorders differ from insecure attachment? To some extent, it is a question of degree: relatively few insecurely attached children have extreme enough problems to meet the diagnostic criteria for an attachment disorder. In addition, a child may be insecurely attached to one key caregiver (e.g. the mother) but not to others (e.g. the father), whereas attachment disorders involve problems that are pervasive as well as severe. Furthermore, insecure attachment does not necessarily result in distress or social impairment, whereas an attachment disorder does. Finally, some 40% of children are classified as insecurely attached by developmental researchers, whereas attachment disorders are rare.

Assessment

Of the child

When evaluating a child who may have an attachment disorder, it is not sufficient to carry out one of the standard assessments of attachment security such as the Ainsworth Strange Situation Procedure (see Chapter 27). It is important to take a careful history from multiple informants and observe the child in several settings. The main focus is on various aspects of attachment.

(1) *A safe haven?* Does the child have people to turn to in times of distress, in order to obtain comfort and renew confidence? Children with an attachment disorder may not seek comfort, or may be ambivalent, or may seek comfort in odd ways, e.g. by backing into the caregiver rather than walking forward and making eye contact.

(2) *A secure base?* Can the child venture out to explore the world, returning to the attachment figure for security when necessary? The child with an attachment disorder may be excessively inhibited about exploring, or may be a disinhibited explorer without due regard for his or her own safety.

(3) *An affectionate bond?* The child with an attachment disorder may show a lack of affection or promiscuous affection.

(4) *Selectivity?* Does the child make use of fairly unfamiliar adults as attachment figures, turning to them for comfort, clinging to them, or showing them inappropriate affection?

(5) *Role reversal?* Does the child act as a caregiver to key adults, or behave in an excessively controlling way to those adults?

A full assessment also needs to determine the age of onset of problems and establish the type and quality of current and previous caregiving. Wider social impairments also need to be considered. For example, how well does the child relate to other children? Does he or she tend to ignore or attack other children when they are distressed? It is also essential to look for evidence of autistic impairments and severe mental retardation. These are possible differential diagnoses and need to be excluded if the diagnostic criteria for an attachment disorder are to be met. Hyperkinesis or brain injury may also need to be considered as an alternative explanation for over-familiarity with adults, disinhibited exploration and poor peer relationships. However, neither hyperkinesis nor brain injury would account for failure to seek comfort from attachment figures when distressed.

Of the care received

A careful history should be taken from birth onwards. The focus should be on the constancy of the chief caregivers versus the number of changes, and on the quality of care given, including warmth, emotional availability, and hostility or abuse. Informants who know the child well should be questioned closely. These may include health visitors and relatives other than the immediate caregivers. Direct observation of the interaction between the child and his or her current caregiver should be carried out, looking for insensitive and inappropriate responding and unusual child behaviours.

Course and prognosis

The natural history of attachment disorders has yet to be formally studied. However, it is possible to draw some provisional conclusions from follow-ups of children who have spent their early years in institutions or who have been insecurely attached. In general, early attachment problems seem particularly likely to interfere with friendships and intimate relationships; somewhat less likely to result in behavioural problems; and least likely to affect cognitive development. The impact of early attachment difficulties is lessened but not abolished when children's social circumstances change for the better, e.g. when adopted by stable and caring families. If they eventually have their own children, will they become neglectful or abusive parents in their turn? This may depend in part on their adult circumstances, and in part on the extent to which they have come to terms with their past, recognising that they were failed by their caregivers and being able to move on from this.

Management

The principal objective of management is to improve the children's caregiving environment. The main contribution of child mental health professionals is often to provide appropriate advice on this to social services and the courts. If a child is currently being maltreated, an alternative placement is obviously needed if the current caregivers cannot be helped to change. If the child has passed through a succession of brief foster placements or has grown up in an institution with rapidly changing staff, he or she needs to be given the opportunity to form lasting attachments, ideally with permanent foster or adoptive parents.

Subject review

Zeanah, C.H. and Emde, R.N. (1994) Attachment disorders in infancy and childhood. In *Child and Adolescent Psychiatry: Modern Approaches*, 3rd edn (M. Rutter, E. Taylor and L. Hersov, eds) Blackwell Science, Oxford, pp. 490–504.

Further reading

Zeanah, C.H. (1996) Beyond insecurity: a reconceptualization of attachment disorders of infancy. *Journal of Consulting and Clinical Psychology*, **64**, 42–52.

17   Enuresis

Though enuresis is sometimes considered a psychiatric disorder, with many parents imagining that it is due to deep-seated emotional problems, it is better seen as a habit or developmental problem than as a mental health problem. Nevertheless, many children do still get referred to child mental health services because of enuresis. In addition, many examiners still consider enuresis to be a child psychiatric topic – hence this chapter! Examination candidates must be careful to distinguish between *nocturnal enuresis* (bed wetting) and *diurnal enuresis* (daytime wetting). Nocturnal and diurnal enuresis differ in several respects and examination questions often seem to be designed to catch out people who confuse the two. Boys are more prone to nocturnal enuresis while girls are more prone to diurnal enuresis. Nocturnal enuresis is commoner than diurnal enuresis and is somewhat less likely to be associated with urinary tract infections or psychiatric disorders (Box 17.1).

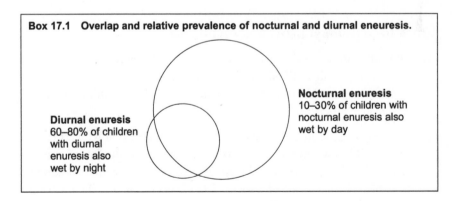

Box 17.1   Overlap and relative prevalence of nocturnal and diurnal eneuresis.

Diurnal enuresis
60–80% of children with diurnal enuresis also wet by night

Nocturnal enuresis
10–30% of children with nocturnal enuresis also wet by day

Primary and secondary

Children are said to have *primary enuresis* when they have never acquired normal bladder control. By contrast, a child who acquires bladder control for at least six months and then loses it again is said to have *secondary enuresis*. This sort of relapse is most likely at the age of five or six and is rare after the age of 11. Having distinguished between primary and secondary enuresis, it is worth emphasising that there are relatively few differences between the two! For example, children with primary or secondary bed wetting are equally likely to have a positive family history or an associated psychiatric disorder. However, the prognosis is worse for secondary enuresis.

Prevalence

Table 17.1 shows the prevalence of nocturnal enuresis in the Isle of Wight study. The emergence of a male preponderance reflects two processes:

(1) Males are slower to achieve dryness (i.e. slower resolution of primary enuresis).
(2) Males are more likely to relapse (i.e. more liable to secondary enuresis).

After the age of seven, secondary enuresis is commoner than primary enuresis.
   Diurnal enuresis occurring at least once a week affects 2% of five-year-olds, with a female excess at all ages.

Table 17.1 Prevalence of nocturnal enuresis occurring once a week or more often (Rutter *et al.*, 1970)

Age	Prevalence (%)	Male:female ratio
5	13	1:1
7	5	1.4:1
9	2.5	1.6:1
14	0.8	1.8:1

Clues to aetiology: proven associations

(1) 70% of enuretic children have a *family history* of enuresis in at least one first degree relative. (The likelihood of a family history is the same for primary and secondary enuresis, and for those with and without associated psychiatric problems.)

(2) Enuresis is associated with *urinary tract infections* (UTIs), particularly in girls. Thus asymptomatic UTIs are present in about 5% of enuretic five-year-old girls, which is some five times the rate in non-enuretic controls. The likelihood of associated UTIs is even higher if the enuresis is diurnal or particularly frequent.

(3) *Stressful life events* at the age of three to four are associated with twice the risk of enuresis. Relevant events include family break-up, separation from the child's mother for at least one month, moving house, the birth of a sibling, admission to hospital, and accidents. Recurrent hospital admission is particularly associated with bed wetting.

(4) Enuresis is associated with *social disadvantage*: lower socioeconomic status, an overcrowded home, and institutional care.

(5) *Other developmental problems*, including language and motor delay, are twice as common among enuretic children as among controls.

(6) Starting *toilet training* after 20 months is associated with a higher rate of subsequent enuresis. Otherwise, the role of specific toilet training practices is unclear. Harsh training is probably undesirable since it causes more upset to the child, but there is no evidence that it results in more enuresis.

Three unlikely causes

(1) In the absence of a clear history of other urinary symptoms, such as continuous dribbling incontinence or very slow stream, it is very unlikely that enuresis is due to a *structural abnormality of the urinary tract* such as a stenosis or an ectopic ureter. Functional bladder capacity may be lower, but this is due to the urge to micturate being felt more readily and not to a less extensible bladder. There is some evidence for delayed maturation of the bladder neck in enuretic children.

(2) Nocturnal enuresis is not a problem of *deep sleep*. Enuresis occurs randomly at any stage of sleep, and there is no evidence that enuretic children sleep unusually deeply.

(3) Though an epileptic fit may involve urinary incontinence, there is no evidence that ordinary enuresis is an *epileptic equivalent*. Enuretic children are no more likely than other children to have an abnormal EEG.

The link with psychiatric problems

An association between enuresis and psychiatric problems has been well demonstrated in epidemiological samples, i.e. the link is not simply an artefact of referral bias. Although the rate of psychiatric disorder is roughly two to six times higher in enuretic children than in non-enuretic controls, it is important to remember that over half of all enuretic children are psychiatrically normal. Predictors of psychiatric disorder include diurnal enuresis, other developmental problems, and female sex. The likelihood of an associated psychiatric disorder is unrelated to the frequency of wetting, to the presence or absence of a family history, or to whether the enuresis is primary or secondary. Among those enuretic children who do have a psychiatric disorder, the type of disorder is not specific: conduct and emotional disorders predominate as in ordinary child psychiatric practice. The link between enuresis and psychiatric disorder could reflect three sorts of causal mechanism:

(1) *Psychiatric problems cause enuresis*. There are some children who are more likely to wet the bed when they are anxious, e.g. after first starting school. On the other hand, some enuretic children may wet the bed less often when they are anxious, e.g. sleeping in a strange bed. One

prospective study did show that children who developed secondary enuresis were more likely than controls to have had emotional or behavioural problems before the enuresis began.

(2) *Enuresis causes psychiatric problems*. Several studies have shown that successful treatment or natural remission of enuresis is accompanied by a decrease in the rate of psychiatric problems. However, children whose enuresis has resolved still have a higher rate of psychiatric problems than controls.

(3) Both enuresis and psychiatric problems result from *the operation of a third factor*, e.g. social disadvantage or biological-developmental problems. Overall, this is the best supported causal mechanism, though the other two probably are important for some children.

Assessment

A detailed history of the wetting and any other urological symptoms is necessary for all cases, as is urinary microscopy and culture. Physical examination and urological investigation are not necessary in straightforward enuresis unaccompanied by any other urological symptom. Enquire about any associated psychiatric problems, and remember to ask specifically about faecal soiling. It is important to enquire about factors influencing choice of treatment. What have the family already tried? How motivated is the child to get dry? Are the parents motivated to participate in treatment e.g. getting up in the middle of the night to supervise the child changing sheets and resetting an enuresis alarm? Is the main concern about nights spent away from home? If so, temporary suppression of enuresis (with medication) may be all that is needed.

Prognosis

Poor prognostic factors in nocturnal enuresis are: male sex, low socioeconomic status, secondary rather than primary enuresis, and nightly rather than intermittent wetting. At puberty 2–5% of children are still enuretic, but spontaneous resolution continues through adolescence; some 1–3% of adults have intractable enuresis.

Treatment

Since uncomplicated enuresis is best seen as a developmental rather than a mental disorder, it is entirely appropriate that professional help usually comes from health visitors, general practitioners and paediatricians rather than from child mental health professionals. Whichever professional is involved, if the child is under the age of five or six, it is often sufficient to reassure the parents that nocturnal enuresis is common and usually outgrown. Common-sense measures include restricting fluids before bedtime or waking the child to use the toilet in the late evening before the parents go to bed. It is not clear, though, how useful these common-sense measures are. In any case, most parents have already tried lifting and fluid restriction without success before deciding to bring their child for professional help.

Both behavioural and pharmacological measures are of proven value in the treatment of enuresis. From a behavioural perspective, it is important that parents do not inadvertently reward and thereby reinforce enuresis, e.g. by letting the child sleep with the parents once the child's own bed is wet. The emphasis should be on praise, attention and other rewards for dry nights rather than on criticism and punishment for wet nights. Keeping a wall chart of wet and dry nights for a month – with the child marking each dry night with a star – is sometimes all that is needed to cure the enuresis. There is no proven value to retention-control training, i.e. training the child to defer micturition for longer and longer.

If the enuresis persists and the family are sufficiently motivated, the most successful behavioural technique for bringing about a lasting cure is an *enuresis alarm*. Urination activates an alarm that wakes the child. Older devices used a pad under the sheet, whereas modern devices use a small pad in the child's pyjamas or underpants, with the alarm being carried in a pocket or on a wristband. When the alarm goes off, the child is expected to get up, go to the toilet, and change pyjamas and sheets as necessary (with parental help if needed). Cure rates of 50–100% are reported, with children typically achieving 14 consecutive dry nights in the second month of treatment (though mentally retarded children may take up to six months). The likelihood of cure is unaffected by whether or not the enuresis is primary or secondary, or by the presence or absence of a family history. The cure rate is lower when there is a high level of family stress, and when the child also wets by day, has a psychiatric disorder, or is unconcerned about the enuresis. Roughly a third of children who do become dry while using the alarm subsequently relapse, returning to wetting the bed again fairly frequently in the year after treatment is stopped. There is some evidence that the relapse rate can be significantly reduced by an 'over-learning' technique, i.e. once the child has learned to be dry at night, the child is encouraged to drink a large quantity of fluids before bedtime, and the enuresis alarm is continued until the child is dry despite the fluid loading.

Why, in behavioural terms, does the enuresis alarm work? There are elements of classical conditioning: the sound of the buzzer (the unconditioned stimulus) leads to waking, and eventually the desire to micturate (the conditioned stimulus) leads to waking too. There are elements of operant conditioning too: the sound of the buzzer is a somewhat aversive stimulus and the child learns to avoid it by not wetting the bed. Finally, social learning theorists would add that the use of the bell and pad helps the family to notice dry nights and to make more of a fuss of the child after dry nights.

If the enuresis alarm does not work, it may be sensible to try the combination of enuresis alarm and desmopressin (see below); or to switch to medication alone, aiming for symptomatic relief rather than for a cure; or to give up for a year or so before trying again. Another option for older and highly motivated children is dry-bed training, which is an intensive form of behavioural therapy that involves hourly waking on the first night, high fluid intake and frequent behavioural rehearsal of proper toileting. Though successful for some otherwise resistant cases, the technique is not suitable for young and poorly motivated children who are likely to see it as a torture.

Many medications have been used in the treatment of enuresis. The first choice should usually be desmopressin (DDAVP), a synthetic analogue of antidiuretic hormone that is probably best reserved for children aged seven or more (and is inappropriate for children under the age of five). The medication is very safe, though it is important to warn patients to avoid large fluid intakes in the evenings in order to reduce the small risk of water intoxication. Given before bedtime, either as a tablet or as a nasal spray, desmopressin eliminates or reduces bed wetting in roughly 70% of children. In most instances, though, the child relapses as soon as the medication is stopped. Despite this reversibility, desmopressin is still a valuable symptomatic treatment that may enable a child to go on school trips or stay overnight with friends without having to face the embarrassment of a wet bed. In addition, the combination of desmopressin and an enuresis alarm may be more successful than an alarm alone, resulting in a higher long-term cure rate. This is particularly true for children with severe wetting or associated behavioural and family problems.

Tricyclic antidepressants in relatively low doses (e.g. 25–75 mg of imipramine at bedtime) have also been shown to be effective symptomatic treatments for nocturnal enuresis. The effect is evident within the first week, and does not seem to be due to the antidepressant, anticholinergic or sleep-altering properties of tricyclics. Enuresis is improved in 85%, with 30% of children becoming completely dry. Tolerance may emerge after two to six weeks on medication, and immediate or delayed relapse on withdrawal of medication is very common. Given the potential toxicity of tricyclics, desmopressin is usually to be preferred.

Anticholinergic medications may be of some use in diurnal enuresis but have not been shown to perform better than placebos in nocturnal enuresis. There is no place for surgical intervention.

Most children with enuresis do not have associated psychiatric problems. In the minority who do have associated emotional and behavioural problems, these problems may need to be assessed and treated in their own right.

Subject review

Shaffer, D. (1994) Enuresis. In *Child and Adolescent Psychiatry: Modern Approaches*, 3rd edn (M. Rutter, E. Taylor and L. Hersov, eds) Blackwell Science, Oxford, pp. 505–519.

Further reading

Rutter, M., Tizard, J. and Whitore, K. eds (1970) *Education, Health and Behaviour.* Longman, London.

Schulpen, T.W.J. *et al.* (1996) Going Dutch in nocturnal enuresis. *Acta Paediatrica*, 85, 199–203. (This brief paper summarises a comprehensive assessment and treatment protocol developed in the Netherlands.)

18   Faecal Soiling

Children have normally acquired bowel control by the age of 3 or 4, though they may still have the occasional accident thereafter. By the age of 11, fewer than 1% of children are soiling themselves once a month or more. By the age of 16, the prevalence of soiling is practically zero. Both epidemiological and clinic series show that soiling is roughly three times commoner in boys than girls.

Faecal soiling may occur for a variety of reasons:

- Constipation with overflow
- Failed toilet training
- Toilet phobia
- Stress-induced loss of control
- Provocative soiling.

Each of these has specific implications for treatment. The term *encopresis* may be used to refer to all varieties of faecal soiling, or may be used more narrowly to refer to the passage of relatively normal stools in inappropriate places, including underclothing. On the basis of a careful history and physical examination, it is usually possible to identify the reason or reasons for soiling and so formulate an appropriate management plan.

Types of soiling and their management

The five types of soiling described below do not always occur in isolation. Children seen clinically commonly have hybrid presentations, showing some of the features of more than one type of soiling. For such children, the different components of their soiling each need to be addressed by the overall management plan. When the symptoms are severe or complicated, or when the soiling does not respond to standard treatment, it will be important for both paediatricians and child mental health workers to be involved.

Constipation with overflow

Children can become constipated for many reasons. A constitutional liability combined with a low-fibre diet is important in some cases. In other instances, an episode of constipation may be initiated by deliberate retention on the part of the child, perhaps because an anal lesion (such as a fissure) makes defecation painful, or perhaps because of a 'battle of wills' over toilet training. Whatever the initiating process, constipation can become self-perpetuating. A large faecal plug is hard to pass and the child may give up in fear of the consequences, promoting further retention. In addition, as the rectum becomes increasingly distended, 'rectal inertia' may set in, with loss of the stretch response that normally results in a sensation of fullness and desire to defecate. Eventually, liquid or semi-liquid faeces may leak round the blockage and overflow.

The appropriate management is to unblock the bowel and re-establish a normal toilet routine. From the outset, the child and family's anxiety and anger need to be defused by adequate explanations of the underlying physiology. Recovery is best promoted by a calm family atmosphere with positive expectations. Clearing the bowel may be possible by using a stimulant laxative such as senna in combination with a stool softener such as lactulose; microenemas or phosphate enemas may be needed initially; bowel washouts are only rarely required. A star chart or similar behavioural programme is used to reward the return to a normal toilet routine. Laxatives are replaced as soon as possible by a high-fibre diet.

Failed toilet training

Some children have never learned bowel control. This can be referred to as primary faecal soiling, by analogy with primary enuresis. Though sometimes attributable to neurological problems or profound mental retardation, primary faecal soiling often seems to reflect inconsistent, insensitive or neglectful toilet training, usually in the context of multiple social and family disadvantages. Suboptimal training may have a particularly marked impact if the child is exposed to chronic psychological stresses during the toddler years when bowel control is usually acquired. Behavioural treatments based on careful record keeping, realistic targets, star charts and appropriate rewards are generally suitable. The most challenging task is often to 'sell' the behavioural package to the family and then ensure that it is correctly and consistently carried out.

Toilet phobia

Some children are scared of the toilet, e.g. fearing that monsters live there, or that a hand will reach up and grab them. Parents are only sometimes aware of these fears, so it is important to explore possible anxieties with the child through conversation, play and drawing. The family can then be helped to discuss the child's fears openly and sympathetically, without ridicule. The fears themselves can be addressed through appropriate reassurance and graded exposure with rewards.

Stress-induced loss of control

Some children acquire bowel control normally but then lose it again after a significant stress, such as a traumatic hospital admission or an episode of sexual abuse. If the child is handled sympathetically, bowel control is usually rapidly regained once the stress is reduced. The primary emphasis of management, therefore, should be on reducing stress and making the child feel safe again.

Provocative soiling

Some children's pattern of soiling seems designed to irritate those around them. For example, they may deliberately defecate into baths or onto furniture, or may smear faeces on walls – subsequently denying that they were responsible for these acts. This covert aggression is often also evident in other aspects of these children's relationships with parents and siblings. Indeed, provocative soiling is usually a marker for multiple problems in the child and family. The child commonly has additional emotional and behavioural problems, and the family as a whole is often severely dysfunctional, failing to meet the child's most basic social and emotional needs. These children and families need help on many fronts, often from social services and education as well as from child mental health professionals.

Prognosis

Whatever type of soiling is involved, persistence into adulthood is very unusual. Resolution is generally more rapid when soiling is the only problem. Both coexistent hyperactivity and nocturnal soiling indicate a poorer prognosis. A chronic course seems particularly likely when soiling is associated with many other problems: behavioural, developmental, scholastic, family and social.

Subject review

Hersov, L. (1994) Faecal soiling. In *Child and Adolescent Psychiatry: Modern Approaches*, 3rd edn (M. Rutter, E. Taylor and L. Hersov, eds) Blackwell Science, Oxford, pp. 520–528.

Further reading

Buchanan, A. in collaboration with Clayden, G. (1992) *Children Who Soil: Assessment and Treatment*. Wiley, Chichester.

19   Psychosomatics

Splitting off the mind as a completely separate entity from the body is often lamented in contemporary times, and its start attributed to the dualism of Descartes (17th century). In fact Plato (4th century BC) said 'This is the great error of our day, that physicians separate the mind from the body'.

Nowadays most paediatricians and child psychiatrists accept the need for a holistic approach, recognising that the physical disorders described in paediatric texts have psychological dimensions, just as the psychological disorders described in this book have physical dimensions. Paediatrics should no more be mindless than child psychiatry should be disembodied!

A list of all the disorders that involved both body and mind would potentially include the whole of medicine. In some instances the direction of effect is primarily *somatopsychic*, with physical antecedents leading on to psychological consequences. In other instances, the direction of effect is primarily from psychological antecedents to physical consequences; this is what most people mean by *psychosomatic*. Distinguishing categorically between conditions that are and are not psychosomatic is bound to be arbitrary and leads, predictably enough, to boundary disputes. In the case of asthma, for example, although it is clear that psychological stress can induce or intensify attacks of wheezing in some predisposed children, many people would resist calling asthma a psychosomatic disorder since stress is just one precipitant among many. More people would agree that children's headaches or stomachaches are often psychosomatic conditions, and yet this may partly reflect our current ignorance of physical predisposing and precipitating factors. It is probably best to speak instead of a *psychosomatic approach* that is potentially relevant to some extent to any condition.

In this chapter, a general introduction to the psychosomatic approach is followed by sections on three illustrative disorders: recurrent abdominal pain, chronic fatigue syndrome, and conversion disorder. Somatopsychic links are the focus of Chapter 24, which describes the common psychological complications of childhood brain disorders; similar considerations also apply to children with a wide range of non-neurological disorders and disabilities as well, though the details vary from condition to condition. For example, the psychological impact of a disorder depends, in part, on whether or not the disorder is (or is perceived to be) life-threatening, and on whether its course is fluctuant, stable, unpredictable or deteriorating.

SOME GENERAL PRINCIPLES

Stress and anxiety can initiate and amplify somatic symptoms

Most readers will know from personal experience or direct observation that stress can induce a variety of somatic symptoms, including headaches, nausea, abdominal pains, diarrhoea, and urinary frequency. It is also common knowledge that an anxious focus on a symptom often makes the symptom seem worse, resulting in increased anxiety, even greater fixation on the symptom, and so on. In addition, a child's anxiety and distress can make the parents feel helpless and panic-stricken. If the parents are unable to hide this, this further fuels the child's anxiety. These vicious cycles, and some of the factors moderating or triggering them, are shown in Box 19.1. Family beliefs about illness play a key role. People differ in the extent to which they make 'normalising' or 'pathologising' attributions about the causes of somatic symptoms: normalising attributions relate the symptoms to environmental or psychological factors (e.g. 'I have a headache because I am under stress and stayed up too late last night'), whereas pathologising attributions focus on organic or pathological causes (e.g. 'perhaps it's a brain tumour'). Normalising attributions are reassuring and can prevent anxiety-related vicious cycles from taking over. Within any one family, the balance of normalising and pathologising attributions will vary over time and according to the nature of the symptom. For example, family stresses may undermine normalising attributions, and having a friend or relative who has recently died of a brain tumour may sensitise parents and children to possible

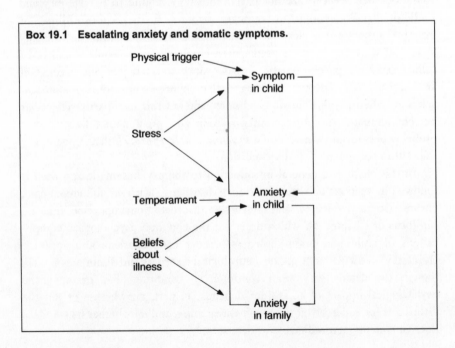

Box 19.1   Escalating anxiety and somatic symptoms.

organic causes of headache. In many instances, anxiety-driven cycles can be interrupted by the reassurance of a trusted doctor who has carried out an adequate investigation. Occasionally, however, doctors are themselves drawn into the vicious cycles of panic and pathologising, with ever more specialist investigations and second opinions reinforcing the family's view that there must be something serious to worry about.

Somatic symptoms can sometimes be a 'mask'

Distress occasioned by psychological or social factors can sometimes be displaced onto a somatic symptom. A particularly transparent version of this can often be witnessed in young children. Thus a child may fight back tears after a quarrel with a friend but then cry inconsolably after a minor fall a short while later. Obtaining relief or sympathy in this way, by focusing on an 'acceptable' somatic symptom such as physical pain, may have the undesirable long-term effect of training the child to somatise psychological distress in future too (Box 19.2). Sensitive parenting can help children learn to disclose their psychological distress without needing to mask it with somatic symptoms (Box 19.3). For both parents and professionals, however, there is also a danger in going to the opposite extreme; psychological probing and psychologising of somatic symptoms can be overdone.

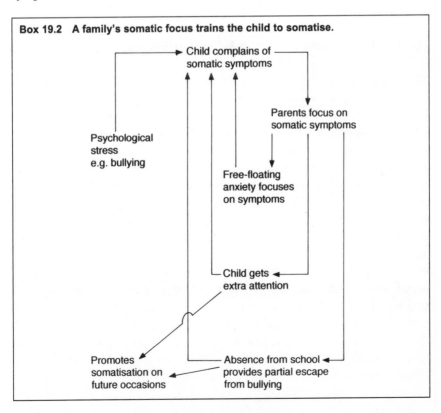

Box 19.2   A family's somatic focus trains the child to somatise.

Child complains of somatic symptoms

Psychological stress e.g. bullying

Parents focus on somatic symptoms

Free-floating anxiety focuses on symptoms

Child gets extra attention

Promotes somatisation on future occasions

Absence from school provides partial escape from bullying

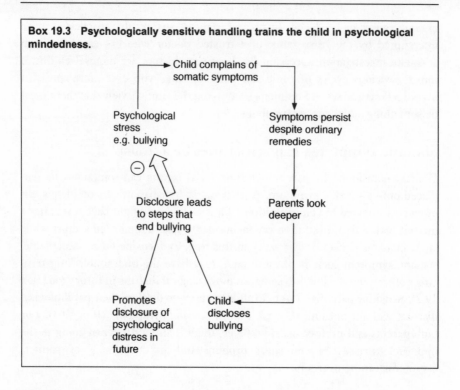

Box 19.3 Psychologically sensitive handling trains the child in psychological mindedness.

Health and illness can each be self-perpetuating

The great majority of ill children want to get better again in order to get back to their friends and resume normal activities. Illness has its attractions too, however, including extra parental attention, sympathy, gifts, and relief from ordinary demands. Although health is usually more attractive than illness, the balance may shift when the child is exposed to acute or chronic life stresses, particularly if the child has no obvious escape other than into illness. Intolerable but apparently inescapable situations can range from undisclosed sexual abuse to being trapped as a high achiever who is doing well at school but cannot sustain the pace or tolerate being overtaken by others. The relative attractiveness of health and illness can also shift after any period of illness, whether purely physical or not. Once someone has been ill for a while, there are fewer reasons to get better again: former friends may have found other people to play with, there is a daunting backlog of school work, and the child may have lost interest or competence in former leisure activities. In addition, prolonged illness may have instilled a liking for the social world of the sick child, whether at home or in hospital. Once the attractions of illness exceed those of health, any move to make the child better may provoke an intensification of symptoms.

An accusatory stance is counter-productive

When children first complain of a symptom, their parents may be able to jolly them out of it or use a 'come off it' approach with success. By the time their symptoms are being presented to health professionals, however, the children would lose face if they got better in response to being told that they were putting it on, or making a mountain out of a molehill, and parents would probably feel foolish and angry too for having been taken in. Predictably enough, 'pull yourself together and stop wasting our time' suggestions may lead to persistence or worsening of symptoms as the children demonstrate that they really are ill. Indeed, it is not just explicitly critical comments that can be counter-productive; the child and family may be very sensitive to any hint that professionals are being dismissive or condemnatory.

Factors in the child

Children with psychosomatic disorders are commonly described as conscientious, obsessional, sensitive, insecure or anxious; these are best seen as personality traits rather than as disorders. Affected children may be temperamentally predisposed to withdraw from new situations, and have sometimes had problems with peer relationships. Only a minority have a coexistent psychiatric disorder, and it is difficult to know how often this is a consequence rather than a cause of their somatic complaints: 'Of course I'm depressed, doctor. Wouldn't you be if you had my symptoms?'

Factors in the family

Family members with somatic symptoms may provide models for the child – in terms of the symptoms themselves, and also in terms of coping style. If relatives have stomach complaints, headaches or seizures, this may sensitise children to these problems or even provide them with a model for conscious or unconscious imitation. If adults in the family typically respond anxiously to their own somatic symptoms, assuming that something beyond their control is seriously wrong, this may well foster anxiety, 'pathologising' attributions, and an external locus of control in the children too.

Although family stresses may initiate or aggravate ill health, there is no convincing evidence that specific types of family stresses are linked with specific types of ill health. 'Psychosomatic' families are sometimes characterised as close families that find it hard to express psychological concerns directly, seeking and providing attention and reassurance through the currency of somatic concern. Other family characteristics that have been said to predispose to psychosomatic disorders are:

- One over-involved parent with the other distant
- Parental disharmony
- Overprotection
- A rigid or disorganised set of rules rather than a stable and flexible set
- Dysfunctional communication without conflict resolution.

Favourable characteristics are said to include warmth, cohesion and satisfactory adaptation to the realities of the family situation. While these suggested risk and protective factors are certainly plausible, they derive primarily from clinical impressions – a potentially fallible guide – rather than from empirical studies.

External stressors

Both chronic adversities and acute life events can play a part. Abuse only seems relevant in a small minority of cases; bullying and academic stresses are probably more common contributors.

Approach to management

Children with somatic symptoms have often been referred to paediatricians in the first instance. Families are better able to accept a psychosomatic approach to assessment and treatment when their family doctor and paediatrician has taken a holistic approach from the outset, considering the interplay of biological and psychological factors from the first assessment onwards. Involving mental health professionals is then just a change in emphasis rather than a complete switch of direction that carries the implicit message: 'We have completed our investigations and there is nothing really wrong with your child, so you had better see the psychiatrists instead'.

The family need to hear from their doctor that the assessment so far has ruled out the dreadful organic diseases that they were worried about – tumours, ulcers, blockages, or whatever. This does not mean that the symptoms are unimportant; it simply means that effective symptomatic treatments can now be deployed without having to worry that there is something more sinister in the background. This message, which helps de-escalate anxious fixation on symptoms, is undermined if physical investigations continue 'just in case'.

There is little to gain and much to lose from trying to force the family to be more psychologically minded than they want to be. If the family continue to feel that physical factors are important, remember that they may be right: current medical views on body and mind will probably seem ridiculously primitive to future generations. It can be useful to emphasise the value of 'mind over matter' and graded rehabilitation approaches. Psychological and behavioural methods can work even when symptoms have a physical cause, which is why these methods are used to help children cope with painful medical procedures or chronic physical symptoms of known organic origin. It is often helpful to teach the child and family techniques such as 'self-hypnosis' or relaxation therapy. These can make them feel more in control of their symptoms. This is treatment for the present episode and prophylactic medicine for the future too. The more psychologically minded families may agree from the outset that psychological stresses could have played a part and need to be explored further. Less psychologically minded families can find this too challenging at the outset, but are sometimes more receptive when 'mind over matter' techniques have started to pay dividends. Children who have a psychiatric disorder, such as depression, in addition to their somatic symptoms may need to have their psychiatric disorder treated in its own right if it does not resolve as a result of the other psychological interventions.

RECURRENT ABDOMINAL PAIN (RAP)

This affects some 10–25% of children, particularly between the ages of three and nine years. Most parents recognise links between the episodes of pain and psychological stresses and provide psychosomatic management without the need for any medical input. Nevertheless, the minority of cases that do get referred on for specialist opinions are sufficiently numerous to account for about 10% of all new paediatric outpatient visits. Even in tertiary paediatric centres, under 10% of RAP proves to be associated with a serious organic disorder. Though there is suggestive evidence that some children are physically predisposed to RAP, psychological stresses are thought to play major roles as precipitating and perpetuating factors.

Factors in the child

Most children with RAP are psychiatrically normal; the slightly elevated rate of psychiatric problems is comparable to that of children with chronic abdominal pain of known organic aetiology. The children are often described as timid, high-strung, over-conscientious children who seek adult approval. Some withdraw from new challenges and others tend to become awkward and irritable when stressed.

Factors in the family

Clinical descriptions of the families emphasise their closeness, their high expectations, and the level of parental concern about the child. Family members have an elevated rate both of emotional symptoms and of somatic complaints, particularly gastrointestinal complaints, some with known organic bases and some not. It has yet to be established whether this familial aggregation reflects modelling, genetic transmission, or shared exposure to adverse environments.

External stressors

There is an association with life events. Most stresses are of an 'everyday' variety, such as a change in school or an impending examination. It is distinctly unusual for sexual abuse to present with RAP without other symptoms of more widespread disturbance.

Natural history

The great majority of children grow out of RAP; very few turn out to have missed organic disorders. In a proportion, it may be a precursor of the irritable bowel syndrome in adulthood.

Treatment

The family need convincing medical reassurance based on an appropriate assessment. Involving the child and family in systematic monitoring and recording of symptoms, antecedents and consequences is often helpful, making the relationship with psychosocial stressors clearer to all concerned. The child can be taught techniques to control symptoms: guided imagery, self-hypnosis, or relaxation techniques. The child should be encouraged to resume normal activities despite any residual pain; parents need to reinforce these activities through praise and attention, simultaneously reducing the extent to which symptoms are rewarded by extra attention. Using these approaches, pain usually disappears or becomes easier to live with if it persists or recurs.

CHRONIC FATIGUE SYNDROME (CFS)

Best known in adults, CFS does also occur in childhood. It is usually defined on the basis of disabling physical fatigue of over six months duration that is unexplained by primary physical or psychiatric causes. It is often accompanied by mental fatigue and by other physical symptoms without a demonstrable organic basis. Low mood is common, with the child and family considering this to be a consequence rather than a cause of the CFS. This low mood is not often associated with self-blame or feelings of worthlessness; a depressive disorder is only diagnosable in roughly a third of cases. As for adult CFS, the evidence for an organic aetiology is weak and inconsistent, but absence of proof is not proof of absence.

This is a disorder where a debate between doctor and family about the relative importance of physical and psychological factors is particularly likely to generate heat rather than light. It is best to remain agnostic, to refuse to be drawn into debates that cannot be resolved on the basis of current evidence, and to get on with treatment. It is helpful to motivate the child and family to beat the problem by harnessing the 'power of positive thinking' and graded rehabilitation approaches. Working with the family, it is usually possible to get the child doing a bit more every day, with a graded return to normal physical activities, leisure pursuits and school. It is worth emphasising that these cognitive-behavioural approaches do help, but that their success does not prove that the disorder was 'all in the mind' in the first place.

CONVERSION DISORDERS

Conversion disorders involve the presence of symptoms or deficits that affect voluntary motor or sensory functioning; these symptoms or deficits suggest an organic disorder but there is no evidence for organic causation and there is positive evidence for psychological causation. These children usually present with a bizarre gait, weakness or paralysis of the legs, funny turns or total incapacitation. Symptoms correspond to the patient's idea of what an illness should look like, only partially matching a doctor's idea; it is these discrepancies that often suggest that the illness is 'hysterical'.

The diagnosis of conversion disorders is fraught with difficulties. A proportion of diagnosed children do eventually turn out to have an organic disease accounting for their symptoms. Apparently bizarre symptoms may prove to be recognised features of a rare disorder that the diagnosing doctor had never considered. Alternatively, the child may have an unusual presentation of a more common disorder. To make matters even more complicated, organic factors may still be important even if psychological factors are indeed responsible for some symptoms. Children whose physical symptoms are not believed may then exaggerate the symptoms in order to be taken seriously. In addition, children may mimic their own episodic disorders, so the fact that a child sometimes has 'pseudoseizures' does not rule out coexistent true epileptic seizures as well.

Despite all these diagnostic pitfalls, most clinicians are convinced that conversion disorder does exist. It can be seen as an (unconscious) enactment of illness in response to an unbearable predicament. Some children respond to stress by acting tough, or grown-up, or pathetic; others respond by acting ill. Doctors need to ensure that they do not make these children worse by initiating a protracted series of investigations and second opinions; they also need to help the child find more adaptive ways of dealing with whatever stresses precipitated the episode.

In developing countries, many reports suggest that conversion disorders are sometimes very common. In Europe and the USA, however, these disorders are encountered less often. Roughly 1% of psychiatric in-patients are diagnosed as having conversion disorders, though the proportion is probably higher among out-patients, particularly those referred by paediatricians. These disorders are rare before the age of five and mostly affect children over the age of 10. Post-pubertal girls may be particularly susceptible.

The child

Premorbid adjustment has often been normal; some have been particularly perfectionist or conscientious students. Only a minority have another psychiatric diagnosis in addition to the conversion disorder.

The family

The family seems normal in most instances; only about a fifth are grossly abnormal. They are usually convinced that the disorder is organic, wanting further physical assessment and resisting psychiatric referral. There is often a family history of physical or psychiatric disorder.

The context and outcome

The child is often stuck in an intolerable predicament, ranging from undisclosed sexual abuse to unsustainably high expectations. The disorder may be precipitated by an adverse life event or by a minor physical illness, although there is sometimes no clear antecedent. In 80% of cases it is possible to identify a model for the symptoms that are enacted: illnesses in the family or the child's wider social circle, or illnesses that the child has previously had. Most recover fully, but a minority run a very chronic course.

Treatment

Physical investigations need to stop. An initial focus on the symptoms rather than on possible psychological stressors may help the family engage. This is a process that may be slow and cannot easily be hurried. A mixture of physical rehabilitation and training in 'mind over matter' techniques provides the child with a way out with honour. The child needs to obtain greater rewards by getting better than by staying sick. This can sometimes be done by altering the family's behaviour, but may sometimes need an in-patient admission. When a child is stuck in an intolerable predicament, this needs to be recognised and addressed. In the longer term, the child needs to learn more adaptive ways of dealing with stresses.

Subject reviews

Garralda, M.E. (1996) Somatisation in children. *Journal of Child Psychology and Psychiatry*, 37, 13–33.

Goodyer, I.M. (1986) Monosymptomatic hysteria in childhood: family and professional systems involvement. *Journal of Family Therapy*, 8, 253–266.

Lask, B. and Fosson, A. (1989) *Childhood Illness: The Psychosomatic Approach*. Wiley, Chichester. (This is a book of clinical wisdom rather than a comprehensive research review.)

Further reading

Sokel, B. *et al.* (1991) Getting better with honor: individualized relaxation/self-hypnosis techniques for control of recalcitrant abdominal pain in children. *Family Systems Medicine*, 9, 83–91.

Taylor, D.C. (1982) The components of sickness: diseases, illnesses and predicaments. In *One Child, Clinics in Developmental Medicine, No. 80* (J. Apley and C. Ounsted, eds) SIMP/Heinemann, London, pp. 1–13.

20 Preschool Problems

Though many preschool children have emotional or behavioural problems, these are often hard to classify. Only a minority have one of the well recognised syndromes described elsewhere in this book, e.g. autism or an attachment disorder. More often, the child has just one area of problems – such as sleep problems, or tantrums, or fears – or a few such problems that do not add up to any recognised diagnosis. For the most part, therefore, the assessment of a preschool child generates a list of problem areas rather than a specific diagnosis. This is a useful exercise though it may not excite the diagnostician who revels in pattern recognition and syndrome spotting!

Common problems

The classic community study of preschool problems and their consequences is the 'Preschool to School' study (Box 20.1). Preschool children can present with the same sorts of symptoms that commonly bring older children to psychiatric attention: worries, fears, misery, aggression, tantrums, overactivity, inattention, and so on. As shown in the box on the Preschool to School study, age trends differ by symptom. Thus as children mature, overactivity and fears become less common, worries become more common, and the likelihood of being difficult to control is almost the same at all three ages.

Developmental or habit problems are also particularly common among preschool children. Delays in toilet training are very frequent, as are comfort habits such as rocking, thumb sucking, head banging, masturbation or hair sucking. Other common difficulties include poor appetite, faddy eating, difficulty settling to sleep at night, and frequent night wakening. As shown in the box on the Preschool to School study, maturation leads to the resolution of many developmental and habit problems. Once they know this, many parents are willing to wait for their child to grow out of these behaviours. If the family do want help, advice on behavioural management, whether from a health visitor, a family doctor, a paediatrician or a mental health professional can be the answer.

Natural history

Though some preschool problems are transient, others persist. The chronicity

Box 20.1   The Preschool to School Study (Richman et al., 1982).

Method

A random 1 in 4 sample of three-year-olds from an outer London borough was studied. A two-stage design (see Chapter 3) involved an initial screening interview, followed by detailed assessments at three, four and eight years of age for all 'screen positive' children and a matched sample of 'screen negative' children.

Main findings at three

Moderate or severe behavioural problems were present in 7%, with mild problems in a further 15%. There was a slight male excess. Boys were more hyperactive; girls were more fearful. Psychiatric problems were more common in the presence of specific language delay or adverse social and family factors, including marital discord, low warmth, high criticism, maternal depression, large family size, and high-rise housing.

Main findings at eight

Of the three-year-olds with problems, 73% of boys still had problems five years later, as did 48% of girls. Overactivity and low intelligence predicted persistence in boys but not in girls. Overactivity predicted conduct disorder; fearfulness predicted emotional disorder. Adverse family factors were more relevant as predisposing than as maintaining causes, i.e. they predicted the onset of new problems but were not good at predicting whether established problems would persist or not.

Percentage with some specific problems at different ages.

	3 years	4 years	8 years
Fears	10	12	2
Overactive, restless	17	13	11
Worries	4	10	21
Difficult to control	11	10	11
Soiling ($\geqslant 1$/wk)	16	3	4
Many comfort habits	17	14	1
Waking at night ($\geqslant \times 3$/wk)	14	12	3

of some preschool problems is evident both prospectively and retrospectively. Prospectively, follow-up studies such as the Preschool to School study have shown that a substantial proportion of severely troubled preschoolers do develop clear-cut conduct, emotional and hyperactivity disorders as they grow older. Retrospectively, this continuity is often evident when assessing the psychiatric problems of schoolchildren, with parental accounts making it clear that the problems go back to the preschool years. Many children with oppo-sitional–defiant disorder have always been irritable and prone to temper tan-trums; many children with separation anxiety disorder have always been very clingy and fearful; and many children with attention-deficit/hyperactivity disorder (ADHD) have always been overactive and inattentive.

Why, then, is it so rarely possible to diagnose conduct, emotional and hyperactivity disorders with confidence in three-year-olds? In part, it seems to be a signal-to-noise problem. For example, although many three-year-olds are very active and find it hard to settle to tasks, most of them develop adequate attention and activity control by the time they start school; only a small minority have persistent problems that eventually warrant a diagnosis of ADHD. Detecting early ADHD (the 'signal') is hard when there is so much background 'noise' in the form of self-limiting overactivity and inattention. There is an urgent need for assessment techniques that can predict which preschool problems are the first signs of chronic disorders. These children could then be targeted for continuing extra help before they run into serious problems. By contrast, reassurance or a brief intervention may be all that is needed for preschool problems that are likely to be outgrown.

Treatment

When preschool children have one of the psychiatric syndromes covered elsewhere in this book, treatment generally follows the standard lines discussed in the relevant chapter. Liaison with the education authority is particularly important for children with chronic disorders such as autism. It is helpful for the education authority to know in advance about emotional, behavioural and learning problems that are likely to require special educational provision. Early warning may also allow the child to be placed in an appropriate playgroup or nursery school, which will often help not only the child but also the worn-out parents.

If the assessment identifies one or more problem areas rather than a specific diagnosis, management strategies need to be considered for each problem. In some instances, parents may not feel that any treatment is necessary once they have been reassured that a problem is common and likely to be short-lived (and told how and when to get back in touch in the unlikely event that the problem does persist). When treatment is indicated, behavioural approaches are often particularly valuable. For example, if temper tantrums or night wakening are being reinforced by parental attention, the solution may be to pay less attention to the problem. The behavioural programme needs to be tailored to the characteristics of the parents as well as those of the child. For example, if parents do not have nerves of steel, they may find it hard to 'extinguish' night wakening by completely ignoring their child's calls or cries in the middle of the night. A more 'softly, softly' approach may suit such parents better, e.g. paying progressively less attention each successive night. It is important to remember that a behavioural programme that the parents cannot carry through to completion is worse than nothing, since it demoralises the parents and trains the child to hold out against any subsequent attempt to tackle the problem behaviour.

Subject reviews

Douglas, J. (1989) *Behaviour Problems in Young Children*. Tavistock/Routledge, London.

Richman, N. and Lansdown, R. (1988) *Problems of Preschool Children*. Wiley, Chichester.

Further reading

Campbell, S.B. (1995) Behavior problems in preschool children: a review of recent research. *Journal of Child Psychology and Psychiatry*, **36**, 113–149.

Minde, K. & Minde, R. (1986) *Infant Psychiatry*. Sage, Beverly Hills. (A book on the problems of children aged under three.)

Richman, N., Stevenson, J. and Graham, P.J. (1982) *Preschool to School: A Behavioural Study*. Academic Press, London.

21   Disorders in Adolescence

Since adolescence falls between childhood and adulthood, it is not surprising that most of the psychiatric disorders of adolescence are either continuations of childhood disorders or early manifestations of adult disorders. But adolescence is not just a blend of childhood and adulthood; it is a stage with unique biological and social characteristics of its own, that colour both normal and abnormal behaviour during the teenage years. Before focusing on abnormal behaviour, it is important to consider the uniqueness of the world the adolescent lives in, as well as the processes of internal mental and physical maturation particular to this stage of life. The behavioural problems that peak in the teenage years such as delinquency, substance abuse, deliberate self-harm, and anorexia nervosa often involve exaggerated and unresolved versions of the ordinary trials and tribulations of adolescence.

A potted history of adolescence

Although puberty is a biological process, adolescence as we currently know it is a relatively new social phenomenon. In the developing world, most people leave school and begin work before or during puberty; physical maturity develops in step with economic and social maturity. The same was true in the developed world until fairly recently, when the combination of earlier puberty (reflecting better nutrition and health) and prolonged education resulted in a 'no man's land' opening up between childhood and adulthood. This is the prolonged period when teenagers acquire adult bodies but not adult roles, rights or financial independence. Of course, this is an oversimplification, but it points to the need to think of adolescence (and indeed every other stage of life too) as culturally as well as biologically determined.

Rules and autonomy

During adolescence there is a shift from accepting rules and boundaries imposed by others to setting them oneself, substituting self-imposed control for externally imposed control. Young people face a demanding task as they try to exercise their growing capacity and desire for self-determination within limits acceptable to their parents and society as a whole. Not surprisingly, surveys confirm that the commonest causes of arguments with parents in this period are issues relating to rules and autonomy. At the more disturbed end of the spectrum, 'out of control' teenagers pursue their own desires while paying little or no heed to society's rules and other people's needs. It is a simultaneous absence of externally imposed and self-imposed control that makes these adolescents particularly difficult to manage for all those involved, including parents, social workers and psychiatrists. When parents can no longer cope, simply taking these youngsters into care in a children's home may only aggravate the problem since the lack of containment in many children's homes is reflected in high rates of various 'out of control' activities. These activities can include precocious and unprotected sexual activity, overdoses and wrist-cutting, drug taking, running away for days at a time, and theft.

Biological and social influences interact

Biological factors contribute to the pubertal upsurge in sexual and aggressive behaviours in humans as in other animals; the consequences of delayed puberty bear this out. However, different cultures channel these biological predis-positions in different ways, amplifying some features and suppressing others. Common sense notions to the contrary there is no convincing evidence that hormone levels are abnormally high among extremely aggressive delinquents or multiple sex-offenders, and the efficacy (let alone desirability) of 'chemical castration' in these circumstances remains controversial. Pathological variations in post-pubertal sexual and aggressive 'drives' seem more related to social and psychological variables than to biological variables.

The interplay of biological and social factors in adolescent development is well illustrated by the findings of a Swedish study of the consequences of early puberty for girls. Roughly 10% of a large and representative sample of girls entered puberty at least two years earlier than average. As adolescents, these early-maturing girls were more likely than their contemporaries to smoke, drink, steal, play truant, disobey their parents, and leave school at the earliest opportunity. These differences stemmed from the tendency of the early-maturing girls to associate with older girls, perhaps particularly with disaffected older girls who were doing poorly at school. A biological difference (early puberty) led on to a social difference (choice of peer group), and it was the social difference that affected adjustment; early-maturing girls without older friends were not at increased risk of norm breaking.

Cognitive development

In many respects, teenagers from the age of 14 or 15 have comparable cognitive capabilities to adults, e.g. on tests of abstract reasoning or 'frontal lobe' func-tions. Conflicts can easily arise from the fact that teenagers are the equals of their parents or teachers in these respects while differing enormously in experience and power. Adults may underestimate teenagers' ability to think things through for themselves; teenagers may underestimate the value of experience.

Just as people vary considerably in the age at which they reach their adult height, it seems likely that people vary widely in the age at which they reach their adult cognitive potential, with this variation having important consequences for psychosocial adaptation. Some studies of juvenile delinquents indicate they are behind their peers in the development of conscience and altruism, although this has proved hard to measure.

Identity

In principle, our society offers youngsters a bewildering variety of possible adult roles: 'you can be anything you want if you really work at it'. In practice, most youngsters' options are restricted and unglamorous. This tension adds to the difficulties of adolescence as the young person attempts to work towards a sense of identity that bridges internal aspirations and external realities. A sense of confusion about personal identity can sometimes be so marked that it largely prevents a young person from functioning. DSM–IV provides a coding for *Identity Problem* under the rubric of other conditions that may be a focus of clinical interest. ICD–10 does not have a comparable category.

There are different risks associated with accepting and rejecting the identities offered by the adult world. Accepting an unglamorous identity that falls well short of previous aspirations may undermine self-esteem and predispose to depression. At the other extreme, some youngsters seem to define their identity primarily in terms of their rejection of adult authority and adult norms, predisposing them to delinquency and substance abuse. An identity based on the rejection of adult values sometimes seems to reflect the cumulative impact of criticism by parents, failure at school, and subsequent identification with a delinquent peer group.

Sexual identity may not be completely clear to young people; surveys suggest that while at least 3% are unambiguously homosexual, at least the same number go through a period of bisexuality, which for the majority is transient.

Solving problems and weathering stress

Though childhood has its own stresses, the transition to adulthood can bring on many more: examinations, broken hearts, unemployment, or intensified arguments with parents. Children who have not learned adaptive ways of relating to others and dealing with crises, perhaps because their parents also lacked the relevant skills, are likely to find the new stresses of adolescence particularly hard to cope with. Violence, substance abuse and self-harm can all be ways of defusing stress or temporarily dealing with problems that cannot be solved more adaptively.

Epidemiology of adolescent psychiatric disorders

The Isle of Wight study of 14 and 15 year olds remains the 'classical' epidemiological investigation of adolescent psychopathology (Box 21.1). Though the main conclusions of this study have stood the test of time, many subsequent studies have found somewhat higher rates of adolescent depression (ranging up to 8%). There has also been growing interest in a 'two population' model of adolescent conduct problems, involving a 'hard core' of individuals who are behaviourally disordered before, during and after adolescence, plus a larger number of previously well-adjusted individuals who go through a relatively transient phase of rule-breaking and antisocial behaviour during adolescence.

Emotional and conduct disorders are the most common diagnoses in adolescence as in middle childhood. These are covered in the relevant chapters,

---

Box 21.1   The Isle of Wight Follow-up (Rutter *et al.*, 1976).

Method

A total population sample of 2303 adolescents living on the Isle of Wight were studied using a two-stage design (see Chapter 3). All subjects were assessed by behavioural screening questionnaires completed by parents and teachers. Full psychiatric assessments were carried out on all 'screen positive' individuals and a random sample of 'screen negative' individuals. Most of the subjects had also been studied four years earlier in the original Isle of Wight study (see Chapter 3), though some were newcomers.

Main findings

(1) Judging from the information gathered from parents and teachers, definite psychiatric disorders were present in roughly 10% of the sample – only slightly higher than the rate in middle childhood. In addition, another 10% of adolescents reported marked internal feelings of misery and worthlessness that were not accompanied by significant outward changes. Was this covert depression? Only long-term follow-up can answer the key question as to whether covert adolescent misery is the precursor of overt adult depression.

(2) Of the disorders that were evident to informants, most were emotional and conduct disorders. Depressive disorders were more common than at ten – 2% rather than 0.2%. (Self-reported misery was even more common: 48% of girls, 42% of boys). School refusal was also more common at 14 than at ten, occurring as part of wider anxiety and affective disorders.

(3) Just under half of the children with disorders at 14 had already had a disorder when assessed at ten. Disorders arising for the first time after the age of ten differed in three main ways from early-onset disorders: they were *not* associated with educational difficulties; there was only a slight male excess; and adverse family factors were less often present.

(4) Only a minority of adolescents were alienated from their parents (as judged by rows, physical and emotional withdrawal, and rejection). Alienation was particularly common when the young person had a psychiatric disorder (especially if this was chronic). Although alienation dating back to middle or early childhood did seem to be linked to psychiatric disorders beginning after the age of ten, alienation *beginning* in the teenage years was not a common cause of psychiatric disorder.

as are two other problems that peak in adolescence, namely juvenile delinquency and deliberate self-harm. The rest of this chapter is devoted to four
conditions that are not covered elsewhere and that are much more common in
adolescence than in childhood: substance abuse, schizophrenia, anorexia
nervosa and bulimia nervosa.

Specific disorders

Substance use and abuse

In a society that permits adults to use selected psychoactive substances for
pleasure or the relief of stress, it is not surprising that most young people
choose to try psychoactive substances, and that many come to consume them
regularly, often with major public health consequences. In a recent survey of
British 15- and 16-year-olds, over three-quarters had been drunk at least once
in their life, and almost as many had smoked. In the previous month, roughly
half had consumed five or more drinks in a row on at least one occasion, and
about a third had smoked. Almost half had tried illicit drugs at some time: about
40% had used cannabis; about 20% had inhaled volatile substances (glues or
solvents); and LSD, amphetamines, tranquillisers and Ecstasy had each been
used by between 5 and 15% of the sample. Though most such experiments with
illicit drugs do not lead to regular use, it is worth remembering that nearly all
young adults who are drug abusers first began to use drugs in school, with
earlier onset predicting greater persistence.

There is no single or simple explanation for the pattern of substance use and
abuse: availability, pharmacological factors, constitutional predisposition, youth
culture, advertising and adult role-models all play a part. Prior psychosocial
adjustment is one more factor amongst many. Children with conduct disorders
are more liable than other children to become substance abusers as adolescents
and adults. The combination of conduct disorder and hyperactivity carries a
particularly high risk. It has proven difficult to establish how far the social and
psychiatric problems of substance abusers stem from the habit itself, and how
far they are simply continuations of the long-standing adjustment difficulties
that predated substance use.

Inhaling organic solvents – known as volatile substance abuse (VSA) or glue
sniffing – is a pattern of substance use that is particularly associated with youth
and social adversity. In the UK, VSA peaks at around 15 years of age; roughly
1% of British secondary school pupils inhale solvents regularly, with the
prevalence being substantially higher for children who come from deprived
backgrounds. Elsewhere in the world, VSA is the rule rather than the exception
among some particularly deprived groups of children, e.g. among the millions
of street children of Brazil. For the user, inhaling solvents is attractive as a
cheap and readily available means of inducing a 'high', or of escaping from an

intolerable situation; the effects are somewhat similar to alcohol but shorter lasting. Common side-effects include nausea, vomiting, headache, tinnitus, and abdominal pain. Inhaling solvents from a bag may lead to a rash around the mouth or nose. Rarer side-effects include liver and kidney damage, respiratory difficulties and encephalopathy. Death can result from cardiac arrest, inhalation of vomit, or from laryngeal spasm (particularly when lighter fluid or deodorants are sprayed directly into the back of the mouth). In the UK, VSA currently results in about 100 deaths per year in people under the age of 18, accounting for some 5% of all deaths in this age group. Up to a third of these deaths occur in children experimenting with solvents for the first time. Though girls are as likely to have tried solvents as boys, most VSA deaths occur in males, perhaps reflecting sex differences in the frequency of use or choice of solvent.

Schizophrenia

The most important thing to know about schizophrenia in childhood and adolescence is that it is very similar to schizophrenia in adulthood – but rarer. Schizophrenia can occur in children as young as seven, but is very uncommon until after puberty. This rarity of prepubertal schizophrenia is puzzling in the light of growing evidence that schizophrenia is usually a neurodevelopmental disorder, perhaps dating back to the early prenatal period. Why should it take so many years before long-standing neurodevelopmental abnormalities finally result in psychotic symptoms? One plausible explanation is that the underlying brain abnormalities are unmasked by normal developmental processes such as myelination or the progressive 'weeding out' of excessive synapses – processes that continue up to puberty and even beyond.

Genetic factors seem at least as important in early-onset cases as in adults. Though males are generally more vulnerable to early-onset schizophrenia, the sex ratio is reversed in the 11–14 age band, probably because girls are much more likely than boys to be post-pubertal at this age. Schizophrenia beginning in childhood or adolescence is particularly likely to be preceded by premorbid abnormalities in development and social adjustment. Neurodevelopmental abnormalities include speech and language delay, clumsiness, inattentiveness, and lowered IQ (mean around 90). The onset of frank psychosis is often preceded by years of poor social adjustment. Though this premorbid picture is often clear in retrospect, it is not sufficiently characteristic to permit a confident prospective diagnosis of incipient schizophrenia.

Schizophrenic symptoms are fairly similar at all ages. Even young children can have Schneiderian first-rank hallucinations and delusions, as well as thought disorder and negative symptoms such as affective blunting and apathetic social withdrawal. In line with developmental level, delusions in children are generally less complex than in adults, and less likely to have sexual or other adult themes. Passivity phenomena and poverty of thought are less prominent than in adults.

Since age makes so little difference to symptomatology, the standard ICD–10 and DSM–IV diagnostic criteria for schizophrenia can be used at all ages. This works well on the whole, although several studies have shown that manic episodes in adolescence are particularly likely to involve Schneiderian first-rank symptoms, often leading to a misdiagnosis of schizophrenia. Diagnosis can be difficult in younger and more delayed children, particularly if the onset of symptoms is insidious. Distinguishing delusions and hallucinations from exaggerated age-appropriate fears and fantasies can be hard in this group, especially if there is a coexisting language disorder. Distinguishing between autism and schizophrenia (Box 21.2) is not hard, but it is a favourite examination topic!

Box 21.2   Comparing autism and schizophrenia.

	Autism	**Schizophrenia**
Characteristic features	Severe social impairment (aloof or unempathic). Severe communication problems. Rituals and repetitive behaviours.	Hallucinations, delusions, thought disorder, negative symptoms
Onset	Under three years, often from birth	Over seven years, mostly post-pubertal ± premorbid developmental abnormalities (milder and less specific than in autism)
Family history	2% of siblings are autistic, and over 10% have lesser autistic features	Often positive family history of schizophrenia
Mental retardation	Usually	Rarely
Course	Non-episodic, chronic, mostly improving somewhat with maturation	Episodic, often with gradually detriorating social adaptation
Neuroleptics useful	Rarely	Usually
Severe long-term social impairment	Usually	Usually
Need community care and specialist services	Usually	Usually

When schizophrenia begins early in life, the onset is often insidious rather than acute. Psychotic episodes commonly involve between one and six months of hallucinations, delusions and thought disorder. Neuroleptic medication often helps reduce symptom intensity but does not necessarily shorten the episode. Adolescent psychiatrists are making increasing use of newer neuroleptics such as sulpiride, clozapine and risperidone to reduce side-effects, improve negative symptoms, or circumvent resistance to more traditional neuroleptics such as chlorpromazine or haloperidol. At present, this is primarily based on extra-polation from adult studies rather than on studies of adolescents themselves. Resolution of positive symptoms is often followed by a recovery phase of several months during which residual negative symptoms partially or fully resolve. As in the case of adult-onset schizophrenia, it is only a small minority who recover completely and have no further episodes. Family work to reduce negative expressed emotion may play a part in reducing relapses, alongside continuing medication; affected individuals may also need special schooling, social skills training, and phased transfer to adult community psychiatric services. Parti-cularly after second and subsequent episodes, recovery is often incomplete and social functioning may gradually deteriorate. Early onset generally carries a worse prognosis than adult onset. The best predictors of the long-term outcome of early-onset schizophrenia are premorbid functioning and the degree of recovery from the first episode.

Anorexia nervosa

Anorexia nervosa has a peak age of onset in the mid-teens and a female:male ratio of around 10:1. Onset is uncommon before puberty. The prevalence is roughly 0.1% in 11–15-year-old girls and 1% in 16–18-year-old girls. The main diagnostic criteria for anorexia nervosa, which are very similar for both ICD–10 and DSM–IV, are shown in Box 21.3. DSM–IV recognises two subtypes of anorexia nervosa: a *restricting* type in which weight loss involves starvation but not binge-eating or purging, and a *binge-eating/purging* type in which weight loss involves binge-eating or purging as well as starvation. Whether these are really two distinct subtypes as opposed to points on a continuum is still in doubt. Depressive and obsessional features are common, sometimes warranting additional diagnoses.

Box 21.3 Diagnostic criteria for anorexia nervosa.

(1) *Underweight:* < 85% of expected weight for age and height (due to weight loss or, in children, to lack of expected weight gain).
(2) *Caused by:* Deliberate dietary restriction, sometimes combined with excessive exercise, appetite suppressants, or purging (i.e. deliberate vomiting or misuse of laxatives, enemas, or diuretics).
(3) *Associated cognitions:* Intense fear of fatness. Feels fat even when underweight (or only feels about right when very underweight).
(4) *Endocrine consequences:* Amenorrhoea in post-menarcheal females, unless on the 'pill'. (Loss of sexual interest and potency in males. Delayed or arrested puberty in early-onset cases.)

Twin studies suggest that genetic predisposition may be important, parti-cularly for adolescent onset of the restricting type of anorexia. Epidemiological studies suggest that cultural factors are also important. Anorexia nervosa is primarily a disorder of the developed world; elsewhere anorexia nervosa is mainly restricted to the most affluent (and thus most westernised) social strata. The contemporary western stereotype of female beauty involves a degree of slimness that obliges most adolescent girls to diet. Liability to anorexia is particularly high in occupations such as modelling and ballet dancing that particularly emphasise slimness. Though most adolescent dieting is benign, social pressures for dieting and slimness do appear to increase the risk of anorexia. There is no specifically 'anorexogenic' family background; the disorder is associated with an increased rate of relatively non-specific problems with family communication and interaction, and also with a higher rate of weight problems, physical illness, depression and alcoholism among relatives.

The predisposing role of specific childhood experiences, including sexual abuse, is uncertain. In many instances, anorexia does seem to have been precipitated by an adverse life event, though the type of life event does not appear to be particularly characteristic. The weight gain and change in body shape due to puberty itself may also contribute to the onset of the disorder, perhaps particularly when the individual is apprehensive about the shift from childhood dependency to sexual maturity and adult independence.

Although it seems natural to assume that anorexic cognitions motivate anorexic behaviour – for example, that a preoccupation with weight leads to excessive dieting – the reverse could also be true. In some circumstances, self-starving behaviour may take on a life of its own. The constipation and delayed gastric emptying associated with starvation can make the affected individual feel full up despite eating little. In addition, starvation may have its own rewards, perhaps in the form of endorphin release or extra attention. If so, starvation may become a self-perpetuating behaviour, with affected individuals subsequently trying to make sense of their own addiction to starvation by coming up with plausible but irrelevant explanations in terms of feeling too fat. From this perspective, even if weight loss began in response to stress or culturally sanctioned dieting, the process may subsequently become a vicious cycle that is hard to escape.

With suitably trained therapists, the treatment of anorexic children and teenagers who live with their families can usually be managed on an out-patient basis. Gradual but steady weight restoration is the first main goal, aiming for an eventual weight within 10% of expected. This is usually accomplished by eating modest meals more often (four to six times per day). Weight gain is facilitated by some combination of family therapy, behavioural techniques and individual therapy. Family sessions aim to promote a family restructuring that will facilitate recovery, often by putting parents more clearly in charge of dietary intake until normal weight control has been re-established. Behavioural techniques can be used to reward adherence to diet and successful weight gain. Individual therapy can provide a mixture of support, cognitive restructuring, education about diet, insight, and problem-solving skills. A well-executed comparison of family therapy and individual therapy showed that family therapy was superior for patients aged under 19 who did not have chronic anorexia. There is no clear role for neuroleptics or appetite stimulants, but antidepressants may have some effect on weight gain and comorbid depression.

In the long term, roughly 50% of cases recover, while 30% are partly improved and 20% run a chronic course. Mortality is under 5%. A minority may progress from restrictive anorexia to binge-eating anorexia and then on to bulimia nervosa. Factors predicting a poor outcome include greater weight loss, vomiting, binge-eating, greater chronicity and premorbid abnormalities. Possible indicators of a better outcome include early onset, good parent-child relationships, and rapid detection and treatment.

Bulimia nervosa

Bulimia nervosa involves frequent episodes of out-of-control overeating in which large amounts of food are consumed in short periods; the disorder should not be diagnosed on the basis of binges that occur exclusively during periods when the individual also meets the criteria for anorexia nervosa. Binges take place against a background of a persistent craving for, or preoccupation with, food. The individual counteracts the fattening effects of binges by means of deliberate vomiting, purging, periods of starvation, or other means. Body weight is usually close to normal, but concern about body weight is heightened.

The peak age for bulimia is a few years later than for anorexia, but there is the same marked excess of females. Though epidemiological studies suggest that bulimia may be more common than anorexia in the general population, bulimia is underrepresented in clinic samples. Most affected individuals can be treated as out-patients with cognitive-behavioural or group therapy, both of which seem to outperform medication. Bulimia is often episodic with remissions and relapses. In the long term, disturbed eating behaviour often persists and depression is common.

Subject reviews

Farrell, M. and Taylor, E. (1994) Drug and alcohol use and misuse. In *Child and Aolescent Psychiatry: Modern Approaches*, 3rd edn (M. Rutter, E. Taylor and L. Hersov, eds) Blackwell Science, Oxford, pp. 529–545.

Steinhausen, H-C. (1994) Anorexia and bulimia nervosa. In *Child and Adolescent Psychiatry: Modern Approaches*, 3rd edn (M. Rutter, E. Taylor and L. Hersov, eds) Blackwell Science, Oxford, pp. 425–440.

Werry, J.S. and Taylor, E. (1994) Schizophrenic and allied disorders. In *Child and Adolescent Psychiatry: Modern Approaches*, 3rd edn (M. Rutter, E. Taylor and L. Hersov, eds) Blackwell Science, Oxford, pp. 594–615.

Further reading

Esmail, A. *et al.* (1993) Deaths from volatile substance abuse in those under 18 years: results from a national epidemiological study. *Archives of Disease in Childhood*, **69**, 356–360.

Miller, P. and Plant, M. (1996) Drinking, smoking and illicit drug use among 15 and 16 year olds in the United Kingdom. *British Medical Journal*, **313**, 394–397.

Magnusson, E. *et al.* (1985) Biological maturation and social development: a longitudinal study of some adjustment processes from mid-adolescence to adulthood. *Journal of Youth and Adolescence*, **14**, 267–283. (Investigates the effects of early and late puberty in females.)

Russell, G. *et al.* (1987) An evaluation of family therapy in anorexia nervosa and bulimia nervosa. *Archives of General Psychiatry*, **44**, 1047–1056.

Rutter, M. *et al.* (1976) Adolescent turmoil: fact or fiction? *Journal of Child Psychology and Psychiatry*, **17**, 35–56. (This describes the Isle of Wight study of adolescents.)

22 Maltreatment of Children

Maltreatment of children became widely recognised in the USA in the 1960s and since then has been uncovered throughout the world wherever systematic enquiry has taken place. Most definitions incorporate two elements: (1) evidence of behaviour towards the child which is likely to be damaging, and (2) evidence of harm to the child *resulting from this*. Note that intention is not part of the definition; some parents may feel they love their children dearly but nonetheless may harm them, albeit unwittingly. Sometimes maltreatment is easy to recognise, e.g. a girl with scalded buttocks and a parent who confesses to dipping her in a boiling bath to teach her a lesson. At other times it is far harder, e.g. a neglected boy who has conduct disorder and whose parents are of low intellect. How much avoidable harm has been done, or would he have turned out this way even if well looked after? Information is far from precise on how much neglect is required to cause specific, measurable damage.

Abuse and neglect cases can be some of the most disturbing and heart-wrenching experiences in child psychiatry, sometimes evoking horror and a wish to rescue the child immediately. Therefore it is important to keep a sense of perspective on how good the evidence is that abuse is indeed happening, and to have a sympathetic team for emotional support to stop becoming overwhelmed by, or cut off from, what is seen.

Types of maltreatment include:

- *Physical abuse:* Non-accidental injury: head injuries, fractures, burns and scalds, bruises. Munchausen syndrome by proxy (factitious illness by proxy). Non-organic failure to thrive and psychosocial short stature.
- *Neglect:* Lack of physical and medical care, supervision, emotional closeness, stimulation.
- *Emotional abuse:* Hostility, deprivation of attention, threats to abandon, inappropriate demands.
- *Sexual abuse:* Penetrative, non-penetrative; intrafamilial, extrafamilial; of girls, of boys.

Epidemiology

Obviously, ascertainment methods and definitions will strongly influence reported rates. In England, about 3% of children under the age of 13 are brought each year to the attention of professional agencies for suspected abuse. A tenth of this figure, 3 per 1000, are on the official Child Protection Register for the whole age range 0–18 years. This prevalence figure is more than doubled for the first year of life, but then settles down to around 3 per 1000 for children aged 1–16, after which there is a considerable drop. Looked at another way, it is important to note that there is still serious abuse frequently coming to light in the 10–15 year adolescent age group. Fatal abuse occurs in about 1 in 10 000 of the population, with violence induced mental handicap about as common in the first year.

In England and Wales, the most commonly registered category of maltreatment is physical abuse, followed by sexual abuse, then neglect; emotional abuse is seldom registered. However, more common than all of these categories, at about half of all registrations, is the non-specific 'grave concern', used where there is thought to be a serious risk of abuse, e.g. because siblings are known to be abused, or because there is a convicted sex offender living at home, etc.

In the USA the government sanctioned figure for the prevalence of maltreatment in children under 18 was 2.5% for 1988, with neglect predominating, followed by physical abuse, and then sexual abuse. There were over 2000 deaths a year resulting from recognised abuse and neglect, in addition to 6000 homicides per year of children aged under eight, generally by family members.

These figures give the predominant type of maltreatment at the time of registration. However, more detailed studies show there is a large degree of overlap, with multiple forms of abuse being the rule rather than the exception. Thus physical abuse severe enough to reach an official register seldom occurs in the absence of emotional abuse, and there is not infrequently a degree of neglect; intrafamilial sexual abuse tends to occur in an atmosphere of inadequate personal boundaries and emotional distortions; and so on.

Clinical picture

Physical abuse

The child is usually presented with some form of injury. The history from the family may include suggestive pointers:

(1) Delay or failure to seek medical help.
(2) The account of how the injury was sustained is vague, lacking specific detail, whereas the remainder of the circumstances are conveyed in convincing particularity.
(3) The account varies in significant ways with retelling.
(4) The account of the incident is not compatible with the injury sustained – e.g. a child with sharp bruises and fractures is said to have rolled off a bed onto a well carpeted floor.
(5) The parental affect while giving the account is abnormal and does not appear to reflect the degree of concern and anxiety one would expect.

(6)   Parental behaviour during the enquiry is suspicious, with hostility, over-emphatic denial of any anger towards the child despite evidence of his behaving in a difficult way preceding the injury, and attempts to leave hospital early before medical investigations are complete.

(7)   Many abused children look sad, withdrawn and frightened, some show frozen watchfulness.

(8)   The child may say something strongly indicative of abuse.

Examination and investigation may show injuries that are strongly suggestive of non-accidental injury. These are well described in most paediatric textbooks, and include characteristic patterns of fractures (including widespread fractures of differing ages revealed on skeletal survey), retinal and intracerebral bleeds from shaking, burns and scalds (including cigarette burns and scalds from forced immersion), and characteristic patterns of bruising (e.g. due to gripping or throttling).

Other forms of physical abuse include deliberate suffocation and poisoning. Suffocation may be presented as an apnoeic attack or as near-miss or actual sudden infant death syndrome (SIDS). One estimate is that 10% of SIDS are due to suffocation; siblings of children on the child protection register have a far higher rate than controls. Poisoning may be presented as accidental when it is not, or simply as a mystery illness.

Munchausen syndrome by proxy, also known as factitious illness by proxy, refers to a child being presented to doctors by a parent who has induced the illness. The child is usually brought repeatedly by the mother to hospital for investigation, yet when she is away the symptoms and signs abate. The parents deny any knowledge of the cause of the illness. Other siblings have often been subject to fabricated illness too, and indeed one study found that 1 in 10 had died in mysterious circumstances. Forms of fabricated illness include, in descending order of reported frequency, respiratory arrests due to smothering, poisonings, seizures, apparent bleeding from a variety of orifices, skin rashes and other skin conditions, fevers, and high blood pressure. As the mother spends more time on the ward it may become apparent that she enjoys medical attention; often mothers have nursing or other health-related training or experience. Other types of physical abuse such as non-accidental injury and non-organic failure to thrive often coexist.

Failure to thrive refers simply to less than expected weight gain. It is a relatively common presentation in paediatric clinics. In the majority a medical condition is found, which can be very varied including heart disease, lung disease, gut disease, hormonal problems and many more. In a minority, however, no medical cause can be found. This group comprise non-organic failure to thrive (NOFT). A proportion of these will simply have undiagnosed medical conditions, but many arise in the context of deviant parent-child interaction patterns. The deviant interactions are especially common in this group at meal times, with the result that most cases of NOFT end up receiving insufficient nutrition (as do many cases of organic failure to thrive, where parent-child interaction is, by contrast, usually normal). To demonstrate that adverse upbringing is the cause, it is essential to document that the weight of the child catches up when they are placed in a benign environment (e.g. a hospital ward, or with foster parents). Children with NOFT have been shown to be at far higher risk of later neglect and abuse than controls.

Psychosocial short stature refers to the impairment of linear growth in conditions of severe abuse and neglect. It is rarer and more severe than NOFT. There is a background of prolonged gross maltreatment, with severe emotional abuse, neglect, and often sexual or physical abuse. One particularly distinctive presentation, sometimes described as hyperphagic short stature, has the following features. The children are stunted, but not malnourished, having near normal weight for height but immature body proportions. Sleep patterns are irregular and disturbed. These children often take large quantities of food from home and from other children, and may gorge themselves until they vomit. Enuresis and encopresis are common and often appear intentional. Mood is usually depressed with grossly self-deprecating self-esteem. Social relations are very poor with no friends and active rejection by others. IQ tends to be towards the bottom of the normal range, attention span is short, language delayed and school achievements far behind. Growth hormone secretion is generally reduced while the children are exposed to stress, returning to normal or above normal levels on admission to hospital. As with NOFT, most of the clinical features improve markedly with removal from the abusive environment. Initial evidence suggests that hyperphagic short stature is a rare condition that results from the combination of severe abuse and a constitutional tendency to hypo-secrete growth hormone when stressed.

Neglect

This refers to an absence of appropriate care rather than positively inappropriate acts. However, the effects of neglect on children can be just as devastating as the effects of abuse, if not more so. Most areas of care may be involved:

(1) *Lack of physical care*. This includes undernutrition and sometimes NOFT, recurrent infections, unkempt dirty appearance, housing dirty and disorganised.

(2) *Lack of medical care*, with failure to bring the child for immunisations, failure to seek appropriate medical help for illnesses and accidents. This can result in avoidable complications of medical conditions, including defective vision from untreated squints, impaired hearing from untreated otitis, and occasionally death, e.g. from hypothermia.

(3) *Lack of enforced house routines, rules and supervision*. This leads to an increased rate of accidents at all ages, including domestic and road traffic. Younger children frequently wet and soil for no organic reason. Older

children are left to wander away from home and are exposed to a variety of risks, e.g. playing on railway lines, associating with drug users, petty criminals, and sex abusers. There is a failure to learn to conform to social norms with resulting difficulties fitting in with other people and organisational arrangements, notably school rules; behavioural disturbance and conduct disorder are common.

(4) *Lack of emotional warmth and availability*. This often has profound effects on children's ability to enter into rewarding close relationships as they have not experienced a normal reciprocal intimate relationship. Their social and emotional skills and feeling for how to develop friendships are usually impaired, and self-worth as a person is very low, sometimes leading into frank depression, but more often being seen as despondency and lack of social interest and responsiveness. Other emotional disorders such as anxiety and fears are not uncommon. Attachment patterns in younger children as measured on separation and reunion with parents are often abnormal, with a high frequency of the disorganised category being seen (see Chapter 27). Other neglected children are indiscriminately friendly, craving affection and physical contact, putting them at high risk of abuse. School age children are unable to maintain significant friendships. Adults brought up in neglecting and abusive environments frequently exhibit inadequate close relationships. This is reflected in abnormal features in the way they describe their relationships with their parents and other intimates, as elicited by the Adult Attachment Interview (see Chapter 27).

(5) *Lack of cognitive stimulation and encouragement in constructive pastimes*. This leads to delayed language acquisition, short attention span with poor concentration, lower IQ, poor skill acquisition, poor attainments, lack of school and examination success, and a greatly diminished sense of competence and initiative.

Emotional abuse

Although emotional abuse is seldom the main cause for the recording of concern on official child protection registers, in many cases it *is* the predominant form of maltreatment going on in a family. Furthermore, it is almost invariably present in the other registered forms of maltreatment. However, because the immediate manifestations are less dramatic and a causal connection is harder to prove, less is done about it. This is not because it is less harmful – research over the last two decades has increasingly shown the profound and enduring effects on children reared under these circumstances. Elements include:

(1) *Extreme hostility and criticism*. Parents can come to see only the bad qualities in the child, and subject them to a withering fire of critical and demeaning comments which they are not equipped to deal with. Follow-

up studies confirm that children exposed to harsh emotional climates are themselves more likely to be cruel and bully others.

(2)   *Rejection and withdrawal of affection.* No warmth or cuddles are offered to the child, who is continually spurned when he makes overtures. This may lead to desperate emotional frustration and impaired close relationships, sometimes with deep distrust of intimacy and consequent withdrawal, or a desperate need for intimacy at any cost. Often a sibling is treated very differently which exacerbates the feeling of rejection.

(3)   *Deprivation of attention.* The child is ignored, especially when he is quiet or behaving constructively; when he seeks someone to play with or approval for an achievement, it is withheld. This leads to less socially acceptable behaviour, and to more antisocial behaviour and aggression.

(4)   *Inconsistency.* Behaviour which is accepted at one moment receives crushing criticism and heavy punishment the next; a parent who is warm and welcoming in the morning is cold and rejecting in the afternoon. This leads to confusion and inability to predict or trust.

(5)   *Threats of abandonment.* For what may be very minor acts of perceived misbehaviour, the child is threatened with expulsion from the home, and may have his suitcase packed, be driven to social services, and so on. The constant fear of abandonment precludes the development of a secure base for the development of relationships and often leads to anxious attachments.

(6)   *Inappropriate stresses and demands.* A child may see his depressed mother repeatedly being beaten by her partner, or taking an overdose. He may be told he is the reason his parents got divorced, and be used as a football in the ensuing acrimony, being asked to take sides, pass messages, act as peace maker, and give comfort and protection.

Sexual abuse

One definition specifies 'the involvement of dependent, developmentally immature children and adolescents in sexual activities that they do not fully comprehend, and to which they are unable to give informed consent, and that violate the social taboos of family roles'. There is a range of severity of acts with a corresponding range of prevalence. Thus 'non-contact' abuse such as exhibitionism is reported to have occurred at some time in childhood by around half of all women. 'Contact' abuse including fondling is reported to have occurred in childhood by 15–20% of women, whereas penetrative acts with vaginal, anal or oral involvement are reported by around 2%. All of these figures are imprecise because of difficulties in ascertainment. Community surveys suggest that females are more often abused than males, with a ratio of 2 or 3:1, but in clinically referred samples the female preponderance is greater at around 4 or

5:1. In clinical samples of sexually abused children there is a small excess of children from socioeconomically deprived backgrounds, but this gradient is far less marked than for physical abuse and neglect, and is virtually absent in community surveys.

Sexual abuse can come to attention in many ways. The most common is the child disclosing the abuse, usually to another child, a parent or another trusted adult; telephone helplines are increasingly used too. Changes in behaviour are common. Whilst precocious sexualised behaviour should clearly raise the suspicion of abuse, more non-specific changes occur frequently, such as sullenness and withdrawal, increased irritability and aggressiveness for no obvious reason, declining school performance and loss of friends. Older children may take overdoses, run away from home, or abuse other children. There may be presentations directly related to penetrative acts: anal or vaginal bleeding or infections, urinary tract infections, enuresis or faecal soiling, venereal disease or pregnancy.

Risk factors for maltreatment

With physical and emotional abuse, there is no single risk factor which predisposes a carer to abuse a child, but rather a range of influences which make abuse more likely. Broadly, they can be divided into the following:

(1) Poor parenting skills with deficient moment-to-moment interaction patterns – this is the final common pathway through which abuse is transmitted;
(2) Stressful circumstances;
(3) Child characteristics;
(4) Weak parental attachment to the child.

These well-established risk factors are summarised in Box 22.1.

With sexual abuse, perpetrators are most commonly men, although around 10% of sexual abuse is committed by women, who may be co-abusers with men, sometimes acting under duress. The proportion where the perpetrator is a family member varies according to the study from around one third to two-thirds. Within the home, fathers are the commonest perpetrators, accounting for around half of clinically seen cases. Stepfathers are disproportionately commonly involved, accounting for around a quarter of clinical cases. Girls living in a home with a stepfather are around six times more likely to be sexually abused than girls living with both biological parents. When sexual abuse does occur outside the home, the perpetrator is nonetheless still usually known to the child and has been trusted to be left alone with him or her, e.g. a neighbour, friend of the family, friend of the child, teacher, babysitter, club leader, etc. Abuse by strangers is relatively uncommon, accounting for around 5–10% of all abuse. Sex rings are being increasingly recognised. The term refers to a group of adults who are abusing several children. They often initially bribe the

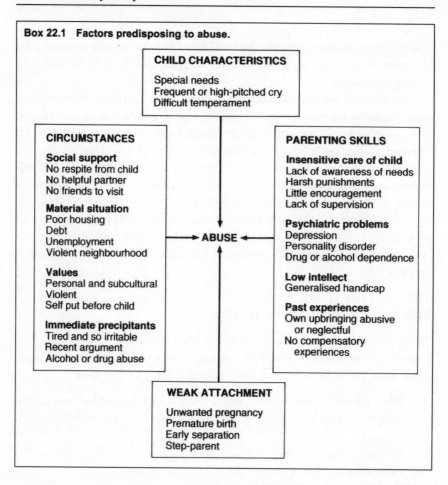

Box 22.1   Factors predisposing to abuse.

CHILD CHARACTERISTICS

Special needs
Frequent or high-pitched cry
Difficult temperament

CIRCUMSTANCES

Social support
No respite from child
No helpful partner
No friends to visit

Material situation
Poor housing
Debt
Unemployment
Violent neighbourhood

Values
Personal and subcultural
Violent
Self put before child

Immediate precipitants
Tired and so irritable
Recent argument
Alcohol or drug abuse

PARENTING SKILLS

Insensitive care of child
Lack of awareness of needs
Harsh punishments
Little encouragement
Lack of supervision

Psychiatric problems
Depression
Personality disorder
Drug or alcohol dependence

Low intellect
Generalised handicap

Past experiences
Own upbringing abusive
  or neglectful
No compensatory
  experiences

→ ABUSE ←

WEAK ATTACHMENT

Unwanted pregnancy
Premature birth
Early separation
Step-parent

children to become involved, but then go on to blackmail them and may use them to make pornographic videos or involve them in child prostitution. The prevalence is unknown, but one survey over two years of an English city of three-quarters of a million inhabitants uncovered 31 child sex rings involving 47 male perpetrators and 334 children ranging from 4–15 years old; 90% of victims were girls; two-thirds had been forced to perform oral intercourse, one third anal or vaginal intercourse.

Effects of maltreatment

To date, few specific outcomes have been linked with specific patterns of maltreatment. This is partly due to the wide overlap of types of maltreatment, so it is hard to study 'pure' abuse of one type. Even when 'pure' forms of abuse are studied, impairments are seen in a wide range of functions. It is plausible that many of these associated impairments are attributable to the maltreatment. This is a causal inference that is supported if the impairments improve or resolve once maltreatment ceases, e.g. because the child is taken into care.

Without this improvement, it is important to consider additional explanations. Thus pre-existing or constitutional impairments may have predisposed the child to being abused. For example, an irritable temperament might be a cause rather than a consequence of abuse. Alternatively, the same genetic or psychosocial factors that predispose the child to abuse may independently have predisposed the child to the additional impairments. For instance, the genetic and psychosocial factors that result in low parental IQ and thereby increase the risk of abuse also increase the likelihood of low IQ in the child whether or not abuse has taken place.

Physical effects   These effects on growth can be marked in severe cases, with NOFT and psychosocial short stature described above.

Emotional regulation   More negative emotions are displayed, and emotional arousal to stressful circumstances happens more quickly and takes longer to calm down. Children may be hyperaroused and hypervigilant. More fear and hostility is shown in response to adult arguments. Four general patterns may be seen:

(1)   Emotional blunting and lack of social responsiveness;
(2)   Depressed affect with sad facial expressions, withdrawal and aimless play;
(3)   Emotional lability with sudden shifts from engagement and pleasure to withdrawal and anger;
(4)   An angry emotional state with disorganised play and frequent outbursts in response to slight frustrations.

Formation of attachments   Maltreated toddlers and infants show a preponderance of abnormal attachment patterns in response to separation and reunion with their parents. Particularly common is the disorganised response, characterised by fear, disorientation, switches between approach and avoidance, odd expressions, freezing, and other bizarre behaviours (see Chapter 27). The abnormal attachment pattern tends to persist through childhood and into adulthood.

Development of self-concept   Maltreated children find it difficult to talk about themselves, and especially about their negative feelings – possibly because they have learned it leads to punishment at home. Measures of how they feel about themselves show low self-worth and low self-competence ratings.

Symbolic and social development   Play is reduced in quantity, and its quality is impoverished, with an increase in routine, stereotyped activity. Social play with other children is impaired. These deficits correlate well with the quality and sensitivity of mother–child interaction. Maltreated children show less sensitivity to the emotions of others, more negative expectations of people, less trust in them, and fewer ideas of how to initiate and maintain a social relationship. They are more prone to construe ambiguous stimuli as aggressive, and respond in kind. Observation of actual peer relationships shows lack of competence, inappropriate aggression in response to friendly overtures, and sometimes a mixed picture of aggression and withdrawal which leads to particularly strong rejection by the peer group. There is some evidence that this represents a disorganised 'fight or flight' response developed in the face of repeated overwhelmingly frightening experiences.

Cognitive development   Both language and non-verbal abilities are less well-developed than in non-abused controls, and school attainments are even more reduced. This may be due to a number of mechanisms, including impaired cognitive development in a home environment lacking in rewarding reciprocal exchanges and stimulation; poor ability to concentrate on schoolwork and organise it; and apathy and lack of motivation.

Emotional and behavioural disorders   These are common in abused children. By adolescence this can result in extreme cases, both of violence with psychopathic personality, and of suicide and deliberate self-harm. An increased incidence of post-traumatic stress disorder is additionally reported in victims of severe physical abuse. Although these findings emerge from studies that compare maltreated children with controls from similar socioeconomic groups and neighbourhoods, the families of the abused children often had disproportionately high levels of ongoing, chronic adversity and deprivation. It is therefore sometimes hard to disentangle the effect of the abuse from the chronic deprivation. Where there are multiple stressors of this kind, the rate of psychopathology may increase disproportionately.

Resilience   How common is it for abused children to be resilient, i.e. to develop normally despite their adverse experiences? Even taking the relatively conservative criterion of absence of significant problems, few abused children get classified as resilient. If competencies are measured across a range of domains, the proportion of resilient children drops still further, to zero in many studies, although many develop normally in at least some domains.

Intergenerational transmission   The proportion of abused children who become abusive parents varies by study, averaging around 30%. Whilst abusive upbringing clearly has a powerful influence, the worst outcomes are by no means inevitable. Even among girls brought up in children's homes because of grossly inadequate parenting, roughly half went on to provide adequate parenting for their own children.

Effects of sexual abuse   As with all types of abuse, it can often be difficult to know how much impairment has stemmed specifically from the sexual abuse, and how much from the generally disorganised and disordered family background. Although outcome studies on clinical samples are likely to miss individuals who were resilient to abusive experiences, they serve to highlight the damage done and typically show a variety of negative consequences that often last for many years.

Emotionally, victims often feel guilt and responsibility for the abuse, especially if they have come to enjoy the sexually arousing experiences. They may experience a sense of powerlessness in response to their inability to stop repeated invasions of their body. They may find it impossible to trust in others, especially older people of the perpetrator's gender. The trauma of the abuse may lead to sleeplessness, nightmares, loss of appetite, other somatic complaints and self-destructive behaviour. Frank symptoms of post-traumatic stress disorder may be present, with intrusive thoughts relating to the actual abuse process and avoidance of any associated people and places. Self-esteem is often very low with feelings of disgust, contamination, dirtiness and worthlessness predominating. Helplessness and hopelessness are frequent, often with an element of anger. The incidence of depression is considerably raised.

Behaviourally, chronic disobedience, aggression, bullying and antisocial acts are seen in both sexes following sexual abuse, but especially in boys. Girls are more prone to self-cutting, burning themselves with cigarettes, and anorectic responses. A proportion of children show inappropriate sexualised behaviour, including sexual contact or play with other adults or children and seductive behaviour towards relative strangers, e.g. staff in residential establishments or in-patient units. There may be persistent overt masturbation in public. As they grow up, a number are drawn to prostitution. Boys who experienced homosexual abuse commonly show confusion and anxiety about their sexual identity. The proportion who go on to be sexually abusive of others is uncertain, but it is clear that a significant minority do.

Factors affecting the impact of sexual abuse include:

- How much coercion and violence were used;
- The duration of the abuse;
- The nature and severity of the abuse, including whether penetration occurred;
- The relationship with the perpetrator, with abuse by a trusted figure such a father being particularly disturbing;
- Subsequent events such as being taken away from the family home to a disruptive residential setting.

Another factor exacerbating the effect of sexual abuse is disbelief by the parent, typically the mother. Around a third of seriously abused girls are not supported by their own mothers, who may deny the abuse ever took place (despite clear evidence to the contrary) and elect to stay with the perpetrators, so rejecting their daughters. Studies of the impact of sexual abuse according to the age at which it occurs do not show any clear period when it is less damaging.

Assessment

The overriding principle in suspected child abuse is to get help. A senior colleague should be informed as soon as possible, and the local social services department consulted. Physical abuse is often picked up initially by paediatricians, and managed in conjunction with social services. Child mental health professionals, however, may see injuries or detect other forms of abuse or neglect while seeing a child for a behavioural or emotional problem. If court proceedings are being contemplated, child mental health professionals may be asked whether significant harm has occurred to the child, what the prospects are for improvement in parenting style, and whether the child should be removed from the family.

A thorough general assessment is very useful because less obvious aspects can be overlooked by an exclusive focus on the circumstances of abuse. It is especially important to see all members of a household, whether or not they are blood relatives, including step-parents, lodgers etc. External reports are essential. GP and health visitor records provide information on regularity of attendance, previous injuries in the index child and other family members, and parental health and behaviour (having obtained parental permission). School reports are equally important. The assessment should cover all the factors depicted in Box 22.1, as well as an enquiry about the possible abusive practices, set within the context of overall parenting and family life. The child should be seen alone, and psychometric tests given if performance is failing significantly at school. Social services should be asked whether they know the family, and whether any of the children is on the Child Protection Register. If abuse seems likely, a child protection conference is likely to be held, to which a range of involved professionals will be invited. Nowadays, the parents are usually invited to attend some or all of the conference. Recommendations are made, which can include placing the child's name on the register and other protective steps.

Investigation of suspected sexual abuse can be carried out as a screening exercise if the level of concern is moderate, or as a full investigative process if suspicion is higher. There are extensive guidelines on how this should be done, and it is imperative to seek advice from a senior colleague with experience in this area. If the child is not overtly disturbed, social workers will often be the agreed party to conduct interviews, but if the child is showing evidence of marked disturbance, or there are special circumstances such as learning disability or very young children, then a child and adolescent mental health professional may need to be involved.

Screening interviews must be carried out with the child alone since if a family member committed the abuse the child is unlikely to reveal this in their presence for fear of the consequences. For example, there may have been explicit physical threats, emotional blackmail, or a fear by the child that if they tell, the family will break up and they will lose a parent. After a general discussion of how things are at home and outside, what the rules and discipline are and who the child likes and who not, it may be helpful to enquire about sleeping and bathing arrangements and how they look after their body. Questions may concern secrets, matters the child has not been able to tell anyone about, whom they would confide in if they had any worries, and whether anybody had done anything to them or touched them in a way they did not like. Asking such specific questions has been shown to increase the rate of disclosure of sexual abuse.

Full investigative interviews are a specialised skill, and are often carried out in conjunction with the police. They are usually videotaped as in the UK and a number of other countries they are admissible as evidence in court, instead of the child having to be a witness and be cross-examined. Anatomically correct dolls may be used, and often help prompt the child's memory. Some young children describe what happened to them and show this in vivid detail with the dolls in a way that is hard to disbelieve. Nevertheless, caution and judgement have to be applied to avoid over-interpreting the child's behaviour and being over-zealous in diagnosing abuse where there is doubt.

Physical examination of the anus and external genitalia is useful but should only be carried out by paediatricians, gynaecologists or police surgeons trained for the purpose. Whilst tearing and bruising are strongly suggestive of abuse, weaker signs may be of uncertain significance, especially as norms are only just being established. Tests for the presence of semen, venereal disease and pregnancy should be considered. Because recovery from the physical sequelae can occur quickly, a negative physical examination does not rule out the occurrence of sexual abuse. In one series where the presence of penetrative abuse was well established, fewer than 40% of the children had physical signs.

Intervention

The management of established abuse is guided by three aims. The first is to prevent further abuse. The second is to mitigate the effects of what has already happened. The third is to meet the child's emotional, social and educational needs in the longer term, which may include deciding whether it is best for the child to live in their own family, making special educational provision, and providing positive social experiences outside the home. A wide range of methods may be used, according to the particular circumstances of the case and resources of the agencies involved. For example, the interventions in one particular case might include:

- A court order forbidding access by the step-father;
- Training in parenting skills for the mother to help her manage her child's conduct problems
- Antidepressant therapy for the mother's low mood
- Individual counselling sessions for the child
- Extra educational provision for the child's learning problems;
- An anti-bullying programme at school;
- An application to rehouse the family in better conditions.

To achieve all this successfully requires good inter-agency liaison.

Management of sexual abuse is guided by the same three aims.

(1) There needs to be an assessment of the likelihood of re-abuse if the child is to remain in, or be returned to, the family where it happened.
(2) Prevention of further abuse may require the removal of the offender or an enforceable system of protection.
(3) The ability of the mother to accept what has happened and protect her child is important, as is the ability of the perpetrator to acknowledge his responsibility.

This is relevant for risk assessment, and to help the child begin to reverse guilt and self-blame; it may pave the way for the perpetrator's eventual reintegration into the family. However, court orders may need to be taken forbidding access if the child is believed to be at risk. Mitigation of the effects of abuse is likely to be helped by skilled therapy. Enabling the child to talk freely about sexual matters can allow them to go on to confront the awful experiences within a safe setting, and so begin to process them emotionally without dissociating and cutting off, or becoming paralysed with fear and anxiety. A variety of psychotherapeutic and cognitive-behavioural techniques may help in this task. Groups may help children achieve cognitive understanding, put their experience in perspective, and receive support from others who have had similar experiences. Meeting the child's longer term needs may include fostering a sense of self-worth and an ability to communicate about emotions and be assertive in threatening situations. An understanding of their own sexual responses and of the boundaries between appropriate and inappropriate sexual behaviour will need to be developed. Family work will need to address whether the mother has resolved the issue of split loyalties between the victim and the perpetrator. Severely affected children with profound mood disturbance, severe self-mutilation, anorexia or other symptoms may need an extensive programme of therapeutic work, often best undertaken in a therapeutic community or residential setting.

When maltreatment was first widely recognised, there was often strong pressure to remove the child from the family, frequently influenced by people's sense of outrage. Subsequent research showed that many of these children did badly, often because the substitute care was deficient. This was particularly the case in some children's homes, where there was a high turnover of poorly trained staff, and where the child was at risk of being abused by care workers or co-residents. Currently, the emphasis is on rehabilitating the child within the family wherever possible. Therefore it is important to be able to predict when this will be successful. In clinical studies where treatment is given and children stay within their families of origin, the overall established rate of re-abuse is 20–40%. Factors predicting outcome are set out in Table 22.1. Parental acknowledgement that abuse has occurred, and a willingness on their part to stay in a treatment programme are two of the most important predictors of successful rehabilitation.

Table 22.1 Prediction of intervention success.

Factor	Better outcome	Worse outcome
Parental	Acceptance of problems	Denial of problems
	Compliance with treatment	Refusal to cooperate
	Normal personality	Personality problems: • antisocial • sadistic • aggressive • abused in childhood
	Supportive partner	Abusive partner
	No psychiatric disorder	Alcohol abuse Substance abuse Psychosis
Characteristics of abuse	Less severe injuries	Severe injuries Burns and scalds Failure to thrive Mixed abuse Penetrative sexual abuse Longstanding sexual abuse Sadistic abuse Munchausen by proxy
Interaction with child	Normal attachment Able to show empathy Responsive caregiving	Disordered attachment Unable to show empathy Insensitive caregiving
	Puts child's needs first	Puts own needs first
Child	Healthy child Resilient response to abuse One nurturing relationship	Special needs – physical or learning problems Extensive psychopathology No positive influence
Circumstances	Good local child care	No facilities
	Informal networks	Social isolation
Professional intervention	Well trained and resourced	Few resources or skills
	Therapeutic relationship	Lack of engagement

Where the chances of improvement are slight, the court may order that alternative care be provided for the child, such as foster or adoptive parents, or in the case of older children, placement in a residential home. In England and Wales, the Children Act (1989) states that

the primary justification for the State to initiate proceedings seeking compulsory powers is actual or likely harm to the child, where harm includes both ill-treatment (which includes sexual abuse and non-physical ill-treatment such as emotional abuse) and the impairment of health or development, *health* meaning physical or mental health, and *development* meaning physical, intellectual,emotional, social, or behavioural development.

The Act puts great emphasis on working with parents voluntarily to maintain the child within the family wherever possible.

Primary prevention of child abuse through intensive home visiting programmes for high risk mothers contacted antenatally has been shown to work, but is not widely deployed.

Subject reviews

Cicchetti, D. and Lynch, M. (1995) Failures in the expectable environment and their impact on individual development: the case of child maltreatment. In *Developmental Psychopathology*, vol. 2. (D. Cicchetti and D. Cohen, eds) Wiley, London, pp. 32–72. (A thorough, well researched review of the impact of maltreatment across different domains of child functioning, and the mechanisms involved in causing it.)

Skuse, D. and Bentovim, A. (1994) Physical and emotional maltreatment. In *Child and Adolescent Psychiatry: Modern Approaches*, 3rd edn (M. Rutter, E. Taylor and L. Hersov, eds) Blackwell Science, Oxford, pp. 209–229.

Smith, M. and Bentovim, A. (1994) Sexual abuse. In *Child and Adolescent Psychiatry: Modern Approaches*, 3rd edn (M. Rutter, E. Taylor and L. Hersov, eds) Blackwell Science, Oxford, pp. 230–251.

Further reading

Cohn, A.H. and Daro, D. (1987) Is treatment too late: what 10 years of evaluative research tells us. *Child Abuse and Neglect*, 11, 433–442. (Sobering review of intervention studies involving over 3000 families in the USA: Over a third of families continued to mistreat their children while in treatment, and over half were believed to be likely to do so after it ended.)

Jones, D.P.H. (1992) Interviewing the Sexually Abused Child: Investigation of Suspected Abuse. Gaskell, London. (An excellent little manual of good practice.)

Kendall-Tackett, K. A. *et al.* (1993) Impact of sexual abuse on children: a review and synthesis of recent empirical studies. *Psychological Bulletin*, 113, 164–180.

Olds, D.L. *et al.* (1986) Preventing child abuse and neglect: a randomised trial of nurse home visitation. *Pediatrics*, 78, 65–78. (Those mothers who received fortnightly visits during pregnancy and for the first two years of their baby's life showed a decrease in abuse and neglect, especially if they were poor, unmarried and teenagers.)

Oliver, J.E. (1988) Successive generations of child maltreatment. *British Journal of Psychiatry*, 153, 543–553. (Shows a few multiproblem families were responsible for a large quantity of severe abuse in Wiltshire, UK, including several cases of violence-induced mental handicap.)

Part III
Risk Factors

23   Mental Retardation

Though somewhat old-fashioned, the term *mental retardation* (MR) is at least understood by professionals and parents throughout the world. The same cannot be said for the alternative terms in current use. Thus *learning disability* means mental retardation in the UK but usually refers to a specific learning difficulty such as a reading disorder in the USA. Conversely, *developmental disability* means mental retardation in the USA but potentially encompasses all manner of developmental problems in the UK. Sadly, widespread prejudice leads to any new term for MR becoming pejorative and stigmatising within a short time. This is likely to persist until society comes to value people with MR.

Definition

For some purposes MR is defined solely in terms of an intellectual disability; for other purposes, social impairment is also essential. Associated educational difficulties are not central to the definition.

- *Intellectual disability*. At its simplest, MR is defined by IQ level alone: an IQ of 50–69 is mild MR; an IQ under 50 is severe MR.
- *Social impairment*. Legal and administrative definitions of MR generally stipulate that in addition to intellectual disability, the individual's level of social functioning is such that they are in need of special care or protection. In English law, this insistence on social as well as intellectual impairment is found in the 1983 Mental Health Act's definitions of mental impairment and severe mental impairment.

Prevalence

(1) *Mild MR*, as defined by IQ criteria, affects about 2% of the general population, as would be expected if IQ is normally distributed. (An IQ of 70 is two standard deviations below the mean and 2.3% of any normally-distributed population falls more than two standard deviations below the mean.) Many of these individuals are never identified by medical, educational or social services – sometimes this is because their social functioning is adequate and they are coping well enough in mainstream

schools, but in other instances they are drowning quietly without the extra input that might have helped them had their MR been recognised.

(2) *Severe MR*, as defined by an IQ under 50, affects about 0.4% of the population, which is some ten times higher than would have been expected if IQ were normally distributed, i.e. there is a small extra 'hump' at the bottom of the normal IQ distribution. Individuals with severe MR are nearly always known to health, education or social services, either because of the severity of their educational difficulties or because of coexisting physical features such as cerebral palsy or epilepsy.

The two population model

It is useful for some purposes to distinguish between two sorts of MR: *organic* and *normal variant* (sometimes described as *subcultural*). The distinction can be clarified by an analogy. The genetic and environmental factors that account for the normal variation in adult height will inevitably result in some adults being in the lower tail of the height distribution. In addition to these individuals with normal-variant short stature, there are other individuals with short stature due to organic conditions, e.g. genetic syndromes such as achondroplasia. The organic group will tend to be shorter and to have more medical problems. The normal-variant group will have many relatives of below-average height (due to shared environment and polygenes), whereas most of the relatives of the organic group will be of around average height because they do not have the same organic syndrome. Using a height cut-off, it would be possible to define very short stature (which is mostly organic), as opposed to moderately short stature (which is mostly a normal variant), but no height cut-off would distinguish perfectly between organic and normal-variant groups.

For MR, the equivalent of a height cut-off is an IQ cut-off – at around an IQ of 50. As shown in Table 23.1, this approach does identify two relatively distinct populations. By comparison with mild MR, severe MR is more often associated with neurological disorder and less often associated with social disadvantage. Only mild MR is associated with a below-average IQ in relatives. Not surprisingly, an IQ cut-off of 50 cannot distinguish perfectly between organic and

Table 23.1 Characteristics of severe and mild mental retardation (Data from Broman *et al.* 1987).

	Severe MR	Mild MR
Major CNS disorder (%)	72	14
Prevalence (%):		
High socioeconomic status	0.4	0.3
Low socioeconomic status	0.8	3.3
Male (%)	63	46
Mean IQ of siblings	103	85

normal-variant cases. Though useful as a conceptual model, the two population model of MR should not be taken too literally: organic and normal-variant causes of MR may coexist, with additive or synergistic effects.

Causes of mental retardation

(1) *Mild MR*. Most mild MR is assumed to be due to the same sorts of polygenic and environmental factors that determine IQ within the normal range. Just as the polygenic component is assumed to be due to many genes, each of which has a small but additive effect on IQ, so the psychosocial component seems to involve many factors such as parental attitudes, positive interactions with the child, or stressful life events, each of which has a small additive effect on IQ. Adverse factors in the physical environment, such as exposure to low-level lead may also add to the effects of genetic and psychosocial factors.

(2) *Severe MR*. The organic causes that account for the majority of severe MR (and a minority of mild MR) are conventionally subdivided according to their time of onset:
   (a) *Prenatal:* e.g. chromosome abnormalities, single gene defects, congenital infections, fetal alcohol syndrome.
   (b) *Perinatal:* e.g. intraventricular haemorrhage in premature neonates, severe neonatal jaundice. Though much used to be made of obstetric complications, it now seems unlikely that these are common causes of MR. If a child has a difficult delivery and subsequently turns out to have severe MR, was the delivery to blame? Not usually. More often, the obstetric complications were either irrelevant or a consequence of pre-existing abnormalities in the unborn child. Thus children with chromosomal problems or prenatal brain damage are at greater risk of an abnormal delivery.
   (c) *Post-natal:* e.g. encephalitis and meningitis, trauma due to child abuse and accidents, severe lead poisoning.

Several syndromes, including the fragile X syndrome and the fetal alcohol syndrome, have already been discussed in Chapter 1. Other relevant syndromes include:

● *Down's syndrome:* affects up to 1 in 600 births, with older mothers at much greater risk. This is the commonest single cause of severe MR, accounting for up to a third of all cases. 95% are due to an extra chromosome 21 resulting from non-disjunction, which is more common in older mothers; 4% are from translocations, which are familial; and 1% are mosaics. Physical features include: small head; round face; upslanting eyes; epicanthic folds; large fissured tongue; low-set simple ears; short stature; single palmar crease; incurved little fingers; and hypotonia. Cardiac and gut malformations are common.

- *Single gene disorders:* There are many rare genetic disorders that sometimes or always cause MR. As a rule of thumb, assume that these disorders are autosomal recessive unless you know otherwise. There are a few exceptions: the Lesch-Nyhan and Hunter (but not Hurler) syndromes are sex linked; and tuberous sclerosis and neurofibromatosis are autosomal dominant.

- *Sex chromosomal anomalies:* individuals with the common anomalies – XO (Turner's syndrome), XXY (Kleinfelter's syndrome), XXX and XYY – are usually of normal or low-normal intelligence, though there is some excess of mild and severe MR.

Diagnostic assessment of MR

Children with severe MR are usually referred to a paediatrician because of associated physical abnormalities, or because of slow development, either noted by parents or picked up on developmental screening. Mild MR may not be noticed until learning difficulties become apparent in school. Parents and teachers are usually fairly accurate judges of a child's ability level. If asked, they are often able to give a good estimate of the child's mental age. Nevertheless, even experienced parents and teachers sometimes grossly misjudge a child's intelligence. Thus a child with autism and normal intelligence (as judged by non-verbal tests) may be thought to be severely mentally retarded on the basis of his poor performance in verbal tests and his lack of 'common sense'. This kind of misjudgement may lead to an inappropriate placement in a school for severe learning difficulties. Even more commonly, children with mild MR are believed by their teachers to be of near average ability, with poor academic performance being attributed to lack of effort, emotional problems, or social disadvantage. Once again, the misjudgement leads to inappropriate academic provision and pressure. Given this, it is sensible to supplement parent and teacher reports with formal psychometric testing. Besides measuring IQ reliably, a detailed psychometric assessment generates a useful profile of the child's cognitive strengths and weaknesses. For children of school age, the Wechsler Intelligence Scale for Children, 3rd edn (WISC–III) or the British Ability Scale, 2nd edn (BAS-II) provide a suitably wide-ranging battery of verbal and visuospatial tests.

Diagnosis of the underlying cause of MR is based on:

(1) A thorough *history*, with particular attention to family history, prenatal infections and prenatal alcohol exposure.
(2) A careful *physical examination*, particularly for neurological signs, dysmorphic features and the skin signs of the neurocutaneous syndromes (see Chapter 1).

(3)   Selected *special investigations*, particularly for the fragile X syndrome, chromosomal abnormalities and metabolic diseases.

Although very few treatable causes will be found, the search for a cause is valuable for genetic counselling and because many parents are relieved by a diagnostic label (partly because this opens the way to joining the relevant parent self-help group). In the UK, diagnosis and counselling usually involve paed-iatricians rather than psychiatrists.

Prevention of MR

Many approaches can reduce the prevalence of the organic syndromes that sometimes or always result in MR. Thus, widespread rubella vaccination can prevent congenital rubella. Folic acid supplementation given around conception and in early pregnancy can prevent neural tube defects, and advice on alcohol consumption in pregnancy can prevent the fetal alcohol syndrome. Prenatal diagnosis of organic syndromes is increasingly possible on the basis of blood tests, ultrasound scans, chorionic villous sampling and amniocentesis. Specific treatments are rarely available, but parents may opt for termination of pregnancy. Continuing advances in obstetric and neonatal care may further reduce the rate of early brain damage, e.g. by reducing the rate and complications of premature birth. Neonatal screening for phenylketonuria, galactosaemia and hypothyr-oidism permits early treatment before irreversible brain damage has occurred. Immunisation can protect children against diseases that cause meningitis (e.g. *Haemophilus influenzae* type b) and encephalitis (e.g. pertussis). Measures to reduce the rate of domestic accidents, road traffic accidents, and physical abuse can reduce brain damage secondary to head injury.

Less progress has been made in reducing the rate of normal-variant MR. Some interventions have targeted the infants of mothers with MR in socially deprived neighbourhoods. These can result in significant increases in scholastic achievement and measured IQ, at least in the short-term. Continuing input in the school years may help maintain these gains in the long term. Just as there is no one critical period after which environmental damage is irreversible, so there is no one therapeutic window after which environmental enrichment is no longer necessary. It is important, though, not to overestimate the likely effect of environmental interventions. One adoption study that compared the effect of being raised by parents from the highest and lowest socioeconomic groups found that it resulted in an IQ difference of around 12 points. A lasting effect of this size is well beyond anything that intervention projects have yet achieved.

Provision of services for children with MR

Service provision is generally governed by a philosophy of 'normalisation', i.e. the promotion of as ordinary a life as possible in the community.

Social provision

Children develop best if they grow up as part of a family. Nowadays, most children with MR live with their biological family. This can be a very positive experience for parents and siblings, but there is often a substantial burden of care too, particularly with severe MR. However, this burden can be eased by extra assistance and support, e.g. mobility allowances, respite care (usually arranged by social services). If the family's capacity to cope is overwhelmed even with maximum respite care, placement in an alternative family setting is highly desirable, either by adoption or long-term fostering. Rarely, a child will require a specialist residential placement.

Educational provision

No matter how severe their learning difficulties, all children are entitled by law to an appropriate education. No child can be denied all schooling on the grounds that they are 'ineducable'. It is increasingly possible for children with mild MR to receive the extra help they need within mainstream schools. Children with severe MR generally attend special schools. Reports from doctors and other health professionals can help education authorities identify special needs and provide for them accordingly.

Medical provision

Appropriate medical care generally involves the family practitioner and the paediatric team based at a child development centre. Involvement of child mental health services is not routinely necessary, but may be helpful for the high proportion of mentally retarded children who have coexistent psychiatric problems.

PSYCHIATRIC DISORDERS IN CHILDREN WITH MENTAL RETARDATION

In the multiaxial schemes of ICD–10 and DSM–IV, MR and psychiatric disorders are coded on separate axes (see Chapter 2). Nevertheless, although MR is not itself a psychiatric disorder, it is a powerful risk factor for psychiatric disorders. Roughly a third of all children with mild MR have psychiatric diagnoses, as do roughly half of all children with severe MR. This compares with some 10–15% of non-retarded children judged by the same criteria. The combination of MR and psychiatric disorder is particularly stressful for families, many of whom find it harder to live with the psychiatric problems than with the problems intrinsic to MR. Psychiatric problems are the commonest reason for family placements breaking down.

Type of psychiatric disorder

Among children with mild MR, the mixture of psychiatric disorders is generally similar to that seen in children without mental retardation, being dominated by emotional, conduct and hyperactivity disorders. In severe MR, the mixture of psychiatric disorder is more distinctive. Thus although emotional, conduct and hyperactivity disorders are still common, so too are autistic disorders, with partial variants of autism being commoner than the full syndrome (see Chapter 4). Thus a substantial minority of children with severe MR are socially aloof or relate to others in a bizarre way. For example, imaginative play is characteristically impoverished; stereotypies can be prominent, and may be exaggerated by boredom, isolation, blindness or deafness. Severe hyperactivity sometimes occurs in association with autistic features or simple stereotypies, and sometimes occurs alone.

Self-injury, such as eye-poking, head banging or hand biting is another behavioural syndrome that is particularly common in severe MR. These behaviours have a functional component that can be shown to vary from individual to individual. Thus in different individuals, self-injury may serve to reduce boredom, to attract attention, or to be rid of unwanted attention. Difficulties with the acquisition of self-help skills (including feeding, toileting and dressing) are also common in severe MR, as are sleep problems.

Specific links

Some organic causes of MR are particularly associated with specific psychiatric problems. The Lesch-Nyhan syndrome, for example, is much more likely to lead to severe self-injury than other organic disorders resulting in equally low IQs. When the organic syndrome is genetic or chromosomal, the common behavioural characteristics are referred to as the *behavioural phenotype* of the disorder. Other examples include the social anxiety, gaze avoidance and litany-like speech associated with the fragile X syndrome; and the insatiable overeating associated with the Prader-Willi syndrome. Non-genetic syndromes can also have associated behavioural features, and these too are sometimes referred to as behavioural phenotypes. Thus congenital rubella is associated with autistic features, while the fetal alcohol syndrome is associated with hyperactivity.

Box 23.1 portrays four possible causal pathways that could account for the observed association between MR and psychiatric disorder. For some psychiatric disorders, the evidence supports possibility B, namely that the same biological factors that cause MR also, and independently, cause the psychiatric problems. Take autism, for example. A child with an IQ of 40 and tuberous sclerosis is at high risk of autism, whereas a child with an IQ of 40 and cerebral palsy is at much lower risk. Thus, IQ cannot account for this difference, which is almost certainly related to the different biological substrates of the two sets of disorders.

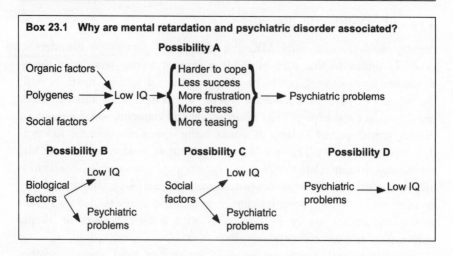

Box 23.1   Why are mental retardation and psychiatric disorder associated?

For some other psychiatric disorders, however, the evidence favours possibility A, namely that low intelligence, whatever its cause, predisposes a child to psychiatric problems. It is certainly plausible that low intelligence and poor academic attainments often undermine a child's self-esteem and result in teasing by classmates. In addition, less intelligent children may find it harder to overcome everyday stresses, and may be more prone to 'act out' when under stress. For all these reasons, lower intelligence could well result in more anxiety, misery and anger. In the case of conduct disorder, possibility A is supported by a fairly linear relationship with IQ. Within the normal IQ range, lower IQ is associated with more conduct disorder even when socioeconomic background has been allowed for. The yet higher rate of conduct disorder among children with MR appears to be a continuation of this trend. It looks as though any cause of lower IQ, whether organic, polygenic or social, increases the risk of conduct disorder.

There is little evidence supporting either of the other two possible explanations for the link between MR and psychiatric problems. The adverse social factors that contribute to low IQ are different from the adverse social factors that increase psychiatric risk (arguing against possibility C). Finally, although psychiatric problems may interfere with school performance, they do not usually reduce measured IQ (arguing against possibility D).

Treatment

Treating the psychiatric disorders of children with MR differs in emphasis but not in principle from treating similar disorders in other children. Behavioural treatment is particularly valuable in building up self-help skills and in reducing undesirable behaviours such as self-injury, stereotypies and frequent night wakenings. To be effective, behavioural therapy must be carefully tailored to the individual child. For self-injurious behaviour, for example, advice to ignore the child during episodes of self-injury may be appropriate for a child who uses the behaviour primarily to attract extra attention. However, it would only succeed in reinforcing the self-injurious behaviour if applied to a child who primarily uses the behaviour to be rid of unwanted attention. In addition to behavioural therapy, a wide range of other therapies can be deployed, including family therapy, cognitive therapy and supportive psychotherapy (depending on the nature of the problem and the age and cognitive level of the child).

The role of medication in the treatment of psychiatric problems associated with MR remains controversial. In the short-term, neuroleptics do reduce serious aggression and may therefore be useful in an emergency. The benefits soon wear off, however. It is then tempting to increase the dose to gain another temporary respite. Unless this temptation is resisted, the dose is likely to escalate progressively, leaving the child on high-dose long-term neuroleptic medication with all its attendant hazards (see Chapter 31). The pointlessness of this long-term medication is often only evident when the medication is finally withdrawn: aggression typically worsens for a while and then returns to its previous level. Challenging behaviour requires social and psychological management, not pharmacological treatment. With this reservation, medication can be useful at times. Moderate doses of neuroleptics can sometimes reduce stereotypies, hyperactivity, self-injury, and agitation, perhaps particularly in adolescents with MR and autistic features. Stimulants may sometimes improve the hyperactivity of children with IQs of around 40 or more, but rarely work for children with lower IQs. At any IQ, stimulants may exacerbate coexistent ritualistic and repetitive behaviours.

Subject review

Scott, S. (1994) Mental retardation. In *Child and Adolescent Psychiatry: Modern Approaches*, 3rd edn (M. Rutter, E. Taylor and L. Hersov, eds) Blackwell Science, Oxford, pp. 616–646.

Further reading

Broman, S. *et al.* (1987) *Retardation in Young Children: A Developmental Study of Cognitive Deficit.* Lawrence Erlbaum, Hillsdale. (This study uses the epidemiological data from the National Collaborative Perinatal Project (NCPP) to examine antecedents and consequences of mental retardation.)

Flint, J. (1996) Behavioural phenotypes: a window onto the biology of behaviour. *Journal of Child Psychology and Psychiatry*, 37, 355–367.

24   Brain Disorders

The preceding chapter considered the psychiatric complications associated with mental retardation, with and without known brain disorders. This chapter is primarily concerned with the psychiatric effects of brain disorders on individuals who are not also mentally retarded.

A rare risk factor

Unequivocal brain disorders are relatively rare in childhood, e.g. about 0.5% of children have epilepsy and 0.2% have cerebral palsy. Current evidence suggests that these brain disorders are usually due not to perinatal complications, as used to be thought, but to genetic factors, prenatal insults and post-natal insults.

There is only very limited support for the notion of a 'continuum of reproductive casualty'. This theory suggests that while severe obstetric and neonatal complications can result in death, cerebral palsy or mental retardation, mild obstetric complications more often result in hyperactivity, specific learning problems or clumsiness, sometimes referred to as 'minimal brain damage'. Since children from socially disadvantaged backgrounds are more likely to have experienced obstetric and neonatal complications, it is essential to adjust for social background when investigating the possible impact of these complications. Having done so, most studies suggest that obstetric and neonatal complications rarely, if ever, cause psychiatric problems in children who do not have overt brain disorders. One possible exception to this rule is an increase in hyperactivity in neurologically intact children who were of low birth weight (usually as a result of prematurity).

A powerful risk factor

When present, overt brain disorders are powerful risk factors for child psychiatric problems, having an impact well beyond that of other physical disorders. This is well illustrated by epidemiological data from the Isle of Wight neuropsychiatric study (Table 24.1). The particularly high rate of psychiatric problems associated with cerebral damage cannot be explained simply by the degree of disability or stigmatisation; there is convincing evidence of direct brain–behaviour links as well. It is striking, for example, that over half of a large

Table 24.1   The Isle of Wight Neuropsychiatric Study (Rutter *et al.*, 1970).

Children with:	Proportion with psychiatric disorder (%)
No physical disorder	7
Physical disorder not affecting the brain	12
Idiopathic epilepsy	29
Cerebral palsy and allied disorders, IQ > 50.	44

epidemiological sample of children with hemiplegic cerebral palsy had psychiatric disorders, despite the fact that the physical disability was typically mild and that most children were of normal intelligence and attending mainstream schools.

At risk for which psychiatric disorders?

As a first approximation, the psychiatric problems of children with brain disorders are similar to the psychiatric problems of other children; conduct, emotional, and mixed disorders are common in both groups. There is no single 'brain damage syndrome'. Moving beyond this first approximation, there are some differences in emphasis. Though all psychiatric disorders are more common in children with neurological problems, autistic and hyperactivity disorders seem to be particularly over-represented. For example, in the Isle of Wight study, hyperkinesis accounted for 19% of psychiatric disorders among children with cerebral palsy, but only 1% of psychiatric disorders among neurologically intact children.

Parents and teachers frequently comment on the oppositionality and irritability of children with brain disorders. Although these are often marked enough to warrant a diagnosis of oppositional-defiant disorder, it is relatively unusual for these children to develop the more seriously antisocial behaviours that are characteristic of severe conduct disorder. Anxiety as well as irritability can contribute to outbursts of rage or distress. Children with neurological problems can easily become overwrought when faced with demands they have difficulty meeting. Episodic outbursts are far more likely to be behavioural than epileptic, although the latter possibility may need to be considered, particularly if the episodes are completely unprovoked or accompanied by other pointers to epilepsy, such as altered consciousness or a subsequent need to sleep.

Specific neurological disorders may be associated with especially high risks for particular psychiatric problems, e.g. Sydenham's chorea has been linked to an unexpectedly high rate of obsessive–compulsive disorder. Some of the behavioural consequences of childhood brain disorders only become apparent in adulthood, e.g. the high rate of adult-onset schizophrenia in individuals with developmental abnormalities of the temporal lobes. The current evidence suggests that there are few differences in the psychiatric consequences of left-

and right-sided brain lesions. Studies of childhood head injuries have not revealed consistent effects of locus or timing of injury on rate or type of psychiatric problem.

Interaction with other risk factors

Having a brain disorder does not generally render children immune to the adverse effects of 'ordinary' psychiatric risk factors, such as exposure to marital friction. There is continuing controversy as to whether children with brain disorders are *more* vulnerable to ordinary risk factors or simply *as* vulnerable.

Mediating links

There are many possible mediating links between brain and behavioural disorders, though the relative importance of different links remains to be established. In some cases, the link may be relatively direct, e.g. autistic impairments may simply reflect damage to the brain systems involved in communication and social interaction. In other cases, psychosocial factors, such as poor self-image, unrealistic family expectations, or peer rejection play an important part too. Specific learning problems and below-average IQ are common consequences of brain abnormalities. When present, these problems add to the stresses on the child, particularly if their special educational needs are unrecognised or unmet (as is all too often the case). Treatments for the physical disorder may also contribute to the psychiatric problems. Anticonvulsants can have adverse psychiatric consequences; regular physiotherapy can lead to considerable resentment because of lost play time; and repeated hospitalisations can disrupt family interactions.

Prognosis

Is the prognosis for any given psychiatric disorder worse if the child also has a brain disorder? Clinicians and parents often suppose so, and this pessimism may be self-fulfilling if it leads to inappropriately low expectations or half-hearted therapy. The evidence is so limited at present that it is often preferable to work on the more optimistic assumption that the prognosis of the psychiatric disorder is independent of the presence or absence of coexistent neurological problems. Indeed, the families of children with brain disorders are often particularly receptive to professional advice, and may consequently be easier to help than the average family seen by child mental health services.

Treatment

The psychiatric problems of children with brain disorders can be treated in just the same ways as the psychiatric problems of neurologically intact children.

Biological treatments are neither more nor less useful than in ordinary psychiatric practice. However, remember that anticonvulsants may have behavioural effects, so a change in dose or type can sometimes be helpful. Individual, family, and school-based treatments can all be useful. Parents are often helped by hearing that their child's problems are common consequences of neurological damage. The energy previously locked up in self-blame can then be diverted into more profitable channels. Access to a parents' support group for children with the same disorder can reduce the family's sense of isolation and powerlessness. Neuropsychological assessments of the child's cognitive strengths and weaknesses can provide a helpful basis for advice to the school and education authority. The child's emotional and behavioural problems often improve dramatically when unrecognised learning problems are finally addressed, whether by provision of extra help in a mainstream school or by transfer to a special school.

Some specific points about particular brain-behaviour links

(1) A variety of rare dementing disorders present in childhood with loss of established skills and a variety of additional emotional and behavioural abnormalities. The same symptoms can be due to purely psychosocial problems (such as sexual abuse), but you need to consider a dementing disorder in any child who presents with loss of skills. A full physical examination is mandatory, and special investigations may be indicated. The presence of psychosocial stressors does not rule out an organic disorder (e.g. a child who has been sexually abused, or who has a drug-abusing mother, may also have HIV encephalopathy).

(2) Frontal lobe seizures are easily misdiagnosed as pseudoseizures: movements, postures, and vocalisations may be bizarre; episodes may be brief; the termination may be abrupt with prompt return to responsiveness; and ordinary EEGs may be unhelpful. Combined video and EEG monitoring can be extremely useful.

(3) It is not yet clear if mild head injuries (which are very common in childhood) have adverse psychiatric consequences. It is clear, however, that serious cognitive and psychiatric sequelae are common after severe head injuries (e.g. closed head injuries resulting in at least two weeks of post-traumatic amnesia). Though the psychiatric disorders of head-injured children mostly involve the sorts of emotional and conduct problems that dominate ordinary child psychiatric practice, severe closed head injury sometimes results in a distinctive syndrome of social disinhibition (resembling the adult 'frontal lobe syndrome').

Subject review

Goodman, R. (1994) Brain disorders. In *Child and Adolescent Psychiatry: Modern Approaches*, 3rd edn (M. Rutter, E. Taylor and L. Hersov, eds) Blackwell Science, Oxford, pp. 172–190.

Further reading

Goodman, R. and Graham, P. (1996) Psychiatric problems in children with hemiplegia: cross sectional epidemiological survey. *British Medical Journal*, **312**, 1065–1069.

Rutter, M. *et al.* (1970) *A Neuropsychiatric Study in Childhood: Clinics in Developmental Medicine, No 35/36*. SIMP/Heinemann, London.

Rutter, M. *et al.* (1983) Head injury. In *Developmental Neuropsychiatry* (M. Rutter, ed) Guildford Press, New York, pp. 83–111.

25   Language Disorders

Many specific language impairments are associated with increased rates of child psychiatric problems. This is not surprising for three reasons. Firstly, language impairments and psychiatric problems may sometimes share a common origin in brain abnormalities that interfere with 'higher functions'. Secondly, language dominates our lives: it is a powerful tool for thought and problem-solving; it is our primary means for obtaining what we want from others; and it plays a key role in social cohesion, with human conversation functioning rather like mutual grooming among chimpanzees. Consequently, language impairments are likely to be frustrating and isolating. Finally, the same disorder of social communication may be construed as a language problem by a language therapist and as a psychiatric problem by a mental health professional; the timber merchant, the botanist and the artist do not see the same tree.

Epidemiology

Estimates of the prevalence of specific language impairment diverge widely, largely reflecting differences in the definition employed. At one extreme, severe and persistent disorders that result in substantial social impairment and occur in children of normal intelligence are quite rare, with a prevalence that is probably under 0.1%. At the opposite extreme, the prevalence of broadly defined language disorders may be as high as 15–25%, though many of these children have relatively minor delays or articulation problems that result in little or no social impairment and resolve without treatment. Between the two extremes, significant language problems may be present in roughly 1–5% of schoolchildren. No matter what definition is used, there is a marked male excess for all developmental language disorders, with two or three affected boys for every affected girl.

Varieties of developmental language disorders

Several different aspects of language can be affected by developmental language disorders (see Box 25.1). The two main groupings within the developmental language disorders are:

Box 25.1 Different aspects of language.

- **Phonology/articulation** refers to the production of speech sounds.
- **Prosody** refers to the expression and comprehension of those aspects of communication mediated by tone of voice and inflexion.
- **Syntax** refers to the production and comprehension of grammatically correct sentences.
- **Semantics** refers to the ability to encode meaning into words and decode meaning from words.
- **Pragmatics** refers to the ability to use and decipher language in a way that is appropriate to the wider social-interpersonal context, e.g. drawing on knowledge of the context to grasp a message that is implicit but not explicit in the words themselves.

---

(1) *Phonologic-syntactic disorders* involve problems in the form but not the content of language. The child wants to communicate and says appropriate things, but there are problems with articulation or syntax or both. Some children have *pure articulation problems* without any other language problems. Delay or deviance in speech–sound production makes these children harder to understand, and may lead to teasing. In cases of *expressive language disorder*, speech develops late and syntactic structures are several years behind age level. Articulation is often faulty too, but comprehension is within normal limits. *Receptive language disorder* is rarer, and nearly always involves a mixture of problems with language comprehension, language expression, and articulation.

(2) *Semantic-pragmatic disorder* refers to a recently delineated and rather poorly defined set of problems concerning the use and content rather than the form of language. In a typical case, articulation and syntax are normal and the child scores well on formal tests of language, but there are problems with everyday conversation and comprehension that parents and teachers find hard to describe. Understanding is highly literal, and the child fails to use knowledge of the context to make sense of what is said. The child's own attempts to explain things or to tell a story do not make allowances for the listener's point of view, they miss out key details, or fail to organise the account into a coherent sequence. The child's speech may be dominated by rambling monologues or repetitive questioning. Prosodic impairments are common, e.g. a monotonous tone of voice or an abnormal inflexion. The degree of overlap between semantic-pragmatic disorder and the autistic disorders is uncertain. There is no doubt that some children with semantic-pragmatic disorder meet all the criteria for autism or Asperger's syndrome (in terms of associated social impairments, rigidity etc.), but there are other children with semantic-pragmatic disorder who seem relatively normal in other respects.

Prognosis for language development

The prognosis for language development depends both on the type of language disorder and also on the presence of associated cognitive impairments. When a language disorder is associated with low IQ, the prognosis is generally worse. Within the phonologic-syntactic disorders, the chances of a complete recovery are highest for children with pure articulation problems and lowest for children with a receptive language disorder. A child with a receptive language disorder and a normal IQ is likely to make enough progress by adult life to communicate fairly well, but some noticeable language deficits usually persist. There is little information on the prognosis of semantic-pragmatic disorder, but studies of autism and Asperger's syndrome suggest that deficits in language use and content can be very persistent.

Associated scholastic difficulties

Severe and persistent language disorders are associated with a substantial risk of scholastic difficulties, even if the child is of normal intelligence (as judged by non-verbal IQ). This risk is mainly for reading and spelling problems, though maths problems may also occur. Children whose language catches up completely do not seem to be at increased risk. Expressive and receptive language disorders carry a higher risk than articulation problems. Indeed, pure articulation problems may not result in any increased risk of scholastic problems.

Associated psychiatric and personality problems

Many studies have shown that children with language problems are at increased psychiatric risk. In some instances, the psychiatric risk may stem directly from the language disorder itself, e.g. as a result of the teasing, frustration, and social isolation engendered by communication difficulties. In other instances, however, the language and psychiatric problems may both stem from a single underlying cognitive or neurobiological disorder.

Children with language disorder are primarily at risk for anxiety disorders, problems with social relationships, and attentional deficits. These problems are often more obvious in older children than in younger children. There is little or no excess of conduct problems. The rate of psychopathology is particularly high in children of low IQ, but the rate is also substantially increased in children of normal IQ. Psychiatric risk is primarily associated with expressive and receptive language problems, although children with pure articulation problems may be more liable to emotional problems.

Children with receptive language problems often show some degree of autistic-like social impairments. These seem to become more evident as the child grows older. One follow-up study of children with receptive language problems and normal IQ found that over half had major problems with social relationships in adult life. In many instances, the failure to make friends or love relationships seemed to reflect a primary lack of social interest and skill rather than a secondary consequence of the social restrictions imposed by communication difficulties.

Though these findings suggest some sort of continuum between classical autism and receptive language disorder (in addition to the likely continuum between autism and semantic-pragmatic disorder), another follow-up finding points to differences rather than continuities between autism and receptive language disorder. Autism does not appear to be a risk factor for subsequent psychosis, whereas receptive language disorder (with or without some autistic features) does seem to carry an increased risk of florid paranoid psychosis in adolescence.

Subject reviews

Bishop, D.V.M. (1994) Developmental disorders of speech and language. In *Child and Adolescent Psychiatry: Modern Approaches*, 3rd edn (M. Rutter, E. Taylor and L. Hersov, eds) Blackwell Science, Oxford, pp. 546–568.

Rapin, I. (1996) Developmental language disorders: a clinical update. *Journal of Child Psychology and Psychiatry*, 37, 643–655.

Further reading

Bishop, D.V.M. and Adams, C. (1989) Conversational characteristics of children with semantic-pragmatic disorder. II: What features lead to a judgement of inappropriacy? *British Journal of Disorders of Communications*, 24, 241–263. (This paper is full of examples of the sorts of language abnormalities found in semantic-pragmatic disorder.)

Rutter, M. and Mawhood, L. (1991) The long-term psychosocial sequelae of specific developmental disorders of speech and language. In *Biological Risk Factors for Psychosocial Disorders* (M. Rutter and P. Casaer, eds) Cambridge University Press, Cambridge, pp. 233–259.

26　Reading Disorders

Reading disorders affect up to 10% of children and are of particular interest to psychiatrists because of the relatively strong links between reading problems and behavioural problems. Nearly all childhood reading problems are developmental in origin, though brain damage in middle or late childhood can result in acquired reading disorders, and childhood dementias lead to progressive deterioration in reading skills.

BACKGROUND INFORMATION ABOUT NORMAL READING

When they start to read, children learn to recognise a small number of very familiar words (such as their own name) on the basis of visual clues from the overall shape of the word. At this stage, they are generally unable to decipher new words. As they come to understand the principles of letter-sound correspondence, they acquire a phonological strategy for deciphering less familiar words. As reading becomes fluent, most words are recognised as a single entity without the need for phonological decoding.

Though many perceptual and linguistic skills are involved in fluent reading, individual variation in reading ability is more closely related to language than to perceptual abilities. In particular, a preschool child's phonological awareness as indexed, for example, by their sensitivity to rhyme and alliteration, is a good predictor of how well they will subsequently learn to read (even when the effect of IQ is allowed for). Improving phonological awareness enhances subsequent reading skill.

Most twin studies suggest that genetic variation accounts for about 30–50% of individual differences in children's reading abilities. Environmental factors, including the amount of parental input and the quality of schooling, also have a major impact.

SPECIFIC READING DISORDER (SRD)

Some children's reading attainments are substantially poorer than would be predicted from their age and IQ – these children are said to have SRD. The relationship at any given chronological age between reading age and IQ is shown schematically in Box 26.1. The correlation between reading age and IQ is fairly substantial (with a correlation coefficient of 0.6). Not surprisingly, brighter children are likely to be reading better. It is worth noting, however, that predicted reading age does not generally equal mental age – there is regression towards the mean. Thus a ten-year-old with a mental age of 13 will not, on average, be reading up to 13-year-old level, while a ten-year-old with a mental age of seven will, on average, be reading at better than seven-year-old level. Roughly 95% of children fall within two standard deviations of their predicted reading age. SRD refers to children, such as subjects B and C in Box 26.1 whose reading attainments are over two standard deviations (SDs) below their predicted reading level. This corresponds, at the age of ten, to being about $2\frac{1}{2}$ years behind the predicted level. Though most children with SRD are reading at well below the average for their chronological age (e.g. subject B in Box 26.1), some very bright children with SRD do have average reading ability (e.g. subject C in Box 26.1). Conversely, being markedly behind in reading attainments (reading backwardness) does not necessarily imply SRD because the child's poor reading skills may be in line with the child's low intelligence (e.g. subject A in Box 26.1).

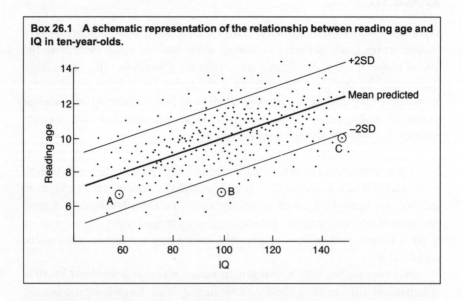

Box 26.1   A schematic representation of the relationship between reading age and IQ in ten-year-olds.

Although it is somewhat arbitrary to define SRD in terms of reading attainments that are at least two SDs below the predicted level, this cut-off does identify a group of children who have a substantial and persistent handicap. These children do seem to represent an extra 'hump' at the bottom of the normal distribution curve of reading ability. Whether such children are qualitatively or just quantitatively different from children who are less far behind with their reading (e.g. only 1 or $1\frac{1}{2}$ SDs behind) has not yet been resolved.

Epidemiology

SRD affects 3–10% of children. Most studies show it to be two to three times more common in males than females. SRD is more common among the children of parents with manual rather than non-manual occupations. The prevalence of SRD at ten years of age was 4% on the Isle of Wight and 10% in inner London; a difference that could be explained by social, school and family factors. SRD appears to be more common among English rather than Italian speaking children, perhaps because English spelling is much more irregular than Italian spelling. Surprisingly, though, similar rates of SRD were found in a comparative study of children from the USA, Japan and China despite the very different natures of printed words in these countries.

Associated features

(1) Spelling is often more severely affected than reading itself, and problems with spelling may persist even if reading becomes reasonably fluent. Arithmetical skills are not typically as far behind as reading skills, though some delay is usual.

(2) Spelling errors are often severe and bizarre. They are commonly non-phonetic (e.g. 'umderlee' for umbrella) rather than phonetic (e.g. 'mite' for might). Reading errors are often based on attempts to guess the word from its shape rather than on faulty attempts to decipher the word phonologically. In both reading and writing, letters and words may be reversed, e.g. 'p' for q, 'b' for d, 'saw' for was, a phenomenon sometimes labelled *strephosymbolia*.

(3) Children with SRD are more likely than other children to have neuro-developmental and neuropsychological impairments, including left–right confusion, poor coordination, poor constructional abilities, motor impersistence and language abnormalities. Whether these associated symptoms delineate as specific dyslexia syndrome is considered later.

(4) Children with SRD span the IQ range from very bright to very dull. The mean IQ of children with SRD is average or slightly below average. Verbal IQ tends to be lower than performance IQ. This may reflect not only the centrality of language rather than visuospatial deficits in SRD, but also the fact that children who read little have less opportunity to build up the skills tapped by the verbal subtests.

(5) Epidemiological studies have not supported clinical accounts that left handedness or mixed dominance is over-represented in SRD. One recent epidemiological study found an excess of both strong left handers and strong right handers among children with SRD.

(6) SRD is more common among children from large families.

(7) SRD is associated with a variety of psychiatric problems, as detailed at the end of this section.

SRD and reading backwardness

Is there any point distinguishing SRD from poor reading that is in line with the child's IQ, e.g. distinguishing between subjects A and B in Box 26.1? The answer is controversial. Some researchers argue that there is little practical justification for the distinction. Others argue that SRD and reading backwardness should be distinguished because they differ in prognosis and associated features (Box 26.2).

Box 26.2   Differences between reading disorder and reading backwardness.

	More strongly associated with:	
	Reading disorder	Reading backwardness
Poor prognosis for reading	√	
Marked male excess	√	
History of relatively specific problems in speech and language development	√	
History of widespread developmental delays		√
Overt neurological disorder		√
Social disadvantage		√

SRD and developmental dyslexia

Is there a subgroup of children with SRD who warrant a diagnosis of developmental dyslexia on the basis that their reading problems are part of a wider neurodevelopmental syndrome that is clearly constitutional rather than environmental? Epidemiological evidence from the Isle of Wight study does not support the notion of a pure dyslexic subgroup. Although children with SRD were indeed more likely to have other neurodevelopmental and neuropsychological problems (poor coordination, constructional difficulties, left-right confusion, etc.), most of the children had only one or two of these additional problems and there was *no* evidence for two distinct groups of children: a dyslexic group with many associated problems and a non-dyslexic group with few or none. Furthermore, whether a child with SRD had many or few associated neurodevelopmental problems made no difference to the child's prognosis, response to treatment, likelihood of associated psychiatric problems, or likelihood of having a positive family history of reading problems.

At present, there is no justification for distinguishing developmental dyslexia from SRD. In an ideal world, it might be best to abandon the term 'dyslexia' altogether. In the real world, however, a label of dyslexia is widely recognised, usually conveys the message that the child's reading problems are not due to stupidity or laziness, and sometimes results in important practical benefits for the child (e.g. extra time in examinations). Given this, there is no reason to deny any child with SRD a label of dyslexia (whether or not additional neurodevelopmental symptoms are present) if this is to the child's overall advantage.

Causation of SRD

SRD is not a uniform condition, though it is not clear if the heterogeneity is best conceptualised as dimensional or categorical. It seems likely that the aetiology and pathogenesis of SRD is also heterogeneous.

In most cases, phonological problems seem central. These make it much harder for affected individuals to increase their reading vocabulary by sounding out new words and thereby familiarising themselves with them. In a minority of cases, visuoperceptual problems may be more important than language-related problems. The significance of abnormalities of ocular vergence control or ocular dominance is controversial.

Twin and family studies suggest that genes may be important, either as single major genes or as polygenic contributors to a multifactorial aetiology. Neurologically impaired children (e.g. with cerebral palsy or epilepsy) are several times more likely to have SRD than ordinary children with comparable IQs. The psychosocial environment is also of great importance, as shown, for example, by the fact that SRD was more than twice as common in inner London than on the Isle of Wight.

Could SRD arise from developmental anomalies in language-related areas of the left hemisphere? There is limited neuropathological support for this, but it is based on so few cases that it is premature to draw any strong conclusions. There is little empirical support for the notion that SRD results from an atypical division of labour between the two cerebral hemispheres (as indexed by left handedness, mixed laterality, etc.). The recent finding of an excess of strong left handers *and* strong right handers among children with SRD is intriguing. Annett's genetic model of handedness suggests that strong left and right handers are mainly homozygotes whereas mild and moderate right handers are mainly heterozygotes. Perhaps there is a heterozygote advantage for reading (analogous to the heterozygote advantage of the sickle cell trait).

Treatment of SRD

Children with SRD are all too often thought to be stupid or lazy by their parents or teachers. These views will tend to aggravate the poor self-image generated by repeated failures at academic tasks. Informing teachers, parents and children that the reading problems are not simply the result of low intelligence or inadequate effort can have a major impact for good, fostering attitudes that are both more realistic and more positive. Since some parents think that dyslexia is a sign of being particularly gifted, it is important to avoid the opposite error of fostering unrealistically high expectations, particularly if the child is of average or below-average intelligence. Listing famous people with dyslexia is not necessarily helpful.

Some children with SRD can receive extra help with their reading and spelling while remaining in mainstream school. In severe cases, and when the child's literacy difficulties are an insuperable block to academic progress in all other subjects, placement in a special unit or school may be helpful. Some schools specialise just in 'dyslexia' while others cater for a range of learning problems, including SRD.

Historically, most interventions to improve reading resulted in short-term benefits but no lasting gains. More recent interventions, combining reading instruction with intensive work on phonological awareness and motivation training, seem more promising. Increasing parental involvement in their child's reading can have marked and lasting benefits.

Prognosis of SRD

It is unusual for children with SRD to catch up entirely and many fall increasingly far behind – not because they are losing skills but because they make less progress each year than their normal peers. The prognosis for reading is improved by high IQ and an advantaged socioeconomic background. Because their academic difficulties persist (with spelling problems often being even more persistent than reading problems), children with SRD typically end up with poor school qualifications even if they have no associated behavioural problems. As a result of their poorer qualifications and continuing problems with literacy skills, they are more likely than their peers to have manual jobs in adult life.

Psychiatric accompaniments of reading disorders

Many studies have shown that SRD is fairly strongly associated with conduct disorder and delinquency. Among ten-year-olds on the Isle of Wight, for example, a third of children with SRD had conduct disorders, and a third of children with conduct disorders had SRD. Recent evidence suggests that the primary link may be between SRD and hyperactivity rather than between SRD and conduct disorder. Since hyperactivity is closely associated with conduct disorder and delinquency, a direct link between SRD and hyperactivity will result in indirect links between SRD and both conduct disorder and delinquency. (The existence of indirect links does not rule out the possibility that there are direct links too, with the frustration generated by learning problems and school failure sometimes fuelling conduct disorder and delinquency.)

Why should reading and conduct problems commonly coexist? There are three possible answers, and each of them may be true, at least in some cases. Firstly, conduct problems may result in secondary reading problems. Though it is certainly plausible that disruptive behaviour in the classroom interferes with a child's academic progress, there is little empirical evidence for this. Secondly, the reading problems may result in secondary behavioural problems. The results of the Isle of Wight study suggested that SRD commonly led to secondary conduct problems, perhaps as a result of the frustration and marginalisation engendered by school failure. Finally, reading and behavioural problems may occur together because they have common antecedents, whether constitutional or environmental. Several studies suggest that hyperactivity may be a key antecedent of both reading and conduct problems. It is relevant that behavioural problems and poor pre-reading skills are already associated in preschool children, i.e. long before the child's behavioural problems could have interfered with school work, and before a child's scholastic problems could have resulted in marginalisation.

Follow-up studies suggest that those children with SRD who are free from additional psychiatric disorders in middle childhood are no more likely than their peers to develop psychiatric problems in their teens (with the possible exception of an increased risk of problems with temper control in adolescent girls with SRD).

When SRD is compounded by conduct problems, the teenage prognosis is worse. These individuals are more likely to leave school at the first opportunity, obtain no qualifications, take up unskilled work, and have a poor work record.

Though SRD is associated with a relatively high risk of adverse psychiatric and psychosocial outcomes in childhood and adolescence, follow-up studies into adulthood suggest that the impact on adult adjustment is far less marked. Though major literacy problems commonly persist into adulthood, adults are able to adjust their choice of occupation and lifestyle accordingly and show no more psychiatric or social problems than controls.

Subject reivew

Maughan, B. and Yule, W. (1994) Reading and other learning disabilities. In *Child and Adolescent Psychiatry: Modern Approaches*, 3rd edn (M. Rutter, E. Taylor and L. Hersov, eds) Blackwell Science, Oxford, pp. 647–665.

Further reading

Annett, M. *et al.* (1996) Types of dyslexia and the shift to dextrality. *Journal of Child Psychology and Psychiatry*, **37**, 167–180. (This paper discusses Annette's genetic model of handedness and brain lateralisation and their possible relationship to reading difficulties.)

Goswami, U. (1994) Development of reading and spelling. In *Development Through Life: A Handbook For Clinicians* (M. Rutter and D.F. Hay, eds) Blackwell Science, Oxford, pp. 284–302.

Maughan, B. *et al.* (1996) Reading problems and antisocial behaviour: developmental trends in comorbidity. *Journal of Child Psychology and Psychiatry*, 37, 405–418.

Snowling, M.J. (1996) Contemporary approaches to the teaching of reading. *Journal of Child Psychology and Psychiatry*, 37, 139–148.

27   Insecure Attachment

Attachment is discussed in detail because it is interesting, important, well-studied, and a favourite examination topic. Attachment disorders are considered separately in Chapter 16.

The nature of attachment

For over 25 years, clinical and scientific thinking about attachment has been strongly influenced by the theories and writings of John Bowlby (1907–1990), a British psychiatrist and psychoanalyst who moved well beyond the traditional limits of those disciplines, drawing heavily on ethology and control theory. Though many disciplines study behaviour, ethologists study animal behaviour (including human behaviour) from a perspective that emphasises ecological and evolutionary considerations. Ethologists consider the function and not just the form of a particular sort of behaviour, asking why that behaviour is adaptive in the ecological niche that the species has evolved to fill. In this context, attachment can best be understood as regulating the balance between security on the one hand and exploration and play on the other. At one extreme, a young primate who always clung to a parent would be relatively secure from predators but would not learn vital independence skills. At the other extreme, an over-independent youngster might acquire many useful skills but meet a premature death. Key adults act as a 'secure base' from which to explore, and as a 'safe haven' to retreat to when the child is threatened and in need of protection.

According to Bowlby, a child's need to be attached to protective figures is as basic and as important as the child's need for food. This contradicted earlier psychoanalytic theories that children became attached because they associated parents with food, the 'cupboard love' theory of object relations. Bowlby's view was supported by Harlow's famous (and heart-breaking) experiments with infant monkeys. When separated from their mothers, the infant monkeys spent most of their time clinging to a cloth-covered model rather than the wire model that they got their milk from. The cupboard-love theory predicted the opposite, namely that infants would associate comfort with the wire model that provided them with food.

Bowlby's ideas on attachment were greatly influenced by control theory, which considers the ways in which a system can use information in order to attain its goals. Potential strategies can be illustrated by some of the different ways a heating system can be designed to maintain a relatively constant indoor temperature: the controlled variable. A thermostat inside the house provides *feedback* information on the controlled variable, boosting the heating when the indoor temperature is too low. The feedback completes a loop: the heating system influences the indoor temperature and, by means of the feedback, the indoor temperature influences the heating system. An alternative control strategy is to use information from predictor variables, sometimes referred to as *feedforward*. One instance is a heating system that is turned on in the autumn and off in the spring – a crude method favoured by many UK hospitals. A more sophisticated system could use an outdoor thermostat that turned the heating up when it was cold outside. The information from predictor variables is not part of a loop: although the season and the outdoor temperature influence the heating system, the reverse does not apply.

In order to maintain an optimal security-exploration balance, attachment behaviour is regulated in response to information about predictor variables. Thus it makes good evolutionary sense for children to move closer to a protective adult when they are ill, or when strangers are around, or when it is dark. Other control strategies use feedback. For example, if you watch young children exploring in the park, you will see that they usually behave as though they are attached to their caregiver by a long piece of elastic, venturing away on their own, but then moving back towards the caregiver again. The behavioural system that keeps the child from straying too far can be thought of as a feedback system in which the controlled variable is the distance between caregiver and child. Thus too great a distance between child and caregiver activates the child's attachment behaviour and brings the child back to the optimum distance again, in much the same way that too low an indoor temperature activates a feedback-controlled heating system and brings the temperature up again.

A wide variety of attachment behaviours can serve the purpose of keeping the child close enough to a caregiver (just as a wide variety of heaters can serve the purpose of keeping a house warm enough). The child's ability to crawl or walk towards an adult is the most obvious sort of attachment behaviour, but calling out, smiling sweetly, or crying are also effective methods for bringing a caregiver closer. A child's anger at being separated from a caregiver can also serve a similar role: angry outbursts may motivate caregivers to maintain even closer contact in future to avoid further outbursts. Anger is rather a risky strategy, however, since it may make a reluctant caregiver even less likely to stay close to the child in future. A better strategy in these circumstances may be for the child to keep demands to the minimum since a reluctant caregiver is better than no caregiver at all.

Children generally develop clear attachments to a relatively small number of people, *attachment figures*, in the second half of their first year of life. Many children have a hierarchy of attachment figures, e.g. a child who is attached to both parents may usually turn to the mother rather than the father for comfort and security if both are present. While separation from familiar caregivers is relatively well tolerated in early infancy if the substitute care is good, separation from attachment figures at later ages is more stressful, particularly for children aged between about six months and four years. The impact of separation from, or loss of, an attachment figure is discussed in the next chapter.

Attachment is not the only component of parent-child relationships; other components include play, teaching and limit-setting. The relative prominence of these different components varies between and within cultures.

Bringing together elements from cognitive psychology and psychoanalytic object relations theory, Bowlby proposed that young children internalise their experiences with attachment figures to generate *internal working models* of themselves and others, and of the relationship between themselves and others. Children who have experienced sensitive and responsive caregiving typically come to see others as caring and reliable, and themselves as lovable and worthy of care. Conversely, children who are rejected or ignored typically come to see others as uncaring and unreliable, and themselves as unlovable and unworthy. In later childhood and adulthood, the individual's behaviour to others will often create new relationships in line with prior expectations. Individuals may also selectively attend to and remember precisely those aspects of their experience that reinforce their internal working model, ignoring or forgetting contradictory experiences. The notion that internal working models play a key role in linking early attachment experiences to later social and psychological sequelae is clinically appealing but, for the present, largely unproven. However, there is much research currently being conducted on the topic.

Secure and insecure attachment

Although nearly all children develop attachments, the quality of these attachment varies greatly. Much research on this subject has used the Strange Situation Procedure (SSP) devised by Mary Ainsworth to investigate the attachment of 12–18 month old children. In this procedure, an infant is observed via a one-way screen or television camera while spending about 20 minutes in an unfamiliar room. One of the child's attachment figures and an unfamiliar adult enter and leave the room in a predetermined sequence (Box 27.1). This highly artificial procedure is not supposed to be representative of the child's ordinary experiences. Just as cardiologists and endocrinologists use 'stress tests' to unmask pathology that may not show up in ordinary circumstances, so the SSP is a stress test designed to show how the child copes with the triple challenge of a strange setting, the presence of a stranger, and separation from the attachment figure. When the SSP was first introduced, a lot of emphasis was placed on how distressed the child became during the separations (phases 3 and 5 in Box 27.1). It has subsequently become clear, however, that the degree of distress about separation is primarily related to the child's temperament and not to the security of the child's attachment. Consequently, more attention is now paid to the child's response to the reunions (phases 4 and 7 in Box 27.1).

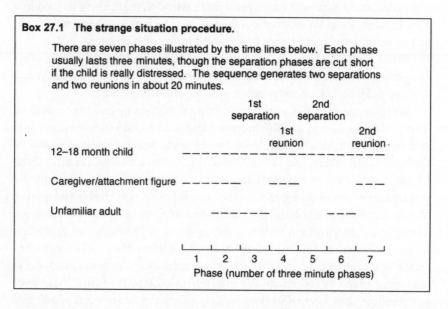

Box 27.1   The strange situation procedure.

There are seven phases illustrated by the time lines below. Each phase usually lasts three minutes, though the separation phases are cut short if the child is really distressed. The sequence generates two separations and two reunions in about 20 minutes.

The original ABC classification used information from the SSP to classify children as securely or insecurely attached to that particular caregiver: type B is secure attachment, while insecure attachments are divided into type A (avoidant) and type C (resistant-ambivalent). (Mnemonic: Ay for Ay-voidant). More recently, an additional variety of insecure attachment has been recognised (type D = disorganised-disorientated); the children who are now included in this new category were previously scattered among the A, B and C categories. The characteristic child behaviours seen with each type of attachment are shown in Table 27.1. The table also shows the approximate frequency of each type in normative American samples, the most commonly associated caregiving styles, and the likely classification of the caregiver's own attachment type, as revealed by the Adult Attachment Interview (see below).

A secure attachment is obviously better than an insecure attachment – or is it? It is true, as discussed later, that a secure attachment does promote subsequent happiness and social success, at least in middle-class America. From an evolutionary point of view, though, it is important to remember that insecure attachments may well be adaptive responses to unfavourable circumstances, in much the same way that restricted growth (stunting) is an adaptive response to chronic malnutrition. If a caregiver is rejecting, an avoidant (type A) attachment may be the child's most adaptive strategy for getting some care without risking total abandonment. 'Half a loaf is better than no bread.' Conversely, if a caregiver is preoccupied and tends to ignore the child, exaggerated (type C) attachment behaviour may be the child's most adaptive strategy for getting his

Table 27.1   The ABCD classification of attachment.

Type	Characteristic child behaviour (SSP)*	Approximate (%) in non-clinical sample	Likely caregiving style	Caregiver's probable attachment type (AAI)**
A = Avoidant	Explores with little reference to caregiver. Minimally distressed by separation. Avoids or ignores caregiver or reunion.	15	Actively rejecting of attachment behaviour or insensitively intrusive. Lack of tenderness. Suppressed parental anger	Dismissing
B = Secure	Uses caregiver as a secure base to explore from. May be distressed by separation. On reunion greets caregiver positively, may seek comfort, then gets on with play/exploration again.	60	Sensitive to child's signals. Responsive to child's needs. Prompt response to distress, buffering negative affect.	Autonomous
C = Resistant-ambivalent	Minimal exploration. Highly distressed by separation. Hard to settle on reunion, with ambivalent mixture of clinging and anger.	10	Minimal or inconsistent responsiveness.	Preoccupied
D = Disorganised-disorientated	Lack of coherent pattern in exploratory or reunion behaviours. Fear or confusion in the caregiver's presence is suggested by disorganised and disorientated behaviours, e.g. rocking, covering face, freezing, unexpected alternation of approach and avoidance.	15	Parental behaviour is frightening or unpredictable. Not responding to infant's cues. Overrides infant's communications and goals. Sends infant double messages, e.g. holds out arms and backs away.	Unresolved

* SSP = Strange Situation Procedure
** AAI = Adult Attachment Interview

or her needs met. 'The squeaky hinge gets the oil.' Whether a disorganised (type D) attachment is ever adaptive is not yet clear.

The relative frequency of the ABCD attachment types as assessed by the SSP varies between and within cultures. To some extent, this may be an artefact of the assessment procedure. Thus although a higher rate of resistant attachment has been described in Japan, this may be because young Japanese children are so rarely separated from their mothers that the SSP is far more stressful for them than for their American or European counterparts. Thus, it is far more likely to elicit marked and prolonged clinging. Such artefacts seem less likely to account for two other cross-cultural differences. In north Germany there is a higher rate of avoidant attachment, perhaps reflecting a cultural push towards early independence; and in Israel there is a higher rate of resistant attachment on kibbutzim where young children sleep in a children's house, a setting where crying or distress may need to be intense and prolonged before a caregiver responds. Many American studies of infants who spend much of their week in non-maternal care also report an elevated rate of insecure attachment, perhaps reflecting the poor quality of some of this non-maternal care.

The rate of insecure attachment is increased by adverse family factors such as maternal depression, maternal alcoholism, or child abuse. This is most obvious for disorganised attachment, which is the sort of insecure attachment that best predicts future problems (see below). Thus the rate of disorganised attachment varies from around 15% in two-parent middle-class samples to over 80% in maltreating families.

The ABCD classification generated by the SSP is specific to the child-caregiver pair that is assessed. A child who is shown to be securely attached to one parent might, if reassessed with other caregivers, turn out to be insecurely attached to the other parent, to a nanny, or to a day care worker. Thus while some young children are similarly attached to all their caregivers, others have a mixture of secure and insecure attachments. For this latter group with mixed attachment types, the current evidence suggests that subsequent development is particularly affected by the quality of attachment to the most important caregiver. Which caretaker is most important? The amount of contact seems relevant since several studies have shown that when infants spend most of their waking time in day care, their development is better predicted by the quality of their attachment to day care staff than by the quality of their attachment to parents. One important implication is that 'quality time' with parents may not entirely offset the ill effects on infants of prolonged low-quality day care.

Attachment throughout life

While the SSP tests the attachment security of children aged 12–18 months, two newer assessments are designed for children aged 3–4 years and 5–7 years. These newer assessments also generate ABCD categories on the basis of the child's response to reunion with a caregiver.

A child's attachment classification is generally stable. One explanation for this stability is that a child's internal working model of relationships is determined early in childhood and is then resistant to change. An alternative explanation is that family circumstances are generally stable, e.g. a mother who is sensitive and responsive to her infant is still likely to be sensitive and responsive to the same child several years later, thereby promoting secure attachment at each age. One way these alternative explanations can be distinguished is by studying what happens when family circumstances change markedly for the better or for the worse. For example, what happens if the caregivers of insecurely attached infants are taught to be more sensitive and responsive? Does this have no effect because early experience has already irreversibly moulded the child? Or do the children become securely attached because what counts is current rather than previous caregiving? What limited evidence there is favours an intermediate answer, namely that early attachment experiences do typically have lasting effects that cannot simply be attributed to the continuity of the environment. However, these effects are not totally irreversible and can be attenuated or even reversed by radically altered life circumstances.

There has recently been an explosion of interest in attachment in adult life. Close adult relationships commonly have an attachment component, providing security, comfort, and a source of confidence. In adulthood, unlike childhood, the relationship is often a reciprocal bond between equals, with each adult being an attachment figure to the other, and commonly a sexual partner too. Research on attachment quality in adult life has drawn heavily on the Adult Attachment Interview (AAI) developed by Mary Main. This interview asks adults for descriptions and evaluations of their childhood attachment relationships, and also enquires about any separations or losses, and the effect these had on the respondent's development and personality. The respondent is asked to provide specific biographical episodes to substantiate global evaluations. The aim is not to reconstruct exactly what happened many years ago but to establish, through discourse analysis, the respondent's current state of mind with respect to attachment. Four categories have been identified, each of which has an association with one of the child ABCD categories (see Table 27.1).

(1) *Dismissing*. The respondent can recall few affectively charged memories from childhood. Closeness and attachment are not valued. An idealised picture of parents is at odds with the specific details recalled. These respondents resemble children with type A attachments – attachment behaviours and feelings are denied, restricted or repressed.

(2) *Autonomous*. The respondent values attachment relationships and either gives a convincing history of emotionally supportive relationships in childhood or has come to terms with a childhood lacking them. Typically self-reliant, objective, and non-defensive. These respondents resemble children with type B attachments – attachment feelings and behaviours are expressed in open and balanced ways, with appropriate dependency and confidence in the attachment figure.

(3) *Preoccupied*. The account of childhood relationships is confused, incoherent and unobjective. They are still caught up in childhood events and unable to move beyond them. Anger at parents is unresolved. These

respondents resemble children with type C attachments – attachment feelings and behaviours are exaggerated and ambivalent.

(4) *Unresolved-disorganised*. Discussions of potentially traumatic events are marked by striking lapses in the monitoring of reasoning or discourse, suggesting dissociated memory systems or abnormal absorption in traumatic memories. These respondents resemble children with type D attachments – disorganised.

Given the complexity and seeming subjectivity of this rating scheme, it is truly remarkable how well parent and infant attachment status correspond. When the parent's attachment type is classified using the AAI (whether before or after the child's birth), and when the infant's attachment to a parent is classified as A, B, C or D using the SSP, then roughly two-thirds of infants match their parents in attachment type.

Consequences of secure and insecure attachments

Many studies have compared the social and psychological development of securely and insecurely attached children. The picture that has consistently emerged is that securely attached children do much better on average. However, not all securely attached children do well, and not all insecurely attached children do badly. It is still unclear whether this group difference arises because insecure attachment is itself the key risk factor; the alternative is that insecure attachment acts as a marker for wider-ranging family abnormalities that have the adverse long-term effects.

Whether the link is causal or not, a secure attachment does increase the likelihood of the child subsequently forming harmonious relationships with adults and children. This is most evident for close relationships with family members and friends. Securely attached children are more cooperative and responsive with their mothers, more likely to comfort younger siblings, and more likely to have good friends. They are less likely to be non-compliant with parents, quarrelsome with siblings, or controlling with friends. The benefits of secure attachments are also evident with familiar but less intimate social partners. On average, securely attached children are less emotionally dependent on teachers and are better able to ask for a teacher's help when they face a challenge they cannot manage alone. Typically, they are also more popular with classmates and less often victimised, perhaps because they show more empathy for peers and engage in less conflict when playing. Attachment security has least influence on the quality of social interactions with unfamiliar adults or children. Such interactions are primarily influenced by the child's sociability, which is a moderately heritable temperamental trait. Conversely, genetic factors seem less important in determining the quality of close relationships.

Early studies, using the ABC classification of attachment, particularly emphasised the link between type A (avoidant) attachment and externalising problems such as aggression. It now seems likely that the more recently recognised type D (disorganised) attachment is the strongest predictor of externalising problems. For example, one study showed that disorganised attachment at 18 months predicted a six-fold increase in serious aggression towards peers in nursery school. Though the disorganised attachment often included avoidant elements, it was noteworthy that those children who had purely avoidant (and not disorganised) attachments were not subsequently more likely to be unusually aggressive towards peers. Perhaps severe family adversity launches children onto a developmental pathway characterised by disorganised attachment and dysphoria in infancy, oppositional defiant disorder in middle childhood, and more severe conduct disorder and juvenile delinquency in adolescence.

An increasing number of studies have used the AAI to investigate the attachment classification of adults with mental illnesses or personality disorders. In clinical samples, the likelihood of an autonomous (i.e. secure) attachment is only about 10%, as compared with roughly 60% in low-risk samples. The remaining 90% of clinic patients are split fairly evenly between the three insecure attachment categories: dismissing, preoccupied and unresolved. So far, there are only hints of links between particular psychiatric diagnoses and specific types of insecurity, e.g. between borderline personality disorder and preoccupied or unresolved attachment.

Subject review

Belsky, J. and Cassidy, J. (1994) Attachment: theory and evidence. In *Development Through Life: A Handbook For Clinicians* (M. Rutter and D.F. Hay, eds) Blackwell Science, Oxford, pp. 373–402.

Further reading

Journal of Consulting and Clinical Psychology (1996) (Issues 1 and 2 of Volume 64 each contain a special section on attachment and psychopathology with many excellent articles.)

Main, M. (1996) Overview of the field of attachment. *Journal of Consultant and Clinical Psychology*, **64**, 237–243.

Parkes, C.M., Stevenson-Hinde, J. and Marris, P. (1991) *Attachment Across the Life Cycle*. Routledge, London.

28 Nature, Nurture, and Family Adversities

Until recently, most studies of children exposed to family adversities assumed that poor outcomes were due to the unsatisfactory conditions in which the children were raised. In fact, the picture may be much more complex. Consider, for example, possible interpretations of the finding that children who are poor readers are more likely to come from homes where they do not spend much time reading to their parents. This finding would lead many to conclude that the children's lack of interest and ability in reading stemmed from a lack of parental attention and encouragement (one can almost hear the cries of 'that's only common sense'). However, there are many other plausible interpretations. One possibility is that although the parents love books and are good readers themselves, the child may have some constitutional reading difficulty ('dyslexia') which means that he finds being encouraged to read very unpleasant, as he cannot do it nearly as well as his younger sister. His parents will soon learn to back off to avoid the whining, resentment and misery they cause! Another possibility is that the parents and child all have genetically determined reading difficulties so that they all avoid anything to do with reading. A third possibility is that both parents and children could easily read if they had the opportunity, but live in an environment where there are no books and the video is king.

Sorting out what is cause and what is effect is no mere academic matter. If we are trying to help people's lives, it is essential we get it right. At an individual level, there is no point, for example, in trying to teach a 'refrigerator mother' holding techniques to 'get through' to her autistic son if in fact he has a genetically determined inability to communicate which has consequently led his entirely normal mother to give up trying. At a policy level, there is little point in rebuilding a sordid estate in order to eradicate the high rate of child abuse and schizophrenia found there, if in fact the reason people with these difficulties have ended up living there is because of their multiple social handicaps which they will take into any new situation, and which should be addressed in their own right. (It might be a good idea to rebuild the estate for lots of other reasons though.) Before reviewing a number of commonly encountered family adversities, it is important to consider some general principles which help disentangle nature from nurture.

GENERAL PRINCIPLES

Association is not the same as causation

Many family factors are associated with an increase in the rate of one or more child psychiatric disorders. It is all too easy to fall into the trap of assuming that association implies causation. If a family characteristic (F) is associated with a child psychiatric disorder (C), it could be the case that F causes C, but two alternative explanations also need to be considered: that C is causing F, which is known as *reverse causality*; and that both C and F are due to the operation of a *third factor* or *confounder*.

Reverse causality

It is plausible that a psychiatrically disturbed child can influence family characteristics. For example, a disturbed child could plausibly evoke parental depression, anger, criticism, coldness, overprotection, punitiveness or disengagement. Some of the most powerful evidence for such effects comes from intervention studies. For example, one study showed that if stimulant medication reduced a child's hyperactivity, this often led to a reduction in maternal criticism of the child, greater maternal warmth towards the child, and an increase in the time the mother spent with the child (see Chapter 5). Of course, it could still be the case that the parental negativity evoked by a child's hyperactivity is also damaging to that child's development.

Third factors

If a parent and child are both particularly fearful of spiders, it seems natural to assume that the child has learned the anxiety from his or her parent. An equally plausible alternative is that the parent's fear and the child's fear have a common origin: perhaps parent and child share a genetic tendency to be fearful, or perhaps they have both watched the same horror film about spiders. Conceptually, adoption studies provide the most straightforward evidence for genetic third factors. If arachniphobia were completely genetic, then adopted children would resemble their biological parents but not their adoptive parents in this respect. Other approaches are needed to identify environmental third factors. For example, if having seen the same film accounts for parents and children both fearing spiders, then an epidemiological approach should be able to show that the association between parents' fears and children's fears disappears once allowance has been made for the effect of film viewing.

Children inhabit three rather different social worlds: the family, the classroom and the peer group. Though distinct, the three worlds are related. Thus children who come from disadvantaged and disharmonious families are also more likely to be attending poor schools and playing with disruptive peers. This can make it very hard tell if an association is causal. For example, if children from disadvantaged families are more often truants, is this because a disadvantaged family environment directly fosters truancy, or is the family disadvantage simply a marker for poor neighbourhood schools that foster truancy? To complicate matters further, adverse factors cluster together within each of the child's social worlds. At home, for example, overcrowding is linked to unemployment, poverty, parental mental illness and a host of other possible risk factors. If overcrowding is associated with delinquency, is this a direct effect of overcrowding, or is overcrowding simply acting as a marker for other risk factors? There are research designs and statistical techniques for trying to answer this sort of question.

Genes, shared environment and non-shared environment

For characteristics that run in families, behavioural geneticists have developed techniques for looking at the relative importance of genes and environment. The *variance* of a trait is a measure of how much that trait varies between people in the population being studied. *Heritability* refers to the proportion of the variance explained by genetic factors. Thus a heritability of 25% for a particular trait means that a quarter of that population's variability on that measure is attributable to genetic differences between people. The rest of the variance is conventionally divided between two environmental components, shared and non-shared environment. Roughly speaking, *shared or common environment* refers to environmental factors that affect the whole family, such as poverty, damp housing or air pollution. *Non-shared or unique environment* refers to environmental influences that are not shared by relatives living together, e.g. being knocked down by a bus, or having a best friend who is a drug addict. The relative importance of genes, shared environment and non-shared environment is usually estimated from twin or adoption studies, though increasing use is now being made of comparisons of full-siblings, half-siblings and step-siblings growing up in reconstituted families. Box 28.1 summarises the twin and adoption findings for three traits: a trait that is entirely genetically determined, a trait that is entirely determined by shared environment, and a trait entirely determined by non-shared environment. In practice, most traits are mixtures of these.

Genetic influence

Most psychological traits have been found to have a heritability of around 50%, i.e. genetic differences between individuals account for roughly half of the observed variance in a given population. Conduct problems are one likely exception to this rule, with most (but not all) studies showing a relatively small

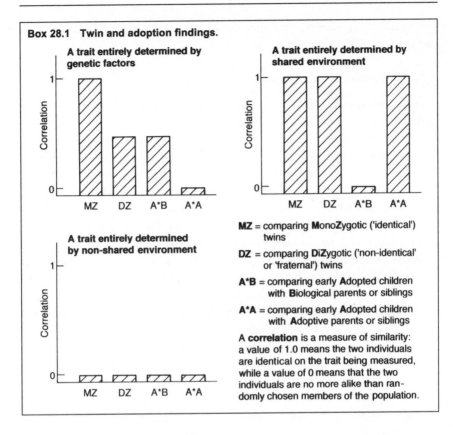

Box 28.1 Twin and adoption findings.

A trait entirely determined by genetic factors

A trait entirely determined by shared environment

A trait entirely determined by non-shared environment

MZ = comparing MonoZygotic ('identical') twins

DZ = comparing DiZygotic ('non-identical' or 'fraternal') twins

A*B = comparing early Adopted children with Biological parents or siblings

A*A = comparing early Adopted children with Adoptive parents or siblings

A **correlation** is a measure of similarity: a value of 1.0 means the two individuals are identical on the trait being measured, while a value of 0 means that the two individuals are no more alike than randomly chosen members of the population.

genetic contribution to this sort of behaviour. At the opposite extreme, liability to autism may have a heritability of over 90%.

Effects of shared environment

Over recent years, behavioural geneticists have made the dramatic claim that shared family environment has little if any effect on most psychological traits. In a landmark review of the area, Plomin and Daniels (1987) state the matter particularly forcibly: 'What parents do that is experienced similarly by their children does not have an impact on their behavioural development'. The gist of the argument is that twin and adoption findings show that family resemblances are almost all attributable to shared genes rather than shared environment; adoptees resemble their adoptive relatives at almost the level expected by chance. Conduct problems stand out as important exceptions to the general rule, with most studies suggesting that shared environment is the main reason for these problems running in families. In addition, even if psychological development is not greatly affected by ordinary variation in the shared family environment, perhaps because most families are 'good enough', the same may not apply to extreme variations. A grossly understimulating or neglectful family environment may be rare, but it may also have a marked impact on all or most of the children in the household.

Effects of non-shared environment

If genes typically explain about half of the variance for most psychological traits, and if shared environmental effects are often weak or absent, what explains the rest of the variance? The popular answer at present is 'non-shared environment', emphasising that children are particularly influenced by the experiences that they do not share with their siblings. It is certainly plausible, for example, that when parents pay more attention to one sibling than another, this is more wounding than when both siblings get less parental attention than the 'average child'. Mental health professionals have long been interested in the effects of scapegoating and favouritism, which are specific instances of non-shared environmental effects. Focusing on each child's unique experience of the family environment can be very helpful clinically. At the same time, it is unclear how powerful these non-shared environmental effects really are. It is wrong to suppose that if genes and shared environment only account for half of the variance on any given psychological trait, then the impact of non-shared experiences must account for the other half. Some of the unexplained variance may be due to measurement error, which is often greatly underestimated, and some may be attributable to the role of chance in brain development. The role of non-shared experiences needs to be assessed directly. It cannot simply be equated with the 'error' term in behavioural genetic analyses.

SPECIFIC INSTANCES

Separation and loss

Since attachment is such an important theme in developmental psychology and psychiatry (see Chapter 27), it is not surprising that many studies have examined what happens to children when their attachment bonds are temporarily disrupted by separations, or permanently broken by losses. There is no doubt that children often find separations and losses very upsetting, but it is less clear whether these unpleasant experiences have serious long-term consequences. Of course, it is highly desirable to prevent or reduce children's short-term distress whether or not that distress has adverse long-term consequences. Nevertheless, the issue of long-term outcome is important.

Do traumatic separations or early losses predispose an individual to persisting psychiatric disturbance? In trying to answer this sort of question, it is crucial to allow for 'third factors'. For example, when studying the effects of divorce on children, it is important to ask how far any adverse effects are due to prior and continuing family discord rather than to separation from one of the parents. In this regard, it is striking that long-term psychiatric problems are more likely to follow the loss of a parent through divorce than through death. This suggests that the antecedents and consequences of loss are more important than the loss itself. Similarly, when children are taken into foster care, the poor quality of their previous care is more important as a predictor of future problems than the fact that they have been separated from their biological parents.

It is also important to remember that separations and losses may set in motion a series of adverse events that have lasting consequences of their own. For example, divorce may be followed by parental depression or less effective parental supervision, a change to a worse school, and less money for leisure activities. These changes may have long-term effects on the children's behaviour even if the divorce itself does not.

Taking these various issues into account, most research findings suggest that separations and losses are not in themselves major risk factors for persistent psychiatric disturbance – though their antecedents or consequences sometimes are.

Hospital admission

Since pain and illness activate a child's drive to stay close to an attachment figure, being admitted alone to hospital is a particularly stressful sort of separation experience. Over the course of several days or weeks, such children may go through sequential phases of *protest, despair and detachment*. This reaction to separation is often observed most clearly when children are aged between six months and four years of age. Though a single separation due to a hospital admission is not associated with an increased risk of subsequent child psychiatric disorder, multiple admissions are associated with higher rates of later problems, mainly conduct disorder and delinquency. This increased risk is far more marked in discordant families, suggesting that many of the harmful long-term consequences of multiple hospital admissions may be mediated by an adverse impact on subsequent family relationships. Though separations are painful for the child, most families are able to buffer the child's distress during and after hospital admissions and thereby minimise the long-term consequences.

Studies carried out at a time when children's wards generally discouraged parental contact showed that the harmful effects of hospital admissions could be reduced by increased parental contact. Fortunately, as awareness of children's attachment needs has grown, hospital policies have shifted markedly so that parents are now usually encouraged to stay with their child for as long as they can, or even to 'room in' with them. For somewhat different reasons, the parents of premature babies on intensive care units are also encouraged to have frequent contact with their children. Though the babies are too young to be specifically attached, increased contact promotes more sensitive and responsive parenting subsequently. Hopefully, this will help counteract the raised risk of child abuse after premature birth.

Bereavement

The death of a parent is typically followed by a brief period of considerable distress that progressively diminishes. Distress may show itself through emotional symptoms, conduct problems, or a mixture of the two. The severe depressive withdrawal seen in some adults is rare in children. A year later, overt distress is generally much less evident, although other manifestations, such as disinterest in school, may persist. There is certainly not a strong link with depression in subsequent adult life; whether there is a weak link remains controversial. If there are adverse effects on psychosocial outcome in adult life, these seem likely to stem not from the bereavement itself, but from indirect consequences such as poverty, chronic depression in the other parent, or negative experiences with a step-parent.

Divorce

This tends to be the consequence of years of decline in the parental relationship, and this needs to be borne in mind when comparisons are made between children from divorced and intact families: the differences may in part be due to the pre-existing discord etc. Parents tend to feel anxious, depressed, angry, rejected and incompetent during the first year after divorce, with these responses diminishing in the second. The divorced parents frequently remain ambivalent about their relationship with each other, often with resultant conflict; both the strong positive and negative feelings reduce if parents find another partner. Inconsistent parenting of children is frequent, especially of sons by mothers. Conversely, mothers may be greatly harassed by their sons, who may blame them for the loss of their fathers. Practical difficulties such as having enough money and getting all the household chores done loom large.

The children show similar changes. Both at home and at school, social interactions become markedly disrupted. There is much fantasy aggression, opposition and fearfulness with a need to seek help from, and proximity to, adults; boys especially seek help from adult males. By comparison with other children, they are more negative and less positive to adults. Younger children usually hope desperately for a reconciliation even if predivorce life had been characterised by severe discord. There is great fear that the father might be replaced through remarriage. Later follow-up shows that though most of the children become well-functioning individuals, the divorce had a big effect on their lives. They become very concerned about the chances of the same thing happening again. If parents remarry, the children have to make further adjustments. While young children often show good relationships with their stepfathers, older children frequently do not. On average, boys are more distressed than girls by the divorce, while girls are more distressed than boys if their mothers remarry.

Family discord

There is a marked association between child psychiatric disorder and being reared in a disharmonious home. Discord, angry arguments, hostility, and criticism are related to conduct disorder in boys, and to emotional disorders in both sexes. Is discord a risk factor in itself? Or is it simply a marker for other risk factors such as poverty, lack of rules or poor supervision? There is quite a lot of evidence that discord is important in its own right. Thus discord is a powerful predictor of child psychiatric problems even in well-off households. The absence of warmth in family relationships is not as relevant as the presence of discord. Family discord is so often connected with poor discipline that it has been hard to tease apart their respective impacts.

In discordant households, children may learn that aversive behaviours are a particularly effective way of getting parental attention. In young children, this effect may be relatively situational, with children behaving negatively when exposed to discord at home, but relating more normally to people outside the family. With time, however, the negative behavioural style becomes more set; the child appears to have internalised the parents' mode of interaction, repeating the same pattern in other relationships.

Parental mental disorder

The children of mentally ill parents are at increased risk of developing emotional and behavioural problems themselves, with a particularly marked increase in conduct disorders. In some cases, a parent and child will both have psychiatric problems, not because of the way the ill parent is behaving towards the child, but because of shared genes, shared environment, or direct modelling. This may apply, for example, to some families where parents and children have anxiety or depressive disorders. In most cases, however, the adverse effects of parental psychiatric disorder are mediated by the children's exposure to parental hostility and marital discord. These factors increase the risk of emotional and behavioural problems in children in general. Parents with a personality disorder (whether antisocial or otherwise) are even more likely than parents with affective or psychotic disorders to have children who develop conduct disorders. This link primarily reflects the greater tendency of parents with personality disorders to be hostile to their children. Child characteristics may also be relevant since, other things being equal, temperamentally difficult children seem more likely to be the targets of parental hostility than temperamentally easy children.

Family size and birth order

Family size and birth order can be measured so easily and reliably that they are included as possible predictor variables in most studies of child psychiatric problems. Researchers who find an association between psychiatric problems and a family composition variable are likely to report that finding, whereas researchers who find no such association may concentrate on other positive findings and not even report the negative findings. The predictable result is a profusion of reported associations, most of which are not replicated by subsequent studies.

One of the few consistent findings to emerge from this muddled field is that children from large families are at greater risk of conduct problems and juvenile delinquency. Though this may partly reflect an association between large families and social disadvantage, family size probably has a direct effect too – with the number of brothers being a stronger predictor of externalising problems than the number of sisters.

Contrary to popular mythology, only children are not psychiatrically distinctive; children from small families are at relatively low psychiatric risk whether or not the family has one or two children. One important implication for our overcrowded planet is that parents who choose to have just one child need not feel that they are selfishly endangering their child's mental health.

Whereas most 'oldest' and 'youngest' children come from two-child families, 'middle' children must come from families with at least three children. Consequently, the link between larger family size and conduct problems will inevitably make it seem as though middle children have more conduct problems than oldest or youngest children if no account is taken of family size. It is not clear whether birth order has an effect on psychiatric problems once the effect of family size has been allowed for, although there may be a link between school refusal and being the youngest in the family.

Subject reviews

Dunn, J. (1994) Family influences. In *Development Through Life: A Handbook For Clinicians* (M. Rutter and D.F. Hay, eds) Blackwell Science, Oxford, pp. 112–133.

Simonoff, E., McGuffin, P. and Gottesman, I.I. (1994) Genetic influences on normal and abnormal development. In *Child and Adolescent Psychiatry: Modern Approaches*, 3rd edn (M. Rutter, E. Taylor and L. Hersov, eds) Blackwell Science, Oxford, pp. 129–151.

Further reading

Cummings, E.M. and Davies, P.T. (1994) Maternal depression and child development. *Journal of Child Psychology and Psychiatry*, **35**, 73–112.

Fergusson, D.M. *et al.* (1994) Parental separation, adolescent psychopathology, and problem behaviors. *Journal of the American Academy of Child and Adolescent Psychiatry*, **33**, 1122–1133.

Goodman, R. (1991) Growing together and growing apart: the non-genetic forces on children in the same family. In *The New Genetics of Mental Illness* (P. McGuffin and R. Murray, eds) Butterworth-Heinemann, Oxford, pp. 212–224.

Goodyer, I.M. (1990) Family relationships, life events and childhood psychopathology. *Journal of Child Psychology and Psychiatry*, **31**, 161–192.

Plomin, R. and Daniels, R. (1987) Why are children in the same family so different from one another? *Behavioural and Brain Sciences*, **10**, 1–60.

Rutter, M. and Quinton, D. (1984) Parental psychiatric disorder: effects on children. *Psychological Medicine*, **14**, 853–880.

29 School and Peer Factors

Though family life undoubtedly has a powerful influence on many aspects of child development, it is important to remember that most children inhabit more than one social world. Even in the toddler years, experiences in day care can be very different from experiences at home. From the preschool years onwards, peer relationships become increasingly important. Close friendships can buffer children from the impact of other adversities, while peer rejection, victimisation or involvement in a deviant peer group can all contribute to the onset of psychiatric problems. The peer group and the family are two different social worlds; the classroom is a third social world, and it too can influence emotional and behavioural problems for better or for worse. A supportive teacher and success in some area of the school curriculum can promote self-esteem and resilience, while a hostile teacher and school failure can have the opposite effect. A chaotic classroom, like a chaotic family environment, can train children to become coercive and disruptive by rewarding these behaviours through greater attention and fewer demands. It is vital to consider classroom and peer factors when assessing any child, and not just when the child's emotional or behavioural problems are mainly restricted to the classroom or playground. Stresses in one setting sometimes present with psychiatric problems in a different setting; stresses at home (such as sexual abuse) may lead to behavioural problems that are more prominent at school than at home, and stresses at school (such as bullying) may lead to distress or disturbance that is more evident to parents than to teachers.

Bully-victim problems

Bullying refers to repeated and deliberate use of physical or psychological means to hurt another child, without adequate provocation and in the knowledge that the victim is unlikely to be able to retaliate effectively. Most bullying occurs in school rather than on the way to or from school. Bullies and victims are commonly in the same school year. Although children are supposed to be supervised at school, most bullying goes unrecognised by teachers, and the victims commonly feel unable to report the bullying either to teachers or parents. Roughly 2–8% of children are bullied at least once a week, and 2–4%

engage in bullying at least once a week. Less severe levels of victimisation and bullying are substantially commoner. English studies have found similar rates of bullying in primary and secondary schools, though studies elsewhere have reported that bullying declines with age. Most bullies are boys, and there may be a small excess of boys among victims too. Physical aggression is most characteristic of boys' bullying; girls' bullying is more likely to involve social exclusion or whispering campaigns.

Two main types of victim are described: *passive* (or low-aggressive) victims, and *provocative* (or high-aggressive) victims. Passive victims are anxious, insecure, quiet individuals who withdraw when attacked and may cry. They typically lack friends and have very poor self-esteem. Among boys at least, passive victims are likely to be physically weaker than their peers. A cautious and sensitive personality probably predates the victimisation, but many of the other characteristics of victims are as likely to be consequences as causes of victim status. It is uncertain how far physical appearance, physical disabilities, or minority group status influence victimisation. Like passive victims, provocative victims are commonly unpopular with their peers. Unlike passive victims, however, provocative victims show a high level of aggression and aversive behaviour: picking fights, taunting others, getting people into trouble, and being easily angered. Clinical experience suggests that hyperkinetic children are particularly likely to become provocative victims.

While there is no doubt that victims often experience considerable distress at the time, the long-term consequences are less clear. Possible consequences include lasting problems with self-esteem, peer relationships, and intimate friendships.

Bullies are typically aggressive not only to their peers but also to their siblings, parents and teachers. They have a positive attitude towards violence and little empathy for victims. At least among boys, bullies are likely to be physically stronger than their peers. The development of aggressive personality patterns may reflect both temperament and parenting (with the parents of bullies being more prone to use power-assertive child-rearing methods, and failing to provide adequate warmth, control, and supervision). Most bullies are *not* especially prone to anxiety, insecurity, or poor self-esteem (though there may be a minority of anxious bullies who dominate their victims in order to bolster a fragile sense of self-worth). Bullies are not generally unhappy or unpopular at the time. In the long term bullies are at an increased risk of criminality and alcohol abuse in adulthood.

Systematic interventions can reduce the rate of victimisation in schools (by about 50% in one carefully planned intervention in Norway). The unaccept-ability of victimisation has to be made clear to all children, and the policy must be backed up by adequate supervision, and by firm but non-hostile sanctions. Victims need to know that they will get the backing of the school, their parents, and their class if they report bullying.

Peer popularity and unpopularity

The most common technique for assessing peer relationships is 'sociometry', which involves asking each child in a class in private which three children they would most want to play with ('positive nominations') and least want to play with ('negative nominations'). Until very recently, most studies of peer relationships simply distinguished between popular and unpopular children, with the implicit assumption that a low number of positive nominations and a high number of negative nominations were equivalent. More recent studies have treated popularity and unpopularity as different dimensions, generating a wider range of associated categories, shown in Box 29.1.

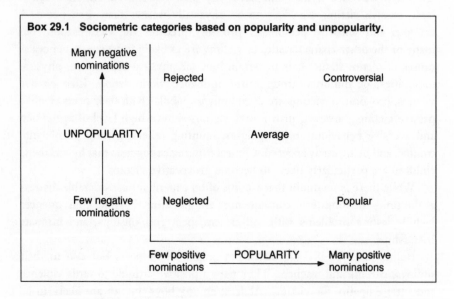

Box 29.1   Sociometric categories based on popularity and unpopularity.

In the past, most studies of 'unpopular' children confounded rejected and neglected children, two groups that differ in several important respects. The peer problems of rejected children are more persistent, and more often associated with aggressive and disruptive behaviours, loneliness, misery, and academic difficulties. In the longer term, rejected children are more likely to drop out of school, engage in delinquent behaviour, and have mental health problems (though it is still unclear whether peer rejection contributes directly to these later problems, or simply acts as a marker for a life-long maladaptive behavioural style). Rejection is probably related mainly to the child's social behaviour, though physical appearance, academic and athletic limitations, and minority group status may all be relevant (and some social groups may need a scapegoat or outcast). An aggressive and disruptive style is the most common identifiable reason for peer rejection. Marked self-isolation, particularly if combined with socially inept or eccentric behaviour, is also liable to result in rejection. Lesser degrees of shyness and withdrawal are more typical of neglected children, and probably do not have serious long-term consequences.

Controversial children are typically characterised by a mixed social style, incorporating both aversive and prosocial elements.

Institutional factors

Rates of child psychiatric problems, absenteeism, and delinquency vary markedly and consistently from school to school, often paralleling differences in examination results. Much of this can be explained by differences in catchment area and intake. Even when intake characteristics are allowed for, however, schools continue to differ markedly in their impact on children's behaviour and academic attainments. These differences can largely be explained by school ethos and organisation. Children are less likely to develop psychiatric problems when they attend a school where they are frequently praised and given responsibilities, where the teachers provide models of good behaviour, and where standards are high, lessons are well-organised, and working conditions are pleasant. These factors seem obvious enough, but it is important to remember that the following equally 'obvious' factors have not been shown to have a marked impact on school effectiveness: size of school, age or layout of buildings, continuity of teaching staff, or type of pastoral care.

Oldest/youngest in class

In most classes, the oldest children are roughly a year older than the youngest children. Though the youngest children are less emotionally and intellectually mature, teachers often fail to adjust their expectations accordingly. This may be part of the reason why one study of London primary schools found that the youngest children (born in the last four months of the academic year) were roughly 30% more likely to have behavioural problems than their classmates. Lesser size and strength may also be relevant, particularly for boys' peer popularity. Being one of the oldest in a class may carry its own risks, such as being bored, or being trained to be coercive (aggressive interactions are more likely to be rewarded when the perpetrator is big and strong).

Subject reviews

Asher, S.R., Eardley, C.A. and Gabriel, S.W. (1994) Peer relations. In *Development Through Life: A Handbook For Clinicians* (M. Rutter and D.F. Hay, eds) Blackwell Science, Oxford, pp. 456–487.

Maughan, B. (1994) School influences. In *Development Through Life: A Handbook For Clinicians* (M. Rutter and D.F. Hay, eds) Blackwell Science, Oxford, pp. 134–158.

Olweus, D. (1994) Bullying at school: basic facts and effects of a school based intervention program. *Journal of Child Psychology and Psychiatry*, 35, 1171–1190.

Further reading

Howlin, P. (1994) Special educational treatment. In *Child and Adolescent Psychiatry: Modern Approaches*, 3rd edn (M. Rutter, E. Taylor and L. Hersov, eds) Blackwell Science, Oxford, pp. 1071–1088.

Mortimer, P. *et al.* (1988) *School Matters: The Junior Years*. Open Books, Wells. (Demonstrates the role of school factors on children's academic and behavioural development. Demonstrates a powerful 'youngest in class' effect.)

Part IV
Treatment

30 Treatment: First Principles

Parents and children come to mental health services for a variety of reasons. They bring with them a number of beliefs and fears about the nature of the problem and what needs to be done. They will be carrying out an assessment of the service they receive from the moment they come through the door.

Engaging the family

If the family feel poorly handled and not understood, they are unlikely to come back again. If this happens, then no matter how thorough and accurate the clinical evaluation has been, the opportunity to do useful therapeutic work will have been lost, and the family may also have been put off seeking help at some later date. Discovering the family's beliefs and fears, and responding to them sensitively is vital to the whole process of engagement. If they feel they are understood, and treated as respected individuals, then the chances of their taking part in treatment will be far greater. This calls for considerable flexibility in response rather than one fixed 'right' way of doing things.

When are labels useful?

It can take considerable courage to walk through a door where the service is for 'mental' problems, and some parents are fearful that you are going to label them or their children as mad, bad, abnormal, or sick in the head. They may be fed up with being made to feel useless by a range of people in authority who tell them that what they are doing is wrong. Under these circumstances being told, for example, that their son has a serious condition labelled 'conduct disorder', and that they need a course of instruction to learn the 'right' way to handle their child may play into their sense of inadequacy and despair. For such a family it might have been more constructive to have said that their child is indeed strong-willed and can behave in an antisocial way at times, but he or she has many strong points that have become obscured by his or her reaction to the stress of school difficulties. The parents clearly are doing their best for their child by bringing him or her to be seen. If they receive support to do more of the useful things they are already doing, there is hope for improvement.

In other families the reverse may be true, and an approach which gives a diagnostic label can take the strain off family relationships and help all involved parties to focus on the child's needs. This can work for a number of reasons:

(1) An official 'label' is, for some families, the single most important thing they take away from their contact with child mental health professionals. Particularly with 'out of the ordinary' disorders such as autism or Tourette's syndrome, it can be an enormous relief to know that the problem has been recognised. It is no coincidence that demons in fairy stories often lose at least some of their power once they have been named. A child and family's sense of isolation is usually lessened once they know that other children and families have similar problems. Professionals should inform families of relevant voluntary groups. There are local and national parents' organisations for some child psychiatric disorders. By joining these groups, families are able to meet other people in similar situations, and may also gain access to newsletters, pamphlets, and lectures.

(2) A diagnosis may also be the 'passport' children and families need to be allowed access to special educational help, extra allowances, special holidays, and so on.

(3) A diagnosis often comes with a prognosis. When the prognosis for natural remission is good, the family may be happy to leave well alone and let time do the work. Indeed, defusing anxiety about the future may hasten spontaneous recovery.

(4) Explaining the implications of a diagnosis is also an opportunity for conveying important information on the nature and origin of symptoms. This too may have therapeutic value, as illustrated by the following three examples. Knowing that autism is not caused by parental unresponsiveness may help parents and others move beyond guilt and blame. Teachers and parents may find it easier to deal constructively with a hyperactive child once they know that he or she is not just being naughty. Knowing that Tourette's syndrome is a neurobiological disorder may help dispel ideas of 'possession'.

Symptoms and social impairments both need to be addressed

Treatment is unlikely to be effective if the problem has not been characterised accurately. The most skilled therapist will not get very far if an important contributory factor has been overlooked and is preventing progress. Therefore, an accurate assessment and formulation is essential before embarking on a management and treatment plan. It is often a mistake to focus exclusively on psychiatric symptoms. As described in Chapter 1, a psychiatric disorder should usually only be diagnosed if two conditions are met: the child has a recognised constellation of symptoms, *and* these symptoms have a significant impact. This adverse impact often takes the form of social impairment affecting home life, school work, friendships or leisure activities. Both symptoms and social impairment may need to be targeted by the intervention plan. Thus with a depressed adolescent, treating the low mood and sleeping problems may not be enough. It may also be essential to decide how to tackle the issue of lapsed friendships, and work out a plan for catching up with missed school work.

Complex problems may need complex solutions

The sorts of problems that present to child mental health specialists are rarely simple. Take, for example, a boy who presents with conduct problems. A careful assessment may suggest that all of the following are relevant:

- An inherited tendency to hyperactivity;
- Dietary intolerance to citrus fruits and additives;
- Specific reading retardation;
- A tendency to see other people as hostile when they are not;
- A family environment that has trained him to act coercively to get attention and avoid demands;
- Inadequate parental supervision;
- Membership of a deviant peer group.

Perhaps tackling just one of these factors can help; the resultant improvements in one area may break a vicious cycle and allow the child to recover. More often, however, clinical experience suggests that it is necessary to target several problem areas at once. Interventions for child mental health problems may target:

- *The child's physiological function* e.g. diet, medication;
- *Parents' and young person's knowledge of a condition* e.g. explanatory leaflets;
- *The external contingencies around the child's behaviour* e.g. parent training programmes, behavioural therapy for specific symptoms;
- *The internal world of the young person* e.g. cognitive therapy, interpersonal therapy;
- *Family relationships and beliefs* e.g. reduction in negative expressed emotion, family therapy;
- *Peer relationships* e.g. social skills training, group therapy;
- *School activities* e.g. extra help with reading, anti-bullying programme;
- *The family's economic and social environment* e.g. change of housing, befriending programmes for isolated families;
- *Alternatives to care in the family* e.g. fostering, admission to a residential community.

These are not mutually exclusive and several may be combined.

Working with other agencies

Many of the children and families seen by mental health services also need special input from other agencies, most notably education and social services. It is essential that each agency defines its role clearly and works in partnership with the other agencies, not at cross-purposes. Liaison meetings should be a means to an end rather than an end in themselves!

Treatment need not mirror aetiology

A disorder caused by physical factors may need psychological treatment, and *vice versa*. It is not always necessary to fight fire with fire; it is sometimes appropriate to fight fire with water! Thus a child's hysterical paralysis may respond better to physiotherapy than psychotherapy. Medication may help a child's hyperactivity even if that hyperactivity is due to being raised in a grossly inadequate orphanage. Equally, a child with genetically caused learning disability may benefit from special education. An adolescent with biologically determined schizophrenia may benefit from reduction of parental negative expressed emotion.

Selecting treatment approaches

The increasing emphasis on evidence-based health provision has much to be said for it. 'Clinical wisdom' and 'common sense' are surprisingly fallible. 'Self-evidently' beneficial interventions may turn out to be worse than nothing. For example, one careful randomised trial of an intuitively appealing package of social and psychological interventions for children at high risk of delinquency showed that the intervention significantly worsened their long-term outcome. Other plausible interventions have also been shown to have little or no effect. Thus conventional tricyclic drugs seem ineffective for depressed children and adolescents (see Chapter 10), and many of the psychological treatments for children administered in everyday clinical settings are ineffective, or almost so.

On the positive side, treatment trials, and meta-analyses based on these trials, have shown that some specific treatments for child psychiatric disorders are effective (see Box 30.1 for examples). But how effective are they? It is not enough to know that a particular treatment makes a statistically significant difference; it is also essential to know whether the size of this difference is large enough to be clinically significant. A tiny effect that is of no clinical relevance could still be statistically significant given a large enough trial or meta-analysis. There are several ways of measuring how effective a treatment is. The commonest one is *effect size*, which expresses change in 'standard deviation' units. For example, if untreated hyperkinetic children are an average of 2.5 standard deviations above the population mean on a measure of hyperactivity, and if treatment with stimulant medication brings them down to an average of 1.4 standard deviations above the population mean, the effect size is said to be 1.1 (i.e. 2.5 minus 1.4). Successful psychological therapies typically have effect sizes of around 0.6

Box 30.1   Examples of effective and ineffective treatments.

There is extensive and sound evidence for the effectiveness of:

- Medication in hyperkinesis
- Parent training in childhood conduct disorder
- Behavioural methods in soiling and enuresis
- Family therapy for anorexia.

There is reasonably sound evidence for:

- Cognitive behavioural therapy for adolescent depression
- Debriefing treatment for post-traumatic stress disorder
- Behavioural approaches to school refusal
- Home visiting schemes for physical maltreatment.

There is evidence that the following have little or no effect, or are harmful:

- Unfocused family work for conduct disorder
- Social skills therapy given in clinic settings for peer relationship problems
- Social work and general support for delinquency
- Medication with tricyclics for depression.

---

to 0.8 when administered in research settings. In ordinary clinic settings, however, the average effect size of psychological therapy may be 0.2 or less. What is this disparity due to? The exclusion of hard-to-treat children and families from research trials is likely to explain part of the difference. There are many other plausible explanations too, though only some are supported by the empirical evidence (see Box 30.2). The overall message for mental health professionals is both sobering and optimistic. It is sobering because psychological therapies as currently used in everyday settings have such a small effect that it seems difficult to justify the cost involved; but optimistic because three

---

Box 30.2   Why is psychological therapy much less effective in routine clinical practice than in research trials (following Weisz et al., 1995)?

Probably relevant:

- Clinics make less use of behavioural and cognitive approaches;
- Clinics rely less on specific, focused therapy methods;
- Clinics are less likely to structure therapy (e.g. through treatment manuals) or monitor therapy to ensure that the therapist adheres to the treatment plans;
- Clinics treat cases with high degrees of comorbidity and families who attend irregularly – both criteria for exclusion from many research trials.

Probably irrelevant:

- Research studies are more recent than clinic studies;
- Some research trials use subjects who are recruited volunteers rather than referred patients;
- Clinic settings are less conducive to success;
- Clinicians are less effective than research therapists;
- Research therapists have had special training in the methods just prior to the intervention;
- Clinics have to provide for a range of children, and a range of problems;
- Clinics are less likely to provide brief interventions.

changes in emphasis could boost effectiveness in future. These changes are a shift in emphasis towards behavioural and cognitive approaches; the use of specific, focused treatment methods rather than vague, diffuse or mixed approaches; and the use of structured therapy methods (e.g. through treatment manuals), with sufficient monitoring to ensure that therapists consistently adhere to treatment plans.

It obviously makes good sense to use treatment approaches that have been shown to work. In practice, though, it is not possible to rely just on published trials and protocols. For example, formal trials are usually on children who meet the full diagnostic criteria for operationalised syndromes, whereas many clinic cases have diffuse or partial syndromes that do not meet these criteria. How should they be treated? In addition, a child or family's circumstances and preferences may make standard protocols unworkable. There is clearly still a key role for clinical judgement and improvisation – extrapolating from published evidence on what works but not following it slavishly.

Modify treatment according to outcome

Having decided on a course of treatment, it is not enough just to give the treatment; it is also important to monitor the outcome. The treatment goals should have been recorded at the outset. Have these been attained? This can be judged clinically, though it is often helpful to seek independent corroboration, e.g. by administering questionnaires to the child, parents or teachers. If the goals have not been attained, it is often sensible to reassess the child and review the formulation before giving up or pressing on with more of the same. Perhaps the child has been resistant to treatment because the initial diagnosis was wrong – a revised formulation may suggest a revised treatment. Even if the original formulation still seems correct, it may be appropriate to switch to a different treatment. Even when trials have shown that treatment X usually works better than treatment Y, a minority of patients may respond better to Y than to X. If the child and family are keen, a second-choice treatment can be tried when the first-choice treatment fails.

Further reading

Garralda, M.E. (1993) *Managing Children with Psychiatric Problems*. BMJ, London.

Kazdin, A.E. (1988) *Child Psychotherapy – Developing and Identifying Effective Treatments*. Pergamon, Oxford.

McCord, J. (1992) The Cambridge-Somerville study: a pioneering longitudinal-experimental study of delinquency prevention. In *Preventing Antisocial Behavior: Interventions from Birth through Adolescence* (J. McCord and R.E. Tremblay, eds) Guildford Press, New York, pp. 196–206. (This careful study puts an end to any notion that common sense interventions are bound to do more good than harm.)

Weisz, J.R. *et al.* (1995) Child and adolescent psychotherapy outcomes in experiments versus clinics: Why the disparity? *Journal of Abnormal Child Psychology*, 23, 83–106.

31   Medication and Diet

MEDICATION: GENERAL PRINCIPLES

Parents often feel uneasy about using medication to alter children's behaviour or emotions; teachers and mental health professionals may feel similarly. These concerns are understandable and partly justified. For example, stimulants are sometimes inappropriately prescribed for children who are disruptive but not hyperactive. Mentally retarded children may be given high doses of neuroleptics for long periods in a futile attempt to suppress their challenging behaviour. Though it is true that psychotropic medication can be used unwisely, it is also important to remember that suitable doses used for appropriate indications can be of great benefit.

Prescribing for children is not simply a matter of scaling adult doses down in proportion to the child's body weight. There are pharmacokinetic and pharmacodynamic differences between children and adults that make paediatric psychopharmacology both quantitatively and qualitatively different from adult psychopharmacology.

Pharmacokinetics

The relationship between the dose administered and the effective concentration in the brain depends on several pharmacokinetic factors (Box 31.1). Developmental considerations are relevant to each of these factors. *Compliance* may depend more on the motivation of parents and teachers than on that of the child. *Absorption* can be influenced by the fact that stomach acidity is generally lower in children. This reduces the rate of absorption of acidic drugs such as tricyclics (since less of the drug is in the lipid-soluble unionised form). Children have particularly active livers, so *clearance* is fast for drugs metabolised by the liver. This results in an exaggeration of the normal 'first pass' effect, i.e. a particularly high fraction of the medication absorbed by the gut is cleared by the liver from the portal circulation before it even reaches the systemic circulation. *Distribution* is affected by the relatively high proportion of extracellular fluid in young children; the greater diversion of medication to the extracellular fluid tends to reduce the amount in blood and brain. The *blood-brain barrier* is more permeable in children than adults so drugs can get through more easily,

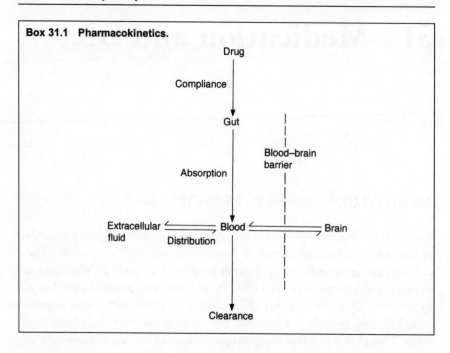

Box 31.1 Pharmacokinetics.

but this easier access to the brain may be partly offset by a higher concentration of drug-binding proteins in the cerebrospinal fluid.

The various pharmacokinetic differences between children and adults pull in opposite directions, with bioavailability being reduced in children by faster clearance, slower absorption and a greater volume of distribution, but increased by greater blood-brain permeability. The effect of rapid hepatic clearance often dominates, with the result that weight-for-weight doses for psychotropics are often 50–100% higher for children than adults. The need for relatively high doses decreases as children get older, dropping fairly sharply around puberty. By mid to late adolescence, drug dosage follows adult norms. Blood levels are useful for adjusting the dosage of some drugs, such as tricyclics and lithium, but are unhelpful with other drugs, e.g. stimulants. Children are very variable in their response to medication and the dosage prescribed needs to be titrated primarily against clinical response, seeing recommended drug dosages (and recommended blood levels) as helpful guidelines rather than set in stone. Because the appropriate dosage is hard to predict in advance, it is sensible to start with a low dose and work up slowly. Once-a-day doses improve compliance but divided doses may be needed to reduce peak and trough effects.

Pharmacodynamics

Once a drug has reached the brain, its effect depends on its interactions with drug receptors. There are major developmental changes in the number and relative proportion of different types of receptors. Since a single drug may activate multiple receptor types, and since these various receptor types may have markedly different effects, developmental changes in the balance of receptor types can result in the same drug having very different effects on children and adults. Perhaps this is why stimulants produce euphoria in adults but not in children – tending, if anything, to make children dysphoric. Psychotropic drugs that work in adults do not necessarily work in children, and *vice versa*. Furthermore, drugs familiar to adult psychiatrists for one set of disorders may be used by child psychiatrists for a rather different set of disorders. For example, tricyclics work well for adult depression but do not seem to be very effective in childhood depression, yet relatively low doses of tricyclics can be used to treat childhood hyperactivity or enuresis.

MEDICATION: SPECIFIC GROUPS OF DRUGS

Stimulants

Methylphenidate or dexamphetamine is usually the drug of choice for the treatment of severe and pervasive hyperactivity. Indications and side-effects are discussed in detail in Chapter 5. Stimulants have a powerful effect, usually reducing hyperactivity by more than one standard deviation. Since most of the children treated with stimulants are two or three standard deviations more hyperactive than average, stimulants typically reduce rather than abolish hyperactivity, emphasising the need for educational and behavioural help too. When hyperactivity is associated with conduct problems, stimulant treatment often improves the conduct problems as well as the hyperactivity.

Hyperactivity in autistic or mentally retarded children may also be helped by stimulants, but sometimes at the cost of a worsening in repetitive behaviours (see Chapters 4 and 23). Since stimulants can precipitate or aggravate tics, most clinicians avoid stimulants for children who have a tic disorder or a strong family history of tic disorders, using clonidine or imipramine instead; stimulants are reserved for severe hyperactivity where these other drugs fail.

The most effective stimulants in the treatment of hyperactivity have mixed adrenergic and dopaminergic actions. Whether this provides a useful clue to the pathogenesis of hyperactivity is uncertain, however, since other classes of anti-hyperactivity drugs have very different pharmacological actions.

Clonidine

This is a specific alpha-2 agonist that can reduce hyperactivity and tics. These effects are not generally marked and can take several months to develop. Sedation and dysphoria can be problematic. Since cardiac effects have been described, ECG monitoring as for tricyclic antidepressants is recommended.

Tricyclic antidepressants (TCAs)

Nocturnal enuresis can be treated with low to moderate doses of TCAs (e.g. 25–75 mg of imipramine nocte), though it is generally preferable to use a behavioural approach or desmopressin instead (see Chapter 17). Hyperactivity can also be treated with low doses of TCAs if stimulants have failed or are contraindicated (see Chapters 5 and 14). In full dosage, clomipramine – a TCA that acts primarily on serotonin reuptake – has been shown to be helpful for obsessive-compulsive disorder (Chapter 13). Judging largely from adult evidence, TCAs may also be useful in panic disorder. Whether TCAs have a role in the treatment of depressed children and adolescents remains controversial: meta-analyses do not support this practice, but many clinicians feel that some severely depressed youngsters do respond well to TCAs (see Chapter 10). The use of TCAs in the treatment of school refusal due to separation anxiety can no longer be recommended (see Chapter 9).

In the low doses used in the treatment of enuresis and hyperactivity, TCAs have relatively few side-effects. With high doses, however, common side-effects include dry mouth, headache, sedation and malaise. There is also a risk of cardiac arrhythmias and sudden death. To reduce this risk, an ECG should be carried out before embarking on anything more than low-dose treatment, to check that there are no pre-existing arrhythmias or cardiac conduction problems. Further ECGs should be obtained as the dose is progressively increased to monitor for the warning signs of prolonged P-R and Q-T intervals.

Selective serotonin reuptake inhibitors (SSRIs)

These are of proven value in the treatment of obsessive-compulsive disorder in young people (Chapter 13). Preliminary evidence also suggests a role in the treatment of depressed children and adolescents (Chapter 10). There are hints that SSRIs may sometimes be helpful for social phobia and elective mutism (Chapter 15) and perhaps for hyperactivity too. Common side effects include gastrointestinal disturbance and restlessness. Though it has been claimed that SSRIs can precipitate severe aggression or self-harm, there is no compelling evidence for this.

Monoamine oxidase inhibitors (MAOIs)

The availability of a selective and reversible MAOI, moclobemide, has made this class of drugs much easier and safer to prescribe since adverse interactions with a normal diet are now very unlikely. MAOIs are of demonstrated value in the treatment of hyperactivity. Their role, if any, in the treatment of depressed children and adolescents is still uncertain.

Neuroleptics

These are particularly useful in the treatment of children and adolescents with psychotic disorders and tic disorders (see Chapters 21 and 14). They are sometimes useful for autistic or mentally retarded children (Chapters 4 and 23), and are third-line treatments for hyperactivity. They are not appropriate long-term treatments for the aggressive behaviour of mentally retarded children (Chapter 23).

Neuroleptics should always be used with considerable caution because of their potentially serious side-effects. Sedation can interfere with learning. In the first few weeks of treatment, neuroleptics commonly cause extrapyramidal side effects such as acute dystonic reactions or parkinsonism. This risk is probably lower with some of the newer neuroleptics such as sulpiride and risperidone. When using more traditional neuroleptics such as haloperidol, there is a case for giving antimuscarinic drugs such as benzhexol prophylactically to prevent extrapyramidal reactions. The antimuscarinic can be withdrawn after about six weeks because it is rarely needed beyond that time and often does more long-term harm than good.

The neuroleptic malignant syndrome is an uncommon but potentially fatal hazard. The four cardinal features of the full syndrome are pyrexia, muscular rigidity, mental changes such as mild confusion, and evidence of autonomic dysfunction, e.g. pallor, sweating or shivering. Blood tests may show raised creatinine phosphokinase and a high white count. Since the early symptoms can progress in less than 48 hours to hyperpyrexia, rigidity, circulatory collapse, and multiple organ failure, it is obviously essential to monitor carefully any child who develops suspicious symptoms while on neuroleptics, discontinuing the medication immediately if suspicions seem confirmed. The full syndrome requires intensive care and muscle relaxants.

Long-term treatment with neuroleptics can lead to the eventual emergence of dyskinesias, which may be irreversible even if medication is stopped. The risk of these tardive dyskinesias is related to the lifetime dose, and may be further increased if antimuscarinics have also been administered for long periods. There is little evidence for the frequent assertion that neurological damage also increases the risk of tardive dyskinesias.

Lithium

This is widely used for the treatment and prophylaxis of bipolar affective disorder in adults, and is probably of similar value in young people. Lithium also has a role in the treatment of severe outbursts of aggression that are triggered by minimal provocation and that have been resistant to appropriate psychological management. Lithium dosage is adjusted to obtain a plasma level of around 0.7–1.0 mmol/litre on samples obtained 12 hours after the most recent dose. Common side-effects include thirst, gastrointestinal disturbance and fine tremor. Since there is a risk of hypothyroidism, thyroid function tests should be carried out before and during treatment. Routine monitoring of renal function is probably unnecessary. Excessive dosage leads to potentially fatal toxicity. The common early signs are coarse tremor, worsening gastrointestinal disturbance, and mild confusion. Since these warning signs of toxicity may be less prominent in mentally retarded children, lithium needs to be used with particular caution in this group.

Anticonvulsants as psychotropics

Anticonvulsants can affect the behaviour of epileptic children for better or worse: reducing seizures may improve behaviour, but anticonvulsants may also produce sedation, irritability or hyperactivity. For children who do not have epilepsy, there is little reason to suppose that anticonvulsants are of value for children's emotional or behavioural problems (even if the children do have minor EEG abnormalities). The one exception is carbamazepine, which can be used instead of lithium to prevent recurrences of bipolar affective disorder.

Benzodiazepines, antihistamines and other minor tranquillizers

Although these are probably the most commonly prescribed psychotropic drugs for children, they are also arguably the least justified. Long-term problems with sleep or anxiety problems are much more likely to respond to psychological approaches. Benzodiazepines may sometimes be useful in the treatment of intense acute anxiety, e.g. before a medical procedure (though it is better still to desensitise children in advance if they are going to encounter feared procedures or situations repeatedly).

DIET

Doctors have been prescribing diets for millennia, and diets are still an important treatment for a wide range of physical problems, including eczema, migraine, phenylketonuria and intractable epilepsy. Specific foods may need to be avoided because they trigger off allergic reactions or because they have other sorts of adverse effects. As one example of a non-allergic effect, fava beans contain oxidising agents that interact with an inherited enzyme deficiency to precipitate haemolytic crises in individuals with favism. When it is unclear how a particular dietary ingredient has an adverse effect, it is better to speak of dietary *intolerance* than of dietary *allergy*.

Does dietary intolerance trigger child psychiatric problems? Feingold suggested that hyperactivity and learning problems were linked to food additives and natural salicylates. The Feingold diet to avoid these substances has been widely adopted, but has not generally proved particularly effective in controlled trials. There is better evidence for the efficacy of an approach based on the 'few foods' diet. Children are initially started out on a very restricted diet that excludes not only additives but also many natural foods, including dairy and wheat products and most fruits. If there is no improvement after two or three weeks, the diet is abandoned. The few foods approach only works for some children.

If behaviour does improve on the few foods diet, the excluded foods are reintroduced one at a time to identify which of them trigger behaviour problems. In some instances, it is possible to carry out double-blind challenges to establish whether a particular food really does make a difference. Controlled evaluations do suggest that this approach can identify foods that worsen children's behaviour. There is no one culprit – different children are intolerant to different foods, and many children are intolerant to several. Additives are common culprits, but so too are dairy products, chocolate, wheat, oranges, tomatoes and eggs. It is unusual for a child to react only to additives; most children who are sensitive to additives are also sensitive to one or more natural foods as well. Although diet is often thought of as a treatment for hyperactivity, the children who respond to the 'few foods' approach typically become less irritable and disruptive as well as less hyperactive. Whether the same approach would help children who were irritable and oppositional but not hyperactive is unclear.

The few foods approach is very hard work for all concerned and not all children and parents can see it through to completion. Cooking a special diet for weeks on end is more than some busy parents can manage and buying special foods can also be very expensive. Furthermore, there is little point embarking on this approach if the child is likely to cheat frequently by stealing from the fridge, buying forbidden foods, or eating other children's school lunches! Is it possible to predict in advance which children are likely to respond to diet? Unfortunately, it is not possible to predict from blood or skin tests (not to mention more dubious tests involving hair analysis or dowsing). Two clinical pointers to a good response are, firstly, that parents have previously noted reactions to food and, secondly, that the children have cravings for particular foods (which may turn out to be the foods that trigger behavioural problems). Parental observations and the child's cravings can be used to design a tailor-made exclusion diet; if behaviour is improved, the excluded foods are reintroduced one by one to identify the culprits. How this 'short cut' compares with the few foods approach has yet to be formally evaluated.

OTHER PHYSICAL TREATMENTS

Electroconvulsive therapy (ECT) is rarely used for children and has not been adequately evaluated. It may be considered when adequate trials of medication have not relieved severe depression or catatonia.

Surgery. Psychosurgery is not indicated for children, but it is worth noting that successful epilepsy surgery may cure children not only of their seizures but also of associated behavioural problems. For example, hemispherectomy for hemiplegic children with intractable seizures often relieves not only seizures but hyperactivity and irritability too. It is unclear whether this behavioural improvement stems from the abolition of seizures, the withdrawal of anti-convulsants, or the removal of dysfunctional brain tissue.

Subject review

Taylor, E. (1994) Physical treatments. In *Child and Adolescent Psychiatry: Modern Approaches*, 3rd edn (M. Rutter, E. Taylor and L. Hersov, eds) Blackwell Science, Oxford, pp. 880–899.

Further reading

Carter, C.M. *et al.* (1993) Effects of a few foods diet in attention deficit disorder. *Archives of Disease in Childhood*, **69**, 564–568.

32 Behaviourally-Based Treatments

Behavioural methods used to be based on the notion that all behaviours are learned, and so can be unlearned. However, a less extreme form of behaviourism states that the expression of most behaviour is influenced by antecedent events and consequent responses. Altering these may change the frequency of the behaviour.

Classical conditioning involves stimulus–contingent effects as described by Pavlov in 1927. A previously neutral stimulus becomes associated with one which triggers the physiological response, and in time the new stimulus alone (now called *conditioned*) leads to a similar response. Treatments based on this model condition new physiological responses such as relaxation to the stimulus. Examples that work well with children and adolescents include systematic desensitisation for traumas and phobias.

Operant conditioning involves response–contingent effects as described by Skinner in 1938. Responses to stimuli, or indeed behaviours of any kind, become more frequent or stronger if they lead to rewarding consequences (*positive reinforcement*), or to escape from unpleasant consequences (*negative reinforcement*). Behaviours become less frequent if previously rewarding consequences are taken away (*extinction*), or if they lead to unpleasant consequences (*punishment*). Treatments based on this model consistently change the contingencies which follow a behaviour. This may be to increase desired behaviour through rewards (a star chart for clean underpants without soiling), or to reduce undesired behaviour through punishment (being made to clean the floor after throwing dinner on it). This approach also includes ensuring that undesirable symptoms or behaviours are not unintentionally rewarded, e.g. ensuring that a child is not rewarded for psychogenic abdominal pain by being allowed to miss school and stay at home.

Social learning theory developed by Bandura in the 1960s led to a general widening of the behavioural model to recognise the primacy of human relationships in influencing learning. In children and adolescents, Patterson confirmed the central role of parental attention in providing rewards, and showed that in families where there is little positive interaction, children may behave antisocially to get attention, even though this may be of a negative kind. Treatments based on this model increase the attention paid by carers to children when they behave desirably (e.g. by speaking warmly to a child who is playing quietly) and withdraw attention when the child is behaving undesirably (e.g. by turning away and stopping talking to a child who is screaming). An example of this approach working well is the use of parent training to reduce a child's antisocial behaviour.

BEHAVIOURAL METHODS IN PRACTICE

Assessment

Rather than initially ascribing meaning to a behaviour, a *functional analysis* is performed. The Antecedents, Behaviour itself, and Consequences (ABC) are carefully characterised in great detail (Box 32.1). Examples of antecedents: Before a tantrum in a four-year-old: mother's nagging demand at bedtime; or, sibling takes toy. Before a panic attack in a 15-year-old: outdoors on a big playing field; in a crowded marketplace. Before psychogenic abdominal pain in a ten-year-old: a row between parents; due to hand in difficult homework. Sometimes changing the antecedents alone ('stimulus control') is sufficient to alleviate the problem.

Box 32.1 An ABC analysis.	
Antecedent events (the setting)	Experiences for child just prior to behaviour People present Places Times of day Situations
Behaviour	Nature: detailed description of what actually happened Onset date Frequency Severity Duration of episodes
Consequences	Changes in demands and expectations of child by others Changes in attention and social set up Attainment of child's immediate goals and wants Impact on siblings and parents

Methods for gathering information include: detailed behavioural descriptions from parents, charts, diaries, visits to home or school to observe behaviour in context, or video of this.

Behavioural analyses thus concentrate on the here and now of what actually happens. The meaning to the parents of the behaviour ('he's becoming a criminal like his uncle'), and their explanations for it ('it's the crisps, doctor') may usefully be explored but are not part of a strict behaviourist approach.

Negotiation of goals with parents and young person

(1) Specify the target behaviours as precisely as possible. Many parents find this difficult, having diffuse concerns: 'he's disobedient', 'he's a Jekyll and Hyde', 'she's sad' etc. The work is to help the parent work out specifically what is worrying.

(2) Assess the impact of the behaviours on the child's life, and on that of the siblings and parents, considering the following domains:
   (a) Emotional/personal impact
   (b) Social
   (c) Developmental
   (d) Learning/competence
   (e) Self-esteem.
   Going through this list often helps the parents review the overall impact from the child's point of view, rather than just their own. For example, they may have arrived concerned by the smell and inconvenience to themselves of a boy who soils. Assessing the impact may make them aware of the social impact on friendships, and emotions. This is often helpful in reducing negativity, and in engaging sympathy and motivation to implement the treatment programme. Parents also become fully aware of the long-term disadvantages of the current situation, rather than just the immediate inconvenience, which may further add to the gains they can visualise from engaging in therapy.

(3) Agree the desired outcome in behavioural terms. Again, this will not be a generality ('he should become nice to me') but specific ('he will dress himself after being asked only once in the morning, without shouting at me; he will be in bed by 8.30 at night'). If a child has frequent major tantrums lasting over five minutes involving kicking and throwing, an appropriate target may be to reduce this to once a week. Total abolition is unrealistic and unnecessary.

(4) Formulate the *positive* behaviours desired. This may not come easily to parents, who are more inclined to think in terms of stopping negative behaviours such as fighting, running, shouting, wetting the bed, etc. The desired behaviours in each case might be: play nicely with your brother, walk calmly, speak quietly, and use the toilet properly. The major part of behavioural work is not the elimination of unwanted behaviour (a child who is only aware of what *not* to do has no help in finding his or her direction, and if totally obedient would stay rooted to the spot) but the promotion of desired behaviour in its place, so the unwanted behaviour simply fades away. Once the desired behaviours have been formulated, it is possible to start planning an intervention plan, with emphasis on how to make it clear to the child what is desired, how to introduce it into the child's repertoire and practice it, and how to reward it once it starts occurring.

(5)   Explain to parents and child:
       (a)   Why the child is behaving this way, in terms of learned habits and circumstances maintaining it, rather than character traits or inner conflicts;
       (b)   That therefore there is a possibility for change, but this will require their change too.

Techniques

To increase desired behaviours:

- *Positive reinforcement:* reward desired behaviour (see below for discussion of rewards).
- *Negative reinforcement:* remove aversive stimulus after desired behaviour has occurred (e.g. stop nagging when child goes to bed).
- *Provide a model* with which child identifies.
- *Train skills* with rehearsal, and role-play.
- *Remove interfering conditions.*

To reduce undesired behaviours:

- *Stimulus change:* remove or change controlling antecedent stimuli.

- *Extinction.* This means removal of previous reward identified with reinforcement of the behaviour, e.g. no longer giving attention to child who is naughty. Parents need to be warned that for a period, the child will work even harder to get back to the previous status quo and behaviour may worsen. Ignoring may mean involving more than just parents, e.g. the aggressive youth getting admiration from his peers.

- *Differential reinforcement* of incompatible behaviour. As noted above, this principle is central to much behavioural work. The desired or prosocial behaviour that should be occurring is identified and rewarded, such as sitting nicely during mealtimes instead of running around, playing cooperatively instead of fighting, spending the night in the bedroom rather than wandering downstairs, etc.

- *Punishment.* This can involve the application of mildly noxious stimuli following inappropriate behaviour. In everyday childrearing this is frequently a telling off or verbal criticism. Mild occasional physical punishment such as a light smack say once a week has not been shown to be deleterious to children, whereas prolonged heavy painful punishment in an atmosphere of cold, hostile rejection is certainly deleterious. Physical punishment is often popular with parents as it may temporarily suppress behaviour, and so be very rewarding for the parent, but often the behaviour re-emerges later and has not been truly extinguished. It may have a role in immediate suppression of damaging behaviour, such as putting fingers into power sockets, or running across the road, but needs to be followed by explanation and plentiful reinforcement of actions incompatible with those being punished. This is very different from the destructive cycles which can occur when desperate parents use harsh physical punishment in extreme, inconsistent, retaliatory ways, without accompanying choices or encouragement for more acceptable alternative behaviours. For all these reasons and because of instances of abuse, application of aversive stimuli is seldom a part of therapeutic programmes, which tend to use other methods, seeing reduced parental use of physical punishments as an index of successful substitution of more appropriate methods.

- *Time out*. This is shorthand for 'time out from positive reinforcement'. Usually it involves taking a child aged around three to eight away from the context where the behaviour occurred, to a dull quiet place for a few minutes. This differs from extinction since the child is removed from all the usual general social stimulation and reinforcement, not just from a specific identified reinforcer. It has the advantage of being a high-impact procedure that is not noxious (although it may well be perceived by the child as a punishment). There are a number of practicalities to setting up a TO programme. These include the following: the rules must be clear, and it should be given for fairly major infractions; a warning and an alternative behaviour should be given to the child before applying it ('please stop hitting and sit down or you'll go to time out'); the child should be taken there in a calm way, using physical force if necessary but not hurting the child; the space or room must be cleared of entertaining items; the parent or teacher must keep an eye on the child but not engage in conversation or recrimination (this would unwittingly be giving attention); and the child must be calm for a minute before coming out.

- *Response cost*. Here specified amounts of reinforcers are withdrawn from the child when he or she displays the unwanted behaviour. This requires that a previous reward system is in place, involving money, points, privileges, etc.; there has to be something positive to withdraw.

- *Overcorrection*. The child is required not only to put right what he or she did wrong, but do more by way of restitution. A variant gets the child to overlearn a response physically incompatible with the original misbehaviour, e.g. repeatedly taking shoes off on entering a house having trailed mud in previously.

- *Desensitisation*. The repeated exposure of an aversive stimulus in a situation where the child is relaxed and reassured. For example, going up through a hierarchy of phobic stimuli while the child is practising relaxation techniques with the mother present.

A note on rewards

- Every child is different. Help parents decide what is motivating, and always check with the child and ask for their suggestions.

- Rewards may be intangible such as time with parents, etc. Tangible rewards do not have to be expensive, they can be sitting in a parent's place at dinner, wearing special clothes, extra TV etc. There are many other alternatives to money and presents.

- They need to be given as soon as possible after the behaviour has occurred (not a bike for Christmas).

- Check what unintended rewards a child is getting for undesired behaviour (e.g. peer approval). Be aware of when desired behaviour is occurring and monitor if it is being rewarded (is the child actually being ignored when she is playing quietly?).

- Check that rewards are being consistently applied.

- Switch rewards every few days. Many parents will say 'I tried that, it worked for a few days then didn't work'. But how many adults would find the same chocolates just as exciting after getting them for ten days in a row?

- When stuck for a reward, consider the Premack principle, which is to use as a reward what a person chooses to spend most of their free time doing. This could be playing on the computer, lying in bed, or whatever is acceptable.

- With older children and adolescents, cultivate self rewarding. Like rewards given by others, these may be intangible, e.g. praising oneself for good behaviour, or tangible, e.g. a treat.

Implementation

To learn a new behaviour, a child must know *what* to do, *how* to do it, and *when* to do it. If a parent is to change the child's behaviour, they too must be equally clear. For the change to occur will require *competence*, or being able to do it, and *performance* repeatedly, which requires the will to do it.

The intervention will only rarely consist of the mechanical implementation of standardised techniques for altering the frequency of behaviours. Rather, most contemporary behavioural therapy draws upon these behavioural principles but adapts them into a wider context. General measures employed include:

- Planning ahead, e.g. reducing school pressures on a phobic girl, avoiding taking a hyperactive boy to the supermarket, taking fight-prone siblings out to the park rather than keeping them indoors.

- Negotiating with the child or adolescent. Many parents make what seem to them to be reasonable demands, only to find them disobeyed, which leads to a major confrontation. Getting parents to negotiate basic situations – bedtime routines, what the family does on Saturdays, for example, – pays big dividends. However, they require the parents to stop and listen to the children and find a compromise which achieves the goal. In return, the young people get to realise their views have been taken into account.

- Addressing beliefs and mood states of both parents and children. Early behavioural programmes were successful, but only in that proportion of cases where the parents carried out the instructions, which was often only half or less of those enrolled. Most practitioners now would spend a considerable amount of time addressing parents' fears and worries ('If I leave him to scream I feel a bad mother', 'I can't bear to ignore crying out at night since it reminds me of being left as a child').

- Adapting the programme according to progress. This is central to behavioural approaches, where success is carefully measured, and if it is not occurring then this is examined in detail and the plan revised, or a new strategy tried, or a course of action more acceptable to the parent found. Rather like a game of chess, particular moves do not produce victory in themselves, but have to be repeatedly adapted as part of an overall strategy to succeed.

EVALUATION OF BEHAVIOURALLY-BASED THERAPIES

Criticisms

Behaviour therapy is soulless and ignores the world of the mind, treating people like dogs or pigeons. Motivation, dreams, fears and beliefs about ways of doing things are ignored.

By concentrating on the presented symptom, a behaviour therapist may entirely miss the broader meaning of the difficulty for the individual and the worries and stresses which led to the difficulty arising in the first place.

By thinking in a 'scientific, logical' linear manner the behaviour therapist may miss the network of relationships and systems in the background which are maintaining the symptom behaviour. A child's tantrums may be the result of a disturbed attachment relationship with mother and require far more than a few star charts to put right.

No place is given for the intangible but essential parts of the therapeutic relationship. Some problems, such as a disability or a bereavement, cannot be taken away. Yet families and children often gain a great deal from being helped to come to terms with these predicaments and can move forward with sympathetic counselling.

It is chiefly effective only for circumscribed complaints, and cannot tackle general relationship difficulties as may occur following sexual abuse or neglectful parenting.

Rejoinders

While early behaviourism in the 1950s and 1960s may have been somewhat mechanical, nowadays it is an approach which is flexible and practitioners take the individual's meanings and beliefs and relationships into consideration. Parents and children like having the opportunity to do something practical to alleviate a problem, rather than just sitting and talking about feelings. Through reductions in problems and increases in good times, whole relationships do change and this is very important. The therapist shares the agenda with the family, rather than making clever formulations hidden from them.

Outcome studies

There have been an enormous number (literally thousands) of well conducted single-case studies, and hundreds of randomised controlled trials of behavioural treatments for children and adolescents. Bodily functions such as eating, sleeping, wetting and soiling have been successfully tackled, with effect sizes of 0.7–1.5 standard deviations. Antisocial behaviour in prepubertal children has repeatedly been shown to be improved, with typical effect sizes of 0.4–0.8 SD. Hyperactivity is helped in the short term while the behavioural contingencies are applied, but the changes are not usually long-lasting and the effect size is only around 0.2–0.4 SD. Emotional disorders such as school refusal and psychogenic pain have responded, but usually with less dramatic improvements.

Subject review

Herbert, M. (1994) Behavioural methods. In *Child and Adolescent Psychiatry: Modern Approaches*, 3rd edn (M. Rutter, E. Taylor and L. Hersov, eds) Blackwell Science, Oxford, pp. 858–879.

33 Cognitive and Interpersonal Therapies

COGNITIVE APPROACHES

These go beyond externally observable behaviour and acknowledge the internal world of thoughts and mental schemas, if not feelings. Cognitions are recognised as having an independent effect on behaviour, and not being just secondary epiphenomena to external events and internal physiology. The mind is recognised as being able to direct behaviour as well as be aware of it.

Behavioural methods are especially useful in situations where:

(1) External contingencies can be controlled, e.g. in a family with parents present for several hours a day, or in a school class.
(2) Individuals have cognitive abilities which are less well developed, e.g. young children, those with low intellect.
(3) Problems are easily identifiable by observable behaviours.

Cognitive methods can be especially useful for situations where:

(1) The individual is less constrained by external contingencies and is relying more on self-direction and choosing their own immediate environment, e.g. out on the street, in the school playground, or alone away from home.
(2) Individuals have the capacity for independent thought which can be translated into action.
(3) Problems are primarily within the mind and not observable to an outsider in terms of behaviour.

Cognitive approaches draw upon the behaviourist tradition of precise measurement and objective empirical validation, and are often combined with behavioural interventions. They are backed by a body of evidence demonstrating cognitive distortions or deficits in various disorders affecting children and young people, including aggression, ADHD, anxiety, PTSD, and depression.

While cognitive approaches designed for specific disorders tend to focus on the content and structure of cognitions within the domain in question, interpersonal problem-solving approaches focus on enhancing the general processes required to generate solutions to everyday social problems. Rather than providing the 'right' way of thinking about the problem, this approach emphasises helping the child generate their own, more useful, solutions.

Cognitive approaches to specific disorders

Depression

Distortions in thinking similar to those found in adults have also been demonstrated in children. Treatment programmes include:

(1) Self-control skills promoting consequences for action (praise self more, punish self less), self-monitoring (paying attention to positive things they do), self-evaluation (setting less perfectionist standards for self), and assertiveness training.
(2) Social skills, including methods to initiate interactions, maintain interactions, handle conflict and use relaxation and imagery.
(3) Cognitive restructuring, involving confronting children about their lack of evidence for their distorted perceptions.

A few randomised controlled trials have shown children who receive CT for depression clearly do better than waiting list controls, and than those receiving traditional counselling. However, only about half respond, and even then the subsequent relapse rate is high, with a further 50% of these becoming depressed again. Nonetheless, this is useful since there is little evidence antidepressants work in children and adolescents. Refinements and adjunctive treatments in addition to the basic CT package are currently being developed.

Anxiety

Again, practice in children has followed that in adults. Similar techniques are used including correction of distortions in thinking, development of positive self-talk, guided imagery enabling mastery over fear-provoking situations, and relaxation during exposure. Randomised trials show good results, with over half of cases being returned to the normal range.

Aggression

Aggressive children have been shown to:

- Perceive far more hostile cues in social situations;
- Attend to fewer cues when interpreting the meaning of others' behaviour;
- Attribute hostile intentions to others in ambiguous situations;
- Underperceive their own level of aggressiveness;
- Generate fewer verbal, assertive solutions to conflict situations but more physically attacking ones;
- Believe this aggression will reduce aversive reactions from others and gain them tangible positive outcomes.

Aggressive adolescents additionally believe aggressive behaviour will increase their self-esteem, and value dominance and revenge more, and social affiliation less, than controls. Interventions usually target these cognitive anomalies, but also address general interpersonal social skills (see below), with a particular emphasis on slowing down automatic, immediate reactions to provocative situations in order to allow more deliberation about suitable responses. Trials have shown significant reductions in aggressive behaviour using these methods, persisting at one and three year follow-ups. Effects in prepubertal children are enhanced by the addition of parent-training programmes.

Attention deficit hyperactivity disorder

ADHD children have short attention spans and difficulty in repressing immediate, often inappropriate, responses to stimuli rather than stopping and evaluating the best course of action. Cognitive therapy should in theory be well suited to address this kind of difficulty. Self-instructional programmes which attempt to slow down cognitive processing to permit examination of alternative courses of action have, however, not been especially effective. It is as if the very nature of the problem means the capacity to activate a different approach to information processing is absent. Behavioural programmes controlling immediate contingencies are more effective, but less so than medication, and with smaller effect sizes than in conduct disordered children.

SOCIAL PROBLEM-SOLVING SKILLS PROGRAMMES

Myrna Shure and George Spivack in the USA have developed perhaps the most comprehensive intervention programme, called Interpersonal Cognitive Problem Solving (ICPS). Many studies have shown that several groups of children and adolescents lack interpersonal skills, especially aggressive children, rejected children, isolated children with few friends, and some depressed children. The ICPS programme concentrates on three core *cognitive processes* that have been shown to be impaired.

(1) *Generation of alternatives:* The ability to come up with several different solutions to a problem situation.
(2) *Consequential thinking:* The ability to see the immediate and longer-term consequences of each line of action proposed, and incorporate this in coming to a decision about the best response.
(3) *Means-ends thinking:* The ability to distinguish the purpose of a plan of action from its content, so ways round an obstacle can be devised if the initial plan fails.

A variety of methods are used to foster these skills, including both individual and group processes with games, discussion, and group interaction techniques.

They can be applied even at preschool level, for example the words '*or*' and '*different*' are taught to help children think about alternative ways to tackle situations, e.g. 'I can hit him *or* tell him I'm cross. Hitting is *different* from telling'. As these programmes have evolved, it has become evident that a number of core skills in perceiving the mental states of others are required to be developed in many children:

(1) *Emotional awareness*. Becoming sensitive to the feelings and wishes of others. In some children, they may even be unaware of their own basic feelings. As these are developed, they can be taught that not everyone feels the same way about things, and that children may feel differently at different times ('I can ask her later when she's feeling better').

(2) *Social information gathering*. Games are played to develop skills in reading situations, listening for clues, and asking others what they mean.

(3) *Understanding motives*. Children are taught to go beyond another person's behaviour to think why they might be acting that way, and to generate solutions appropriate to these motives.

Having developed these skills, most programmes go on to apply them initially in hypothetical situations, and then in real situations. The cognitive steps may be spelt out to the child, e.g. they are encouraged to count off on each finger as they go through the sequence of STOP-THINK-DO-REVIEW in generating and enacting solutions.

Outcome studies show strong effects in hypothetical situations, but more mixed results in real life situations. These programmes are considerably enhanced if adults around the children have been taught the thinking too, and thus can reinforce it in the heat of the moment. Under these circumstances short-term results are good, but long-term follow-ups have not yet been carried out.

INTERPERSONAL PSYCHOTHERAPY (IPT)

This mode of therapy was developed for treating depression by Gerald Klerman and Myrna Weissman in New York, and then specifically modified for use with adolescents. IPT is a time-limited, brief psychotherapy based on the premise that depression occurs in the context of interpersonal relationships. The two main goals are to identify and treat firstly the patient's depressive symptoms and secondly the problem areas associated with the onset of the depression. Five specific areas are reviewed, and one or two worked on. Four are the same as in adult IPT: grief, interpersonal role disputes, role transitions, and interpersonal deficits. A fifth area, single parent families, was added because of its frequent occurrence and the conflicts it engenders for adolescents. The emphasis is on issues in current relationships rather than those in the past. In the initial phase, depression as a clinical disorder is explained, and an effort is made to demystify the experience. The adolescent is encouraged to think of herself as in treatment and is assigned the sick-role. Despite this, the adolescent is encouraged not to avoid the usual social expectations and to see friends, attend school, and behave in the family as normally as possible. Parents are seen and encouraged to be supportive rather than hostile or critical. The school is approached, and the effect of depression on school performance and behaviour explained. In the middle phase the focus is on the problem area(s) selected:

(1) *Grief* is not considered a problem unless it is prolonged or becomes abnormal. The therapist helps the adolescent discuss the loss of a loved one, as well as identify and experience the associated feelings. As the patient begins to grieve appropriately and the symptoms dissipate, the loss should be better understood and accepted and the patient freed to pursue new relationships.

(2) *Interpersonal role disputes* occur where one of the parties has different expectations to the other about the relationship. The therapist helps the young person to identify the dispute, to make choices about negotiations, to reassess expectations for the relationship, to clarify role changes, and to modify communication patterns to enable resolution of the dispute. Parents may be brought in to facilitate negotiations if they are a party to the dispute.

(3) *Role transitions* are when adolescents need to negotiate puberty, cope with sexual desires and the wish for intimate relationships, separate from parents and family, and achieve success in planning work or further education. There may be feelings of loss about letting go of old roles, or fear and inadequacy about their ability to take on new roles. The therapist aims to help the young person to come to terms with these feelings and negotiate a viable future.

(4) *Interpersonal deficits* are apparent when the individual appears to lack the social skills to establish and maintain appropriate relationships within and outside the family. As a result, the adolescent may be socially isolated or lacking close friends, which can lead to feelings of depression and inadequacy. The therapist reviews significant past relationships and identifies repetitive or inappropriate ways of behaving. New strategies are identified and discussed, and the patient encouraged to apply these to current issues. Role play may be used to identify problematic interpersonal situations and enable the adolescent to explore and practice new communication skills and interpersonal behaviours, e.g. learning how to make friends. Practising within the session and in small increments at home can engender a sense of social competence in the young person that generalises to other situations.

(5) *Single parent families* may arise from divorce, separation, imprisonment

of one parent, absence of a parent from the outset, or death of a parent by medical illness or violence. Each of these situations presents unique emotional conflicts for the adolescent and the custodial parent. Therapy aims to help the young person come to terms with the current situation and negotiate appropriate adaptations. There is often a need to grieve for the loss of the previous situation.

In the termination phase, progress is reviewed, often with other family members present. Symptoms and conflicts are presented in four categories: those representing symptoms specific to the depressive episode; those secondary to it; more enduring conflict areas that represent personality style; and those areas of conflict that are part of a normal developmental process. The adolescent will have already addressed feelings relating to termination of contact with the therapist, and a slight increase of depressive feelings following termination is predicted. Trials of IPT suggest it is as effective in treating depression in adolescents as in adults, and has an effect at least as large as cognitive-behavioural therapy.

INDIVIDUAL COUNSELLING AND PSYCHOTHERAPY

There are differing levels, on a continuum from support and counselling at one end to psychodynamic psychotherapy at the other:

- *Support and counselling*. This includes unburdening of problems to a sympathetic listener, ventilation of feelings within a supportive relationship, and discussion of current problems with a non-judgemental helper. Advice may be given. The main aim is to relieve symptoms and restore the status quo prior to the difficulty, or come to terms with an event.

- *Intermediate levels of psychotherapy*. Interpersonal psychotherapy (IPT) as described above is an example of this.

- *Psychodynamic psychotherapy*. Here, a prolonged deep interpersonal relationship is fostered, during which both intra- and interpersonal processes are revealed and analysed. Disturbing early experiences may be re-lived, allowing conflicts which underlie symptoms to be explored and insight gained, and conflicts to be worked through and resolved without handicapping defences. Advice is not given. The aim is thus more than symptomatic relief: it is reintegration and change in personality functioning towards greater wholeness and maturity. Psychoanalytic interest in children's symptoms dates back to Sigmund Freud, who described the case of little Hans in 1909; his daughter Anna Freud in the 1920s elaborated child psychoanalysis, as did Melanie Klein in the 1930s. Later, Virginia Axline developed play therapy more formally.

A major issue in individual work at all levels is the quality of the interpersonal relationship between therapist and patient. Several adult studies show that irrespective of the particular form of personal therapy given, one of the major determinants of outcome is the warmth and empathy of the therapist. One way of addressing the need for this empirically would be to give the same (or as similar as possible) treatment by correspondence or in a manual. In the field of parent-training for child conduct disorder, studies show that these approaches are indeed effective, although less so than when a live therapist is involved.

In child psychiatry, much work for the benefit of the child is done through the parents, and counselling and support is part of many clinicians' basic repertoire irrespective of child disorder. It may be a major component in helping parents come to terms with a diagnosis of mental retardation, or in coping with a daughter's depression. Studies on counselling in these settings suggest parents find the apparent attitude of the clinician to them central ('likes me; likes my child'), and want an informal atmosphere where they can ask questions.

Direct work with children and adolescents differs in a number of ways from that with adults. Firstly, the child may not have wanted to be seen alone; usually they do not have to give consent. Secondly, the method of working with younger children may need to be less talk-based initially, and focus on drawing or play to gain insight. Thirdly, even when therapy can help children come to terms with a difficult situation and offer them the opportunity to mature and change, children are not masters of their own fate in the same way as adults, so they may well continue to be exposed to damaging or harmful influences, for example harsh punishment and neglect within the family, or a mother who is alcoholic. In these circumstances it is essential to try as hard as possible to ameliorate the conditions, and it may be unethical to give individual therapy without so doing.

There have been very few well conducted evaluation trials of individual dynamic psychotherapy, so it is hard to be certain of its effectiveness at present.

Subject reviews

Kendall, P.C. and Lochman, J. (1994) Cognitive-behavioural therapies. In *Child and Adolescent Psychiatry: Modern Approaches*, 3rd edn (M. Rutter, E, Taylor and L. Horsov, eds) Blackwell Science, Oxford, pp. 844–857.

Pelligrini, D.S. (1994) Training in interpersonal cognitive problem-solving. In *Child and Adolescent Psychiatry: Modern Approaches*, 3rd edn (M. Rutter, E. Taylor and L. Hersov, eds) Blackwell Science, Oxford, pp. 829–843.

Trowell, J. (1994) Individual and group psychotherapy. In *Child and Adolescent Psychiatry: Modern Approaches*, 3rd edn (M. Rutter, E. Taylor and L. Hersov, eds) Blackwell Science, Oxford, pp. 936–945.

Further reading

Mufson, L. *et al.* (1994) Modification of interpersonal therapy with depressed adolescents. *Journal of the American Academy of Child and Adolescent Psychiatry*, **33**, 695–705.

34 Family Therapy

BACKGROUND

'No man is an island' wrote Donne, and family therapy recognises this. Whereas psychodynamic therapy and biological psychiatry focus on the individual's internal mental processes and pathology as the root of problems, family therapy arose from the notion that the *family system* exerts a strong influence on all members, and that imbalances in the system can manifest themselves as problems in *the identified patient* who is presented to express the family's *dysfunction* or *disequilibrium*. Children are especially affected by these processes since so much of their lives takes place within the family context. More recent developments in family therapy have acknowledged the influence of family belief systems and the attitudes prevalent in the current social and cultural climate. People's way of functioning is affected by their idea of how they should be. Gender, race and role expectations all influence people's beliefs and behaviour, as do a variety of personal and general experiences ranging from parental demands to TV advertisements. A variety of methods have been developed to make use of these concepts in therapy.

Family systems theory began to develop in the late 1950s and in the 1960s. It recognised limitations in explanations of human behaviour based on *linear causality*, which focus on actions by individuals, and the content of what they say and do. As an alternative, Gregory Bateson, an anthropologist, introduced ideas from *cybernetics* into family therapy. He proposed that *reciprocal determinism* is at work, and that one needs to look at process rather than content. This will reveal the interdependence of family members: one event doesn't lead to another single event; rather, a change in one member affects all other members in differing ways, who then react and impinge upon the first person, and so on. Examination of the process reveals *circular causality*. Systems theory and thinking can equally be applied beyond the family to inform relations between the individual or the family and wider networks and agencies such as other relatives and friends, school, and social services.

Example

- *Linear causality:* a depressed mother has produced a dependent son by failing to get him to leave home, and an uncontrolled daughter by supervising her inadequately.

- *Circular causality:* a mother is unhappy because her husband stays at work for much of the time. She turns to her 18-year-old son for companionship, so excluding her 15-year-old daughter. The son feels her loneliness and stays at home to be with her, and so puts off leaving home and going to college, and becomes increasingly withdrawn. The mother blames the father for being away so much and withholds sexual favours; she becomes depressed. The ensuing coldness between the parents leads the daughter into a series of superficial relationships, in which she seeks but never finds the comfort and warmth lacking at home.

- *Implication:* behaviour is as much determined by the interactional context in which it occurs as by the intrapsychic or emotional processes of any individual person.

Terms used in family therapy

- *Family system.* An entity whose component members influence each other, with relationships organized by family rules.

- *Subsystem.* For example, husband-wife dyad; mother-child, father-child; parents-children; males-females, etc.

- *Family rules.* These regulate and stabilise how the family functions as a unit. Many may be covert: 'if you complain to mother it puts up her blood pressure', 'we never discuss money', 'boys don't show feelings'. Dysfunctional families may follow dysfunctional rules, and helping them become aware of these during therapy may enable them to replace them with more useful ones.

- *Homeostasis.* This term has been brought to family functioning from physiology. It suggests that there are (behavioural) mechanisms to keep relationships controlled within a relatively narrow range. For example, a threat to father's authority by a child's misbehaviour may trigger a look or counterthreat to bring the child into line, which in turn will lead to the child making a small adjustment of his or her behaviour, and so on. The codes to effect this *feedback loop* may be quite subtle and private. In times of transition due to changed circumstances or family life cycle adjustments (see below) these old homeostatic responses may fail and get out of control; sterile, ineffectual patterns may become endlessly repeated. Recognising this can help families develop new, healthier patterns of communication and behaviour.

- *Family lifecycle framework*. This is a further way in which family therapy recognises that external forces influence family and individual wellbeing. The proposal is that there are *developmental tasks* that require mastery at each stage. Failure to come to terms with these changes and to make the necessary adjustments may then lead to strain or dysfunction in the family system and problems or symptoms in one or all family members. Successful negotiation of the transitions may require *first order changes* (defined as within the system but not affecting its structure) or *second order changes* (which require a fundamental alteration in the system's structure and function). Some of the life cycle stages are shown in Box 34.1, though individual, socioeconomic and cultural variations need to be considered, as do the impact of dislocations such as divorce, unemployment, severe illness, etc.

Box 34.1   Life cycle stages.

Stage	Tasks
(1) Leaving home	(a) Develop own identity independent of family of origin (b) Form close peer relationships (c) Gain work and financial independence.
(2) Cohabitation	(a) Form marital system (b) Realign relationships with extended family, and friends.
(3) Family with young children	(a) Adjust marital system to make space for children (b) Join in child-rearing, financial, and household tasks (c) Realign with extended family to incorporate parenting and grandparenting roles.
(4) Family with adolescents	(a) Adjust relationships so adolescent can move in and out of system (b) Refocus on midlife marital and career issues (c) Start joint caring for older generation.
(5) Children leaving home	(a) Renegotiate marital system as a dyad (b) Develop adult-to-adult relations with grown children (c) Accept in-laws and grandchildren into system (d) Cope with disability and death of parents.
(6) Late life	(a) Adjust couple functioning in face of physiological, financial, and work-role decline (b) Deal with loss of spouse, siblings, and friends (c) Accept assistance from children/outside agencies.

Some working practices common to most types of family therapy

- *Seeing as many family members as possible*. This used to be very strongly recommended in order to assess the communication patterns and inter-relationships going on. The concern was that failure to see all members at least once would easily lead to erroneous conclusions being drawn, or to a lack of appreciation of important influences. Nowadays most family therapists will work with whoever can come, while recognising the importance of the family system. It is therefore possible to work in a systemic way with only one person.

- *Drawing a family genogram (family tree)*. This rapidly enables all the family members to be recognised for their influence, including grandparents, aunts and uncles, and deceased relatives. Intergenerational patterns may be revealed, and family stories and expectations brought to light 'he's the black sheep of the family', 'I'm a Daddy's girl', 'All the men in our family die early or drink heavily'.

- *Use of colleagues to observe the therapy process*. This may be through a one-way mirror. The therapist then receives feedback on what is happening in the family and suggestions for interventions, which may be given through an earbug, by a telephone, or by taking a break to talk to them.

Varieties of family therapy

There are many varieties of family therapy, which have evolved over time within themselves and which have influenced each other. Three schools are particularly well known. Confusingly for the novice, all begin with 'S'. *Structural* makes explicit the structure of a family in terms of who holds the power and what the communication patterns are. Therapy attempts to correct any distortions in this structure through practical manoeuvres. *Strategic* makes use of novel practical strategies to help families find a fresh way to break out of ingrained negative cycles of behaviour, without prescribing a 'correct' structure. *Systemic* or *Milan* uses questioning to reveal to family members the forces and beliefs which constrain their behaviour towards each other, enabling them to change these if they are uncomfortable with what is revealed.

Irrespective of the particular type of family therapy, there have been a number of shifts in the way family therapists think about personal difficulties. Prior to systems thinking, the dominant medical or psychodynamic models tended to locate pathology within the person; the cause was frequently seen as beyond the patient's conscious control. Therapy was likely to be targeted on the individual to alter the pathological process.

From the mid 1960s to the mid 1980s, systems thinking and other developments brought about what some have described as a 'second wave' of thinking about personal problems. This way of thinking emphasised that people's behaviour was strongly influenced by their interaction and communication with those around them. Behavioural psychology had already described how the pattern of stimuli and responses could determine an individual's behaviour, but family systems thinkers focused on a more complex set of environmental determinants. The client was seen as a basically healthy person who had run into a problem and was seeking help to put it right. The therapist attempted to alter the family influences on the client, with the result that the whole system shifted, including the personal characteristics and problems of the client. Therapy was carried out in the 'here and now' working on current problems. It did not concern itself with past origins of difficulties, or with behaviour that the therapist but not the client perceived as a problem. The focus was on changing external contingencies rather than on the individual as a conscious agent.

The last decade has heralded what some have described as the 'third wave' of thinking about personal problems. This has recognised the wider cultural context of people's lives, and has focused on what people can do rather than what they cannot. It acknowledges that active conscious processes shape a person's sense of identity. People construct a story about themselves that has to be respected and worked with, using the person's own language rather than imposing professional jargon. The person is seen as having many strengths which may need mobilising to fight the difficulties outside themselves. The therapist focuses on helping the individual to deploy more of the effective strategies that are already part of their repertoire. This may be achieved by helping the person become aware of the 'script' they are living, and enabling them to 'rewrite' a more positive story by which to live their life. Sometimes this is called the *narrative approach* to therapy.

There are also other approaches to working with families which recognise the complexities of wider interrelationships but which did not primarily evolve from cybernetic systems theory. These include psychodynamic family therapy, and behavioural family therapy. The latter has had well documented success in improving the outcome for people with schizophrenia by reducing the number of critical comments by nearest relatives. In childhood, behaviourally based parent training is effective in improving conduct problems.

STRUCTURAL FAMILY THERAPY

Salvador Minuchin developed this approach in the 1960s working with deprived ethnic minorities in the USA. It is geared to the present, and operates in the here and now. Thus there is no discussion of past history, or the origins of dysfunctional relationships. Change occurs through action and not via gaining insight. Problems addressed are in the present day-to-day world, not unresolved past inner conflicts. It is based on a *normative family model* which is functioning well, in which there are *clear and well marked boundaries in relationships*. This is especially true in:

(1) The marital subsystem – protection of spouse privacy;
(2) The sibling subsystem – a hierarchical organisation in which different tasks and privileges are consonant with the age and gender of the siblings, as determined by the family culture;

(3)   The boundary around the nuclear family which is well demarcated, whilst recognising great cultural variations.

It is a fundamental principle that the symptom is the product of a dysfunctional family system, and that if the family organisation becomes more normal or functional, the symptom will disappear. Symptoms are not specific to dysfunctional structures.

Terms

- *Hierarchy*. The relative influence of each family member on the outcome of an activity. This needs to be defined in relation to specific circumstances, as it is not a permanent or invariable concept. For example, parents exercise responsibility and authority. A parentified child is an example of abnormality or dysfunction.

- *Boundary*. An invisible line which demarcates a system, subsystem or individual from its surroundings. It arises from the rules of who participates in an operation and how it is carried out, and from the roles each person takes towards others during a particular family function. The boundary preserves the integrity of the (sub)system so members can carry out tasks without interference, but should be permeable enough to allow inter-dependence. Thus boundaries can be construed along a continuum, with one end too permeable and the other too rigid:
    - *enmeshment* results from boundaries which are undifferentiated, permeable, or fluid. Individuals in the relationship are handicapped by not being able to be autonomous.
    - *clear boundaries* promote healthy relationships
    - *disengagement* results from rigid, impermeable boundaries, and there is little interplay or communication between family members.

- *Alignments*. These occur through the joining or opposition of one member of a system to another in carrying out an operation, they can be positive or negative. Structures observed may include:
    - *Coalitions* of two family members against a third: e.g. father and son against mother. Coalitions vary in how stable they are. Some coalitions are based on detouring, e.g. couple appear to get on, because they detour their problem via the child.
    - *Triangulation* where each parent demands the child be an ally in a conflict with the other.
    - *Alliances* when two share an interest not shared by a third. This is a healthy supportive structure, which is not detrimental to others.

- *Power* refers to relative influence.

- *Identified patient* The person brought for help, although in fact the cause of the problem lies in the interaction patterns at a family-wide level and will be affecting all members in different ways. The task of therapy includes revealing the way the symptoms of the identified patient are used by the family to support its functioning, and how they fit its transactions (Box 34.2).

Box 34.2   The Jones family visit a structural family therapist.

Mr Jones is a maths teacher, and Mrs Jones is a former nurse who looks after their three children. Robert, 15, has incapacitating abdominal pain with no obvious organic cause and has missed most school for the last six months. Jane, 13, has no reported problems and is doing very well academically. John, 10, refuses to do what his mother asks and frequently swears at her.

During questioning it emerges that to make it easier for Mrs Jones to help Robert with his frequent bouts of pain in the night, he sleeps in the parents' bedroom on a camp bed. The repeated night disturbances led Mr Jones to suffer from lack of sleep which was affecting his teaching, so he had moved into the spare room. Most evenings he spends correcting students' scripts in his study, and at weekends he goes fishing alone. He explains that he thinks Robert's problems derive from a delicate constitution worsened by appendicitis three years ago.

The therapist does not respond to this explanation for events rooted in the past, but notices that Mr Jones and Jane sit together on one side of the room, John is in the middle, and Mrs Jones is at the other end sitting very close to Robert and whispering to him. After a while she decides that the boundary between Mr and Mrs Jones is rigid and they are disengaged, whereas that between Robert and Mrs Jones is too fluid and they are enmeshed. She therefore intervenes by altering the seating arrangements so Mr and Mrs Jones have to sit next to each other away from the children and are set the task of finding two practical steps to help Robert back to school for one hour a day. Meanwhile the three siblings are sat in the other corner of the room and instructed collectively to plan a treat for their parents.

These manoeuvres are designed to promote parental authority and strengthen the marital subsystem, and the sibling subsystem. For homework, the parents are instructed to go out one evening a week and to agree a joint implementation of their plan to get Robert back to school. Mr Jones, who hitherto hardly ever did anything with Robert, is instructed to take him fishing with him on Saturdays. In later sessions the sleeping arrangements are addressed, and Mrs Jones is asked what Robert does to get her to mollycoddle him so much. The therapist is thus reframing his behaviour as sympathy-seeking to avoid school rather than illness. Mrs Jones begins to see his role in organising her caring behaviour and gets quite angry at him, with the result that he moves out of the bedroom and Mr Jones moves back in. Both parents are supported in their programme to be consistent in accepting no excuses for not going to school. His abdominal pain ceases to be discussed much at all during sessions and gradually diminishes.

Intervention techniques

The therapist is *active*, and *directive*. She challenges patterns of family interaction and reveals covert rules. This is done through *joining* the family system and *accommodating* to its style, getting to feel what it is like. She will acknowledge the painful situation, but absolve the individual from responsibility, e.g. 'you are quite childish – how do the others manage to keep you that way?' She will *reframe* the symptom as part of the family structure and use the force of her personality, which should be powerful and empathetic, to help bring about change. To do this she may need to *unbalance* the system by exposing dysfunction, and destabilise it to encourage the emergence of a healthier structure. She may get the family to *enact* the problem within the room to see what is going on and provide alternatives, e.g. if the daughter is anorexic, have a family meal.

STRATEGIC FAMILY THERAPY

Here therapists use a range of *strategies* to get rid of the specific set of presenting symptoms. Unlike structural therapists, strategic therapists are not concerned about imposing some predetermined normative structure on the family.

This mode of working arises out of an interactional approach where one communication is seen as arising in the context of another, not in isolation. In the case of children fighting, for instance, it is inappropriate to ask 'who started it', since each party would say that they were only reacting to what the other did. Therefore, it is necessary to take the whole system as the unit of study. Watzlawick stated that 'all behaviour is communication' – just as it is impossible not to behave, so it is impossible not to communicate. For example, the husband who withdraws and 'refuses to communicate' with his wife is in fact speaking volumes about his resentment, anger, and rejection of her. *Paradoxical communication* is confusing, typified by the *double bind*, where the content and form of the message may contradict each other, for example when a mother says to her daughter 'lovely to see you' while giving her a frozen stare.

The current pattern of communication and behaviour is held to maintain the presenting problem; its history and aetiology are seen as irrelevant. As a consequence, this can be a very optimistic therapy where, for example, years of rancorous feelings and despondent explanations can be bypassed in favour of concentrating on what can be done differently from now on.

Jay Haley and his wife Cloe Madanes were major developers of strategic therapy. Haley wrote a number of influential books, including *Problem-solving Therapy* in 1976. He argued that symptoms were not behaviours beyond one's control, but a strategy for controlling a relationship when all else failed. He cited the example of a woman who insisted her husband be home every night or she would have panic attacks. In this way she blamed her control of the situation on the panic attacks. Symptoms are used to control relationships when more up-front methods fail.

Strategic therapists concern themselves with current daily communication patterns as well as with repetitive sequences of interactions between family members. Communication defines the relationship; symptoms are tactics in this struggle. The therapist's goal is to manoeuvre the patient into developing other ways of defining the relationship so the use of symptoms as a method of exerting control will be abandoned.

Techniques

The therapist has to design a strategy for each problem, and is responsible for change. The approach is pragmatic, concerned with what works. The therapist uses his power to overcome 'resistance' of patients, and is 'manipulative', i.e. keeps the rationale for intervention hidden from patients.

- *Relabelling.* This is a tactic to emphasise the positive, making apparently dysfunctional behaviour seem reasonable. For example, Haley describes telling a wife whose husband chased her with an axe that he was trying to get close to her. Thus both sides of a communication are examined, and the less obvious aspect is brought out, sometimes described as 'addressing the meta message', in this case that the husband cared desperately for his wife. Such relabelling can change the context of relationships and lead on to improvement.

- *Directives.* These are assignments set for families to perform outside the session. For example, a mother is told to stop interrupting when father and son are talking together. However, often these directives don't work as the families are resistant and have invested in the status quo.

- *Prescribing the symptom.* This may then be tried as a form of *paradoxical intervention*. The patient is told to keep on doing what they came to therapy to stop doing. This is designed to provoke defiance in the patient, who may come back next time and say they did it far less than previously. If they carry on, they are forced to recognise that they have some control over the behaviour, and confront its unreasonableness and the effect it has on others. The domineering mother may be instructed to carry on running absolutely all the small details of the family's lives and not to let anyone else have the slightest say about anything. A boy refusing school may be instructed never to go out of the house, and not even to look at a book. The issue then becomes one of control, as the patient is told they are in charge of the symptom. The domineering wife no longer runs everything in the house if the therapist is telling her what to do; or if she resists the directive she will be less domineering. The assumption is that if the symptom was presented as a way of gaining an advantage, it will resolve once it puts the patient at a disadvantage (Box 34.3).

- *Humour and metaphor.* These may be used to tap into a family's lighter side, release pressure, and sidestep logical thinking. To get families to break out of fixed patterns may require tangential, indirect 'uncommon solutions'.

- *Provision of alternatives.* Other activities are suggested to replace the problem behaviour.

- *Externalising the problem.* This technique attributes agency to the symptom in a light-hearted way to enable the family to unite against it, and has been well described by Michael White. This places less emphasis on failure, decreases conflict around the symptom, opens up new possibilities for action, and taps into families' lighter side (optimism replaces pessimism). For example, rather than blame a boy for soiling, the trouble is ascribed to 'sneaky poos' who have to be taken on in a battle to beat them. Imaginative charts are drawn to show progress and to make it an epic game where the child is helped to devise creative strategies to win.

Box 34.3   The Jones family visit a strategic family therapist who uses Haley's approach.

The same family described in Box 34.2 is interviewed. However, this time no structural reorganisation of seating arrangements is made. The therapist notes that Robert's abdominal pain serves to keep his mother at home looking after him rather than return to nursing as she says she wants but doesn't seem really to want. The therapist tells the family that the situation is serious and instructs Mrs Jones to increase her surveillance of Robert, checking his pain level every hour for the next fortnight, and under no circumstances is she to leave him unattended in the house. Robert is to report the slightest twinge of pain, being told that otherwise if it is left too long it is likely to get far worse. He must ask his mother to attend to him very closely, irrespective of her sacrifice.

After two weeks of this the family gradually become aware of how dominating Robert's pain is. Mrs Jones gets fed up with waiting on him hand and foot. Robert himself feels constrained as he now has to report sick all the time and isn't allowed out to see his friends in the evenings. A shift of attitude occurs and Mrs Jones responds less keenly to Robert's episodes of pain. He in turn reports less and starts going out more, eventually getting back to school.

Brief solution-focused therapy

This is a variety of strategic therapy developed by Steve de Shazer amongst others. This extends the approach which focuses on success, and typically involves no more than five to ten sessions. Questioning emphasises the exceptions: When was the symptom *not* present? What were you doing at the time? How could you do more of this? Differences are noticed in the severity of the symptom and attention is paid to what was happening at the time. The focus is on what happens when things are going right rather than on when things go wrong. The assumption is that people already know what they need to do to solve their complaints; the therapist has only to help them discover their own creative solutions for coming 'unstuck'. The solution may not be closely matched to the problem and may comprise quite different elements. De Shazer uses the metaphor of coming upon a locked door blocking progress to a more satisfactory life. Rather than spend a long time agonising about why the door is there and who locked it, all that is necessary is for the family to find a set of 'skeleton keys' which will open this door and others blocking their progress.

Techniques

- *Precise description* of the problem is requested: 'How would I know if her depression was getting better? What would I see?' Limited but achievable goals are aimed for, and by focusing on precise descriptions, the families are led to recognise improvements, however small. These then become reinforcing and provide the motivation for the family to keep doing things differently, and so lead on to further change.

- *Miracle question:* what would it look like if you woke up tomorrow and the problem was gone? What precisely would be different?

- *Miracle intervention:* X is to act tomorrow as if he had no problem, Y is to implicitly acknowledge this by her responses, X is to implicitly note these, but there is to be no discussion about it.

- *Focus on successes:* become aware of those occasions when the problem is absent. What is going on at the time? Notice these successes: how on earth did you manage not to do it (the symptom behaviour)? How are you managing not to do it now? So you managed the urge, let's develop your 'urge surfing'. If a strategy works, stick with it; if it doesn't, do something different.

MILAN SYSTEMIC FAMILY THERAPY

Developed by Selvini-Palazzoli, Prata, Boscolo and Cecchin in Milan, Italy, for chronic, resistant cases, this approach concerns itself with bringing out covert beliefs and meanings that constrain a family's behaviour. The model is to recognise and challenge the beliefs, so they can be re-examined and modified to fit what is going on more precisely, and the expectation is that behaviour will then be changed to fit in with the new set of beliefs or priorities. This is the opposite of structural family therapy, where the objective is to change behaviour through direct action rather than as a consequence of adjusting beliefs. According to Milan systemic therapy, there may be several conflicting sets of beliefs regarding a single action which conflict. Regarding a daughter who is staying out late, for example, a parent may feel she should come home earlier as she is at risk of being taken advantage of, but may also feel that if too much discipline is applied, she will run away from home like her older sister. As they are revealed, the beliefs can be tested against other family members' views and interests and be developed accordingly. As with other modes of family therapy, the systemic approach has changed over time, with increasing emphasis on the role of language in shaping beliefs.

The central technique is one of circular questioning, in order to reveal how beliefs relate to the behaviour. Thus, each question follows on from the response to the last, aiming to reveal what meaning this has for other beliefs in the system, and to uncover their interrelationships. Whereas linear questioning proceeds convergently to clarify with increasing detail what the mental state or behaviour is, circular questioning aims to elicit the *connections* to other beliefs, and to other family members. Thus one is aiming to see how experiences are connected to belief systems, rather than find out more and more about the experience. For example, if someone repeatedly brought anger to sessions, rather than continuing to explore the feeling, one would find out what it would mean to take the feeling away. One might discover they would be left believing they're worthless, impotent, a victim, and as this is even more unpleasant, they continue feeling angry.

Techniques

Hypothesising

- This is carried out before the session, before the family can impose its definition of the problem.
- It organises the questioning. It is an evolving process in which hypotheses are tested by gathering information.
- It clarifies the gains and losses the symptom brings to each family member, and how the symptom helps the family which is struggling with the prospect of change.
- In a family experiencing a chronic problem, each member moves to stop change, wishing to reinstate the status quo after the change has happened, and trying to retain old patterns even though they conflict with the new situation. This notion of 'resistance' to change was more characteristic of earlier systemic therapy; now there is a greater acceptance that families really do want to change.

Neutrality

- The therapist avoids getting drawn into the family system or taking sides; she may have a team on the other side of a one-way mirror to help her keep independent.
- Answers are not evaluated or agreed with: understanding is shown, and perhaps empathy, but no family member's view is accepted as right or definitive.
- The therapist remains allied with all family members.
- The therapist tries to understand, and not to prescribe how the family should be – she lets them generate their own solutions.

Circular questioning

- This means that one question leads on to the next in a different direction outwards, rather than linearly towards a definition of phenomena (Box 34.4).
- Individuals are asked to state the problem in behavioural terms, not in terms of mood states.
- The effect of the symptom on relationships is discussed: 'Who does what in response? Who is most affected? Who noticed first? Who is most worried?'

Box 34.4   The Jones family visit a Milan systemic therapist.

The same family described in Box 34.2 is interviewed. This time the therapist asks a series of questions eliciting the differences amongst family members, initially asking the daughter, Jane, 'Who is the most upset that Robert is not going to school?' She says her Daddy. Mrs Jones is asked what would happen if her husband got firm and insisted Robert went. Mr Jones interjects that he would never insist as this would be an authoritarian act, and his own father was a rigid disciplinarian who scarred him for life by his bullying, so no son of his is going be treated the same way. Jane is now asked who would be most upset if Robert *did* go to school. She replies that her Mummy would be lonely. Mrs Jones is then asked again what would happen if her husband got firm and insisted Robert went to school. She replies that Robert is delicate and she is anxious that if he were pushed, he would have a nervous breakdown, just as Mr Jones did when he was 15. The younger brother John is asked what would happen if Robert went back to school. He replies that Jane would be triumphant, as she is clever but Robert failed his mock exams earlier in the year and would be made to look stupid. John says the whole family has had it drummed into them how important school success is. Their father was a dustman's son but through academic success had become a middle-class teacher.

The therapist takes a break to consult her colleagues behind the one-way mirror. They suggest the family seem paralysed by two fear-provoking, conflicting beliefs: if you don't work hard enough you might fail academically; if you work too hard you might have a breakdown. They recommend the therapist ask the family members how each of them sees the future in two years time. On her return to the family, she asks this. Robert says he would like to be free of pain and back to playing football, and grins as he says that by then he won't have to do maths any more. John says he hopes he'll be in the school football team at the secondary school he'll be attending by then. He adds that he wishes that his father, Robert and he could play football together as they used to, stating proudly that his Dad used to be in the university team. Mother says she'd like to be nursing again, and Jane says she'd impressed if her Mum did that. Father says he couldn't wish for any more than they have said, but hopes he won't have to wait two years for a football game with his sons: what about a game tonight? The boys agree enthusiastically.

The therapist says she is impressed by the way the family work together to solve problems. She wonders whether Mr Jones' experience of having had a breakdown and then recovering could be used to help Robert? Mr Jones says it occurs to him that he could go back to helping Robert with maths. He had been anxious not to put pressure on his son but now thinks Robert probably doesn't know where to start, having been out of school for so long. Robert looks relieved. The family carry on discussing what they could do now, in order to get to where they want to be in two years time. At the follow-up visit two weeks later Robert's pain is far less and he has begun a graded reintroduction to school.

- Differences between people are considered: 'Who cares most that Lucy won't eat?'

- Hypothetical scenarios are considered to define the effect of the symptom on relationships: 'If Jim didn't have the problem, who would be closest to him?'

- Timing is explored: What were relationships like before and after the 'problem'? Thinking about the future, 'What would happen if it never got better?'

- Questioning may be triadic, i.e. asking a third person about the relations of the other two: 'How do your brother's tantrums affect your mother?'

- New alternatives are canvassed: 'What would have to happen to stop Jim misbehaving?' Meanings and actions are separated.

- Circular questioning of silent/'mad' family members is used: 'If he were to speak, what would he say?'
- Emotions are treated descriptively, not sympathised with: 'Which of your children understands your depression best?', 'What would have to change to reduce your depression?'
- Information is shown to have different meanings for different family members, thus revealing family relationships.

Positive connotation

- This is more than a form of reframing or relabelling because it tries to address the rules of the whole family 'game', rather than one individual's behaviour.
- Symptomatic behaviour is reframed as good because it helps maintain the system's balance, so facilitating family cohesion and wellbeing. Thus volition is ascribed, and the symptom is seen as helping the family, not as a negative entity.
- The presumed intent is what is positively connoted, not the behaviour: 'Thank you for preventing the outbreak of family strife over your brother's bad behaviour by refusing to eat'. It was believed by early systemic therapists that because positive connotations express approval, families do not resist them. More recently therapists have taken the view that it is not change that is necessarily resisted, but approaches to treatment which do not match the families' beliefs.

After perhaps 30–40 minutes of a session, the systemic therapist often withdraws to confer with her team behind the one-way mirror for ten minutes or so. After this she re-enters the room and gives 'the message' which may be accompanied by a task for family members to carry out. An example of each follows.

Paradox and counterparadox

- A *paradox* is set up by the family's acceptance of the therapist's positive connotation: why does a good thing, family cohesion, require a symptom in its member? The therapist spells out the dilemma the family are in.
- A *counterparadox* may be presented by the therapist as a message designed to help the family find a way out. Rather than saying that the symptomatic patient should change and the rest of the family should not, the counterparadox is designed to break up the dysfunctional, paradoxical pattern, for example by prescribing no change. The family is then left on their own to resolve the paradoxical absurdities after the session.

The invariant prescription

This task was developed by two of the four original Milan four, Selvini-

Palazzoli and Prata. It aims to unhinge collusive parent–child patterns, in which a 'game' is played out by family members and keeps the child symptomatic. This is often achieved by the child siding with the 'weaker' parent and defeating the 'winner' through illness behaviour. The parents are told to plan a few evenings out, departing before dinner without forewarning, leaving only a note saying 'we'll not be home tonight'. On return they are not to give any explanations to their children, saying 'these things concern only the two of us'. Each parent is asked to keep a private notebook of the verbal and non-verbal behaviour which follows carrying out the prescription. This procedure is designed to strengthen the parental alliance and break pre-existing coalitions, blocking 'games' of control which had perpetuated abnormal behaviour.

Narrative approach

This approach to therapy is a recent development that has been adopted by some strategic and systemic therapists. It focuses on the stories people have which guide their lives. John Byng-Hall combines this with an emphasis on attachment theory in his variety of family therapy based on *Rewriting Family Scripts*, the title of his 1995 book. Adults and children in a secure enough setting can construct a new way of seeing their future and be helped to live it, liberated from past constraints and expectations. David Epston uses letter writing as part of the *Narrative Means to Therapeutic Ends*, the title of his 1990 book with Michael White. Often harrowing life-stories and problems are rewritten using the person's terminology, but emphasising how all along they fought the incredible strains they were put under with heroism. Evidence is found of instances when they were not dominated by the problem, and they are encouraged to think about the future from the strong, competent person that has emerged from the interview so far. The person is encouraged to create or seek out a receptive social group from their immediate circle so as to be able to live out their new story and identity.

EVALUATION OF FAMILY THERAPY

Criticisms

Some family therapists have little knowledge of specific syndromes in child and adolescent psychiatry. Rather, all problems are seen as arising from abnormal patterns of relationships. They fail to recognise the contribution of partly or entirely constitutional disorders such as Asperger's syndrome or ADHD. Even with a condition such as conduct disorder where psychosocial factors are highly relevant, a family therapy approach might not pick up the specific reading disorder present in a third of cases, and so fail to address the causal contribution this may be making.

Many family therapists seldom see the child on his or her own. Yet a child interview is often essential to reveal depression, bullying, or abuse. For fear or shame or other reasons, children may not say what they mean in front of other family members.

Families come for help because they feel that their child's symptoms need addressing directly. However, they may be put off by what they perceive as irrelevant intrusion into their private relationships. Some forms, notably Milan systemic, may use a second team to observe the therapist, which is expensive. In Milan therapy, it is hard for a therapist to be neutral if they have statutory obligations to protect the child from abusive practices. The lack of explanation of why the questioning is following this line, and the confusing nature of the intervention, can alienate some families who vote with their feet and don't come back.

Rejoinders

Many if not all of these concerns can be overcome through flexible working. For example, in a multidisciplinary team, it is often possible to have an initial general assessment before proceeding to family therapy, although most family therapists do not work this way. Engaging the family is the art of the therapist, and a skilled one will not lose families by becoming too probing too soon, but will be sensitive to what the family can tolerate. One of the main advantages of having a background in family therapy is to be able to recognise and address intrafamilial influences on behaviour, which a linear 'diagnostic' approach fails to do.

Outcome studies

There have been rather few rigorously controlled outcome studies, or meticulously carried out single case studies. However, randomised controlled trials have shown that family therapy can be an effective therapy for anorexia nervosa and juvenile delinquency. These are both notoriously hard conditions to treat, so the results are impressive, with effect sizes of 0.4–0.7 standard deviations.

Subject review

Gorrell Barnes, G. (1994) Family therapy. In *Child and Adolescent Psychiatry: Modern Approaches*, 3rd edn (M. Rutter, E. Taylor and L. Hersov, eds) Blackwell Science, Oxford, pp. 946–967.

Further reading

Goldenberg, I. and Goldenberg, H. (1991) *Family Therapy: An Overview*. Brooks/Cole, Pacific Grove, CA.

Byng-Hall, J. (1995) *Rewriting Family Scripts*. Guilford, London.

Haley, J. (1976) *Problem-Solving Therapy*. Jossey-Bass, San Francisco.

Minuchin, S. (1974) *Families and Family Therapy*. Harvard University Press, Cambridge, MA.

White, M. and Epston, D. (1990) *Narrative Means to Therapeutic Ends*. Norton, London.

Part V
Multiple Choice Questions and Answers

Multiple Choice Questions

1 Assessment

1.1 *In child psychiatric assessments:*

(a) There is a low level of agreement between parental reports and self-reports of children's emotional symptoms
(b) If psychiatric symptoms cause a child a lot of distress but no social impairment, a disorder should not be diagnosed
(c) It is usually possible to identify the cause of child psychiatric disorders
(d) Identifying the child and family's strengths is useful for planning treatment
(e) Families' and professionals' explanations of symptoms often differ widely

1.2 *When eliciting information from parents:*

(a) Fully-structured interviews give a more detailed picture of child symptoms than do semi-structured interviews
(b) Questionnaires can be a useful screening device
(c) With semi-structured interviews, the presence of symptoms is typically rated according to the interviewer's criteria, not the respondent's
(d) It is usual to see the father separately to elicit his view of the problem
(e) The early childhood history will not be relevant for disorders of adolescence

1.3 *Concerning individual interviews with children:*

(a) It is essential to focus immediately on the emotional or behavioural problems or the children will lose interest
(b) There is little point in directed questioning for children aged under 10
(c) Children rarely volunteer information on obsessions or compulsions unless asked directly
(d) Children's accounts of their peer relationships may differ markedly from that given by their parents or teachers
(e) Children may fear they are going to be given an injection or admitted to a hospital ward

1.4 *In child psychiatric assessments:*

(a) Teachers are not very reliable informants about disruptive behaviour
(b) Teachers may misconstrue specific learning problems as hyperactivity
(c) All children should have a full physical examination including height, weight and cardiac auscultation

(d) Most dysmorphic syndromes will be missed unless the child is seen undressed

(e) A child who has regressed, with the loss of established skills, should have a neurological examination

2   Classification

2.1 *Concerning the classification of child and adolescent mental health problems:*

(a) A categorical approach is almost invariably superior to a dimensional approach

(b) Problems which occur just at home or just at school are less likely to reflect
constitutional factors than problems occurring in both settings

(c) Oppositional–defiant disorder is categorised as an emotional disorder because of
the predominant angry affect

(d) Nearly all adolescent disorders fit into one of the three groupings of emotional,
disruptive or developmental

(e) Current child psychiatric schemes distinguish between disorders largely on the
basis that they have different signs and symptoms, rather than on the basis that
they have different causes

2.2 *DSM–IV and ICD–10 (research version):*

(a) Differ in some details but are similar in overall approach

(b) Only include diagnostic categories that have been validated by epidemiological and
multivariate studies

(c) Use operationalised diagnostic criteria

(d) Include categories for children who do not meet operationalised criteria

(e) Often judge whether a disorder is present or not on the basis of level of distress or
social impairment, as well as on the basis of the symptom profile

2.3 *In the multiaxial schemes of DSM–IV and ICD–10:*

(a) A conduct or emotional disorder is coded on the first axis of either scheme

(b) Reading disorder is also coded on the first axis in ICD–10 but not DSM–IV

(c) Mental retardation and reading disorder are coded on different axes in DSM-IV

(d) DSM–IV includes a separate axis for the highest level of premorbid functioning

(e) Both schemes have an axis for the current level of social impairment/adaptive
functioning

2.4 *Factor and cluster analyses:*

(a) Factor analyses identify dimensions

(b) Cluster analyses classify attributes

(c) The number of clusters is identified from the eigenvalue

(d) Items contributing to the same dimension correlate poorly with one another

(e) The pattern of clustering may depend on which attributes are considered

3   Epidemiology

3.1 *Epidemiological studies of children and adolescents have generally shown that:*

(a) 25–40% have a psychiatric disorder

(b) Autistic disorders are one of the commonest child psychiatric disorders

(c) Children with conduct problems only rarely have emotional problems too

(d) Most children with psychiatric disorders are in contact with mental health professionals

(e) Psychosocial disorders have become less common over recent decades

3.2 *The following are more common in girls than boys:*

(a) Diurnal enuresis
(b) Hyperkinetic syndrome
(c) Delayed speech
(d) Anorexia nervosa
(e) Completed suicide

3.3 *The following occur more in boys than girls:*

(a) Animal phobia
(b) School refusal
(c) Teenage overdose
(d) Selective mutism
(e) Conduct disorder

3.4 *Disorders more likely to present in adolescence than childhood include:*

(a) Enuresis
(b) Anorexia nervosa
(c) Depression
(d) Autism
(e) Selective mutism

3.5 *Social disadvantage is associated with a much higher rate of:*

(a) Truancy
(b) Autism
(c) Mild mental retardation
(d) School refusal
(e) Juvenile delinquency

4 Autistic Disorders

4.1 *Characteristic features of infantile autism include:*

(a) Repetitive and ritualistic behaviours
(b) Phobias
(c) Self injury
(d) Poor communication skills
(e) Lack of social interest or skill

4.2 *The following features are fairly common among autistic children:*

(a) More difficulty mixing with adults than with other children of the same age
(b) Echolalia
(c) Indifference to environmental change
(d) Head circumference above the 97th centile
(e) Gaze avoidance

4.3 *The following features are fairly common among autistic children and teenagers:*

(a) Hallucinations
(b) Hand flapping
(c) Tendency to treat people like things
(d) Seizures starting in adolescence
(e) Overactivity and poor attention

4.4 *Infantile autism:*

(a) Is also known as Asperger's syndrome
(b) Never affects behaviour before 6 months of age
(c) Is prelinguistic schizophrenia
(d) Always begins by the age of 28 months
(e) Loss of language may occur after a period of normal development

4.5 *When assessing a supposedly autistic child, it is important to consider the following differential diagnoses:*

(a) Separation anxiety
(b) Rett's syndrome
(c) Mental retardation
(d) Dyslexia
(e) Developmental dysphasia (language delay)

4.6 *Infantile autism:*

(a) Males and females are equally affected
(b) Roughly 3–5 children per 1000 are affected
(c) Parents are typically of high socioeconomic status
(d) Is often caused by cold mothers who fail to bond normally
(e) Affects 25% of full siblings.

4.7 *The prognosis of autism is worse if:*

(a) IQ is under 60
(b) Clumsiness is present
(c) The child is male
(d) Useful speech is absent at the age of 5
(e) The pattern of rituals changes with time

4.8 *Roughly half of autistic individuals:*

(a) Never acquire useful speech
(b) Die before the age of 30
(c) Lose cognitive skills in late adolescence
(d) Never marry or hold a paid job
(e) Remain markedly aloof in adult life

4.9 *Common cognitive findings in autistic children include:*

(a) Verbal IQ much lower than performance IQ
(b) Loss of previously acquired skills between the ages of 3 and 10 years
(c) Retardation in most areas is mixed with islets of normal or superior ability

(d)   Selective agnosia for high frequency sounds
(e)   A defect in 'Theory of Mind'

4.10   *The following are usual in Asperger's syndrome:*

(a)   Circumscribed interests
(b)   Clumsiness
(c)   Stilted speech
(d)   Impaired social understanding
(e)   Marked language delay in the preschool years

5   Hyperactivity (Hyperkinesis/ADHD)

5.1   *Hyperactivity:*

(a)   Is a common complaint of parents about their children
(b)   Occurs mainly in middle class children
(c)   Affects equal numbers of boys and girls
(d)   Is more commonly diagnosed in the UK than the USA
(e)   Is usually first diagnosed in the 5–11 year old age band

5.2   *Characteristic features of hyperactivity include:*

(a)   Short attention span
(b)   Hand flapping and other mannerisms
(c)   Fidgeting
(d)   Elevated mood
(e)   Lack of selective attachment to parents

5.3   *Characteristic features of hyperactivity include:*

(a)   Distractibility
(b)   Impulsiveness
(c)   Getting up and wandering around when expected to be still
(d)   Sudden, repetitive, stereotyped, purposeless movements
(e)   Calling out in class and not waiting turn in games

5.4   *The following features would cast serious doubt on a diagnosis of hyperactivity:*

(a)   Symptoms reported by parents but not by the child's teacher
(b)   Onset at age 12
(c)   Well behaved throughout a 15 minute mental state examination
(d)   Sleeps soundly at night
(e)   Symptoms worsen after eating tomatoes, oranges or some other natural food

5.5   *Hyperactive children are likely to be:*

(a)   Of above average intelligence
(b)   Disobedient at home and/or disruptive in class
(c)   Popular classmates
(d)   Underachieving at school
(e)   Over-familiar or disinhibited with unfamiliar adults

5.6 *Hyperactivity is:*

(a) Usually associated with a history of parental neglect
(b) Commonly associated with demonstrable brain damage
(c) More frequent in those with epilepsy
(d) Associated with other developmental disorders e.g. language delay, clumsiness
(e) Commoner in children reared in institutions from infancy

5.7 *Natural history of hyperactivity:*

(a) Hyperactive children have often been overactive and inattentive since they were toddlers
(b) Symptoms may not be a cause for concern prior to school entry
(c) Overactivity and inattention typically become less troublesome during the teenage years
(d) A substantial minority remain restless and inattentive in adulthood
(e) Hyperactive children are at increased risk of criminality and substance abuse in adult life

5.8 *Treatment of hyperactivity:*

(a) Hyperactivity is a good target for psychodynamic psychotherapy
(b) Hyperactive children are best placed in a busy classroom environment because the increased arousal improves attention
(c) Barbiturates are contra-indicated
(d) Exclusion of artificial additives from the diet is usually helpful
(e) Imipramine is of demonstrated value in the treatment of hyperactivity

5.9 *Recognised side effects of treating 6–10 year old children with stimulants include:*

(a) Addiction
(b) Repetitive activities or stereotypies
(c) Slowing in growth
(d) A paradoxical increase in appetite and sleep
(e) Tics

6 Conduct Disorder

6.1 *Conduct disorders are:*

(a) Commoner in girls than boys until the age of 7
(b) Commoner in inner city areas
(c) Commonly restricted to one situation e.g. school not home or vice versa
(d) One of the commonest of child psychiatric disorders
(e) Typically more transient than emotional disorders

6.2 *The following child factors increase the risk of conduct disorder:*

(a) Hyperactivity
(b) IQ under 70
(c) Specific reading disorder
(d) Epilepsy
(e) A 'difficult' temperament as an infant

6.3 *The following family factors increase the risk of conduct disorder:*

(a) Marital friction or breakdown
(b) High parental expectations
(c) Parental mental illness
(d) Overcrowding and poverty
(e) Mother goes out to work

6.4 *The following family factors increase the risk of conduct disorder:*

(a) Maternal overprotection
(b) Strict house rules and close supervision
(c) Parent criminality
(d) Large family size
(e) Elderly parents

6.5 *Characteristic features of oppositional–defiant disorder are:*

(a) Repeated shoplifting
(b) Frequent refusal to comply with adult requests
(c) Frequent temper tantrums
(d) Frequently annoys others on purpose
(e) Persistent truancy

6.6 *An 8 year old boy is stealing persistently from home. The following are plausible formulations:*

(a) He is making up for getting less pocket money than his friends
(b) The stealing is part of a grief reaction after a recent bereavement
(c) He needs cash to pay protection money to bullies at school
(d) He feels starved of affection and is stealing for comfort
(e) He has SRMR (specific retardation of moral reasoning) and does not know right from wrong

6.7 *The following features of childhood conduct disorder worsen the prognosis:*

(a) A greater variety of conduct symptoms
(b) Poor peer relationships
(c) Associated hyperactivity
(d) Problem evident in just one setting e.g. school
(e) Late onset

6.8 *Conduct disorder:*

(a) Most adults with antisocial personality disorder had been conduct disordered children
(b) Most children with conduct disorder develop antisocial personality disorder
(c) In childhood, conduct disorder is more often associated with anxiety than depression
(d) Children with conduct disorder are particularly likely to misinterpret the actions of other children as hostile
(e) Conduct disorder increases the risk of depression in adult life, particularly in females

6.9 *Truancy :*

(a) Children who truant are likely to be at home when they are not at school
(b) Severe depression is a recognised cause
(c) Truancy is associated with conduct disorder and delinquency
(d) Most truants are of below average academic ability
(e) Truancy is the commonest cause of absence from school at all ages

7 Juvenile Delinquency

7.1 *Juvenile delinquency:*

(a) Violent offences peak in the mid-teens and then fall throughout adult life
(b) Most juvenile delinquency involves offences against property rather than people
(c) All types of juvenile offences are commoner in males
(d) Middle class youths are less delinquent judging from convictions but not according to self-report
(e) Equally impoverished neighbourhoods may differ markedly in delinquency rates

7.2 *Juvenile delinquency:*

(a) Usually leads to adult criminality
(b) Is associated with criminality in parents and siblings
(c) Is nearly always associated with overt psychiatric disorder
(d) Is highly heritable
(e) Is a common sequel of encephalitis

7.3 *Juvenile delinquency is associated with:*

(a) Below-average intelligence
(b) Characteristic EEG abnormalities
(c) Troublesome behaviour in school from an early age
(d) Extroversion
(e) Poor peer relationships

7.4 *Juvenile delinquency is associated with the following family factors:*

(a) Poverty
(b) Having older brothers
(c) High parental expectations
(d) Erratic or inconsistent discipline
(e) Critical and cold parenting

8 School Refusal

8.1 *School refusal:*

(a) Is commoner at 14 than at 10
(b) Affects girls more than boys
(c) Is the commonest presentation of emotional disorder in childhood
(d) Is associated with low socioeconomic status
(e) Is linked with large family size

8.2 *School refusal:*

(a) Tends to start in early May (before examinations)
(b) Is more common in boys
(c) A precipitating factor can often be identified
(d) Scholastic failure is common
(e) Is the commonest cause of school non-attendance in teenagers

8.3 *In school refusal:*

(a) School factors are unimportant
(b) Depression is a rare underlying cause
(c) Complaints of abdominal pain are unduly common
(d) The child's fear is often of leaving home rather than of going to school
(e) The child may fear other children

8.4 *School refusal:*

(a) The parents are often emotionally over-involved with the child
(b) Is associated with strict discipline at home
(c) The child is usually hyperkinetic
(d) Is often associated with delinquency
(e) Often reflects the family's view that schooling is unimportant

8.5 *School refusal:*

(a) In an 8-year-old may be a manifestation of separation anxiety
(b) In a 15-year-old may be a manifestation of depression
(c) May present as headache
(d) In a 10-year-old is likely to be associated with stealing from mother
(e) In a 14-year-old is usually a forerunner of agoraphobia in adult life

8.6 *In the treatment of school refusal:*

(a) A rapid return to school is generally contraindicated
(b) In-patient treatment is needed in some cases
(c) A change in school is often necessary
(d) Tricyclic antidepressants often facilitate a return to school
(e) Home tuition is usually a helpful interim measure

8.7 *School refusal:*

(a) With treatment, over half return to full-time school
(b) A return to school is more likely for younger children
(c) Often turns into truancy if untreated
(d) Usually followed by persistent neurotic disorder in adult life
(e) Often leads to a lifetime of work refusal

9 Anxiety Disorders

9.1 *Anxiety disorders in childhood:*

(a) Are among the commonest sorts of child psychiatric disorders
(b) Commonly occur together with depressive disorders

(c) Commonly occur together with attachment disorders
(d) Commonly occur together with reading disorders
(e) Occur more often if parents have anxiety disorders

9.2 *Separation anxiety disorder:*

(a) Is mainly a disorder of preschool children
(b) Is a common cause of school refusal
(c) Characteristically involves reluctance to speak except at home
(d) Is likely to respond to tricyclic antidepressants
(e) Often leads on to agoraphobia in adult life

9.3 *Generalized anxiety disorder:*

(a) Is less common after puberty
(b) Involves wide-ranging worries about the past, present and future
(c) Often leads to somatic complaints
(d) Usually occurs together with other anxiety or depressive disorders
(e) Is appropriately treated with cognitive therapy

9.4 *Specific phobias:*

(a) Can only be diagnosed if the child recognises the fear as irrational
(b) Can only be diagnosed if the feared stimulus is either avoided or endured with intense distress
(c) Are equally common in boys and girls
(d) Are appropriately treated by behavioural or cognitive means
(e) Usually follow a traumatic event and resolve within six months

10 Depression and Mania

10.1 *Depressive disorders in childhood and adolescence:*

(a) Are more likely than their adult counterparts to involve disturbed sleep and appetite
(b) Are less likely than their adult counterparts to involve guilt and hopelessness
(c) Are a common cause of school refusal
(d) Are a common cause of enuresis
(e) Are more closely related to school transition than to pubertal status

10.2 *Depressive disorders in childhood and adolescence:*

(a) Are present in roughly 8% of 10-year-olds
(b) Are present in roughly 20% of 15-year-olds
(c) Psychological therapies have a demonstrated role
(d) Tricyclic antidepressants have a demonstrated role
(e) Usually remit within 6 months and rarely recur

10.3 *Mania in childhood and adolescence:*

(a) Becomes much commoner after puberty
(b) Is usually chronic rather than episodic in prepubertal children
(c) Is rarely present at the onset of a bipolar disorder - depression usually comes first

(d) Is often accompanied by 'first rank' hallucinations or delusions

(e) Should not be treated with neuroleptics

11   Suicide and Deliberate Self-Harm

11.1 *Completed suicide in children and adolescents:*

(a) Is almost unknown under the age of 10

(b) Is commoner in females

(c) Self-poisoning is more typical of male suicides than female suicides

(d) Is commoner in countries where hand-guns are easily available

(e) Has been getting rarer for decades, but may now be levelling out

11.2 *The risk of completed suicide in childhood and adolescence is increased if:*

(a) The individual has a disruptive behavioural disorder

(b) Family members have depression and other emotional problems

(c) Family members have alcohol or drug abuse problems

(d) There has been a disciplinary crisis

(e) The individual has been talking about suicide

11.3 *Deliberate self-harm (attempted suicide) in children and adolescents:*

(a) Roughly 14 times commoner than completed suicide

(b) Much commoner now than 50 years ago

(c) Most have a definite psychiatric disorder

(d) Under 5% have a prior history of self-harm

(e) Usually planned for between 6 and 24 hours

11.4 *The likelihood of deliberate self-harm (attempted suicide) in children and adolescents is increased by:*

(a) A history of physical or sexual abuse

(b) Placement in a children's home

(c) Easy access to medication

(d) School or work problems

(e) Recent media reports of attempted suicides

11.5 *The prognosis of deliberate self-harm (attempted suicide) in children and adolescents:*

(a) Roughly 10% will harm themselves again within the year

(b) Extensive family psychopathology increases the likelihood of repetition

(c) Psychiatric disorder increases the likelihood of repetition

(d) Repetition is more likely in females

(e) Roughly 5% will eventually kill themselves

12   Reactions to Stress

12.1 *Grief in childhood:*

(a) The initial crisis response often involves emotional numbness rather than overt distress

(b) Anger and resentment may be more marked than misery

(c) Feelings of hopelessness, worthlessness and guilt are unusual unless the bereavement has triggered a depressive disorder

(d) Children form new attachments very rapidly to make up for the loss of key attachment figures

(e) Progress through the stages of grief is not irreversible - children can go backwards as well as forwards

12.2 *Post-traumatic stress disorder can be triggered off by:*

(a) Medical procedures

(b) Sexual abuse

(c) Life-threatening injuries or illnesses

(d) Rejection by friends

(e) Witnessing one parent attacking the other

12.3 *Characteristic features of post-traumatic stress disorder include:*

(a) Poor concentration

(b) Loss of appetite

(c) Repetitive re-enactment of the trauma in play

(d) Inability to recall an important aspect of the trauma

(e) Indiscriminate friendliness

12.4 *Characteristic features of post-traumatic stress disorder include:*

(a) Exaggerated startle response

(b) Distress at reminders

(c) Enuresis

(d) Destructiveness

(e) Intrusive images

13   Obsessive-Compulsive Disorder

13.1 *Childhood obsessive-compulsive disorder (OCD):*

(a) Affects females more than males

(b) Involves very similar symptoms to OCD in adults

(c) May not involve resistance to obsessions and compulsions

(d) Is often accompanied by anxiety or depressive disorders

(e) Was present in 70% of adults with OCD

13.2 *The causation of childhood obsessive-compulsive disorder (OCD):*

(a) OCD can be part of the congenital cocaine syndrome

(b) Family studies suggest that OCD is genetically related to Tourette's syndrome

(c) CSF studies suggest that OCD is associated with melatonin hypersecretion

(d) Scan studies suggest that OCD involves temporal lobe pathology

(e) OCD can follow acute streptococcal infections

13.3 *The following treatments are commonly helpful for childhood obsessive-compulsive disorder:*

(a) Psychodynamic psychotherapy
(b) Paradoxical injunction
(c) Response prevention
(d) Clomipramine
(e) Fenfluramine

14 Tourette's Syndrome and Other Tic Disorders

14.1 *Tics:*

(a) Are sudden, frequent, stereotyped and purposeless
(b) May be preceded by a premonitory urge
(c) May take the form of complex motor acts
(d) Are reduced or absent in sleep
(e) Affect over 1% of children at some time in their lives

14.2 *Tics:*

(a) May take the form of sniffs, grunts or words
(b) Usually begin by the age of 4
(c) Can usually be suppressed temporarily by an act of will
(d) Are generally worsened by stress
(e) Are rarely present when the individual is alone and relaxed

14.3 *In Tourette's syndrome:*

(a) Prevalence is under 1 per 10 000
(b) Males greatly outnumber females
(c) Phonic tics usually emerge before motor tics
(d) Coprolalia occurs in over 80%
(e) Epilepsy is common

14.4 *In Tourette's syndrome:*

(a) Roughly 30% of affected individuals are mentally retarded
(b) Inattention and hyperactivity are common
(c) Focal neurological signs are present in the majority
(d) Obsessive-compulsive symptoms are common
(e) Symptoms typically worsen progressively throughout adult life

14.5 *In Tourette's syndrome:*

(a) A family history of schizophrenia is commoner than expected by chance
(b) A family history of obsessive-compulsive disorder is commoner than expected by chance
(c) Neuroleptics are a recognised treatment for the tics
(d) Stimulants are a recognised treatment for the tics
(e) Imipramine is a recognised treatment for the tics

15   Selective Mutism

15.1 *Selective mutism is commoner in:*

(a) Males
(b) Only children
(c) Children with below-average intelligence
(d) Children from chaotic or socially disadvantaged families
(e) Children with articulation difficulties

15.2 *Selective mutism:*

(a) Affects under 0.1% of 6–10 year olds.
(b) The child may speak at school but not at home
(c) Children often meet diagnostic criteria for anxiety disorders too
(d) Is usually sudden in onset, often following a definite stress
(e) If it does not resolve within 12 months, it often persists for over 5 years

16   Attachment Disorders

16.1 *Attachment disorders:*

(a) Are one of the few disorders that can be diagnosed in an infant of 6 months
(b) May begin in late childhood if the child is orphaned
(c) Characteristically involve the absence of imaginative play
(d) Can be limited to a seriously troubled relationship with the key caregiver
(e) Are common consequences of lengthy mother-infant separations in the neonatal period

16.2 *Children with a reactive attachment disorder (inhibited type) commonly show:*

(a) Clinginess in infancy
(b) Lack of emotional responsiveness
(c) Ambivalence to caregivers
(d) Misery
(e) A willingness to approach relatively unfamiliar adults for comfort when distressed

16.3 *Children with a disinhibited attachment disorder commonly show:*

(a) Attention-seeking behaviour
(b) Hypervigilance
(c) Reduced need for sleep
(d) Indiscriminate friendliness
(e) Aggression in response to another person's distress

17   Enuresis

17.1 *Epidemiology of enuresis:*

(a) Nocturnal enuresis is about equally common in males and females at the age of 5
(b) Nocturnal enuresis is commoner in males than females at the age of 7
(c) Diurnal enuresis is commoner in males than females at the age of 9

(d) Around 10% or more of 5-year-olds wet the bed at least once a week
(e) By the age of 9, most children who wet the bed have had at least one lengthy remission when they were dry every night

17.2 *Schoolchildren with nocturnal enuresis:*

(a) Are likely to have a family history of enuresis in a first degree relative
(b) Often have structural abnormalities of the urinary tract
(c) Always have a maturational lag
(d) Are at substantially greater risk than other children of asymptomatic urinary tract infections
(e) Commonly have epilepsy or epileptiform discharges on their EEG

17.3 *Nocturnal enuresis is more likely:*

(a) In children exposed to stress before the age of 4
(b) In REM sleep
(c) In children who experienced harsh toilet training
(d) In children who sleep particularly deeply
(e) When toilet training was started after the age of 24 months

17.4 *Psychiatric correlates of enuresis:*

(a) Enuresis is usually part of a wider psychiatric syndrome
(b) Enuresis is typically associated with emotional symptoms rather than conduct problems
(c) Psychiatric symptoms are more likely if the child wets by day and not just at night
(d) Psychiatric symptoms are commoner if the enuresis is secondary rather than primary
(e) Children whose enuresis has resolved are no longer at increased psychiatric risk

17.5 *An assessment of a 9-year-old girl with nocturnal enuresis should include:*

(a) A gynaecological examination
(b) An EEG
(c) Cystometry
(d) Urinalysis
(e) A micturating cystogram

17.6 *Which of the following treatments reduce the frequency of bed wetting:*

(a) Tricyclic antidepressants
(b) Stimulant medications
(d) Desmopressin
(c) Anticholinergic medication
(e) Carbamazepine

17.7 *Which of the following, if used correctly for three months, will usually result in a lasting cure of bed wetting:*

(a) Amitriptyline
(b) Fluid restriction in the evenings
(c) Enuresis alarm

(d) Waking the child to use the toilet after a couple of hours of sleep
(e) Synthetic antidiuretic hormone

17.8 *Nocturnal enuresis is more likely to persist in children who:*

(a) Are female
(b) Have never previously been dry for at least six months
(c) Have a positive family history of enuresis
(d) Grow up in poverty
(e) Wet the bed every night rather than a few nights per week

18 Faecal Soiling

18.1 *Faecal soiling occurs once a week or more in:*

(a) Over 50% of 3-year-olds
(b) Under 10% of 4-year-olds
(c) Around 3% of 11-year-olds
(d) Around 1% of 16-year-olds
(e) Boys much more often than girls

18.2 *Recognised causes of faecal soiling include:*

(a) Inadequate toilet training
(b) A high-fibre diet
(c) Mental retardation
(d) Sexual abuse
(e) Covert aggression towards the family

18.3 *Recognised causes of faecal soiling include:*

(a) Constipation
(b) Fear of the toilet
(c) A family fixation on bowel habits
(d) Diseases of the central nervous system
(e) Threadworm infestation of the gut

18.4 *Children with faecal soiling often need:*

(a) Laxatives
(b) Bowel washouts
(c) Imipramine
(d) Behavioural programmes
(e) In-patient treatment

18.5 *The prognosis is worse when faecal soiling:*

(a) Occurs in girls
(b) Is associated with hyperactivity
(c) Occurs during the day rather than in sleep
(d) Is accompanied by other developmental problems
(e) Is accompanied by social or school problems

19   Psychosomatics

19.1   *Psychosomatic problems in children are more likely:*

(a)   In families that attribute symptoms to environmental or psychological factors
(b)   Among conscientious, sensitive and insecure children
(c)   When children have been bullied
(d)   When relatives have somatic symptoms
(e)   After a period of organic illness

19.2   *Recurrent abdominal pain in childhood:*

(a)   Affects around 3–5% of children
(b)   Peaks at 10–12 years of age
(c)   Has an identifiable organic cause in roughly 40% of cases
(d)   Commonly persists into adult life
(e)   Is commonly secondary to undisclosed sexual abuse

19.3   *In children with the chronic fatigue syndrome:*

(a)   The fatigue typically persists for between 2 and 6 months
(b)   Low mood is common
(c)   Self-blame and feelings of worthlessness are common
(d)   Treatment hinges on families accepting that the problems are not organic
(e)   The treatment of choice is usually graded rehabilitation

19.4   *Conversion disorder in childhood:*

(a)   Is mainly a disorder of 5–10 year olds
(b)   Affects boys more than girls
(c)   Is usually modelled on illnesses the child has observed
(d)   Usually occurs together with a depressive disorder or another psychiatric diagnosis
(e)   Mostly affects children from apparently normal families

20   Preschool Problems

20.1   *Common problems in 3-year-olds include:*

(a)   Worrying
(b)   Waking at night
(c)   Autism
(d)   Overactivity
(e)   Fears

20.2   *Factors predicting more behavioural problems in 3-year-olds:*

(a)   Mother in paid employment
(b)   Male
(c)   Specific language delay
(d)   Maternal depression
(e)   Marital discord

20.3 *Concerning 3-year-olds with moderate or severe behavioural problems:*

(a) Problems resolve within 5 years in over 75% of children
(b) Resolution of problems is commoner in boys
(c) Family factors are good predictors of the chronicity of established problems
(d) Early overactivity is a predictor of conduct disorder in middle childhood
(e) Early fearfulness is a predictor of emotional disorder in middle childhood

21   Disorders in Adolescence

21.1 *In a representative sample of adolescents with psychiatric disorders:*

(a) About half have long-standing disorders that have persisted since middle childhood and the other half have new-onset disorders
(b) Long-standing disorders are mostly conduct and emotional disorders
(c) New-onset disorders are mostly eating and psychotic disorders
(d) Adverse family factors are more often associated with new-onset than with long-standing disorders
(e) Educational difficulties are more often associated with new-onset than with long-standing disorders

21.2 *Concerning adolescent drug use:*

(a) Ecstasy is the drug most used by adolescents
(b) 60% of teenagers who experiment with drugs continue to use them regularly
(c) Most young adults who are drug abusers first began to use drugs in school
(d) A history of conduct disorder is associated with a higher rate of drug use in adolescence
(e) A history of school refusal is associated with a higher rate of drug use in adolescence

21.3 *Common side effects of volatile substance abuse ('glue sniffing') include:*

(a) Asthma
(b) Nausea and vomiting
(c) Headache or abdominal pain
(d) Erosion of dental enamel
(e) Rash around nose or mouth

21.4 *Deaths from volatile substance abuse ('glue sniffing'):*

(a) Commonly result from laryngeal spasm
(b) Commonly result from status epilepticus
(c) Mostly occur in males
(d) Only rarely occur in first-time users
(e) Account for around 25% of deaths in childhood

21.5 *Schizophrenia in childhood and adolescence is:*

(a) Very rare before the age of 7
(b) Commoner in males at all ages
(c) Less genetic than adult-onset schizophrenia

(d) Commonly preceded by difficulties in social adjustment

(e) Associated with a worse prognosis than adult-onset schizophrenia

21.6 *Recognised symptoms of schizophrenia in childhood and adolescence:*

(a) Affective blunting

(b) Auditory hallucinations of other people making critical comments

(c) Insistence on sameness

(d) Pronominal reversal

(e) Thought disorder

21.7 *First psychotic episodes in childhood and adolescence:*

(a) The onset is characteristically acute

(b) The episode usually lasts between one and six weeks

(c) Apathy and social withdrawal typically resolve faster than delusions

(d) The majority have no further episodes if the initial episode is treated promptly

(e) Psychosocial functioning prior to the episode is one of the best predictors of long-term outcome

21.8 *Anorexia nervosa in children and adolescents:*

(a) Female:male ratio of around 3:1

(b) Roughly equal prevalence throughout the world

(c) Affects around 2–4% of 15-year-olds

(d) Uncommon before puberty

(e) Early onset may lead to delayed or arrested puberty

21.9 *Anorexia nervosa in children and adolescents:*

(a) Onset may be precipitated by adverse life events

(b) Family therapy is of demonstrated value

(c) Adequate weight gain is rarely possible without hospitalisation

(d) Within 5 years, 90% have fully recovered

(e) Greater initial weight loss predicts poorer long-term outcome

21.10 *Bulimia nervosa:*

(a) Commonly associated with depression

(b) Has a peak age of onset in the early teens

(c) Typically involves a body weight over 25% above that expected for age and height

(d) Often episodic with remissions and relapses

(e) Is more likely than anorexia nervosa to come to professional attention

22 Maltreatment of Children

22.1 *Regarding maltreatment and abuse:*

(a) The great majority of cases occur before the age of 5

(b) The most commonly registered category in the UK and USA is emotional abuse

(c) In the USA there are around 600 homicides a year of children under 8

(d) A common presentation of Munchausen syndrome by proxy is respiratory arrest

(e) Most cases of Munchausen syndrome by proxy are perpetrated by the child's step-father

22.2 *Non-organic failure to thrive (NOFT):*

(a) No medical cause can be found for the low weight
(b) Deviant parent–child interactions are common at meal times
(c) Is associated with a greatly increased risk of later neglect and abuse
(d) Catch-up weight gain if the child is admitted to hospital is strongly suggestive of NOFT
(e) Is rarer than psychosocial short stature

22.3 *Recognised risk factors for physical abuse include:*

(a) Lack of social support for the mother
(b) Severe disability in the child
(c) Father drinks 4 units of alcohol per week
(d) Premature birth of child
(e) Father unemployed

22.4 *Recognised risk factors for physical abuse include:*

(a) Full-time working mother
(b) Excessively close supervision of the child
(c) Child aged less than one year
(d) Parent has a personality disorder
(e) Grandparents live in the same house

22.5 *Regarding emotional abuse:*

(a) It affects around 30% of children who are also being physically or sexually abused
(b) It is less damaging than most other forms of abuse
(c) It is associated with autistic problems
(d) Threats of abandonment can lead to anxious attachment patterns
(e) Extreme hostility and criticism by parents increases the chance that the children will be bullies themselves

22.6 *Regarding the sexual abuse of children and adolescents:*

(a) Penetrative abuse is reported retrospectively by about 1 in 200 women
(b) Boys are less commonly affected than girls
(c) The commonest presentation in girls is with a urinary tract infection
(d) Irritability and aggression may be the only presenting symptoms
(e) Community surveys show that it is much rarer in the highest socioeconomic groups

22.7 *Regarding the sexual abuse of children and adolescents:*

(a) Over 5% of reported cases are committed by females
(b) Stepfathers are disproportionately common perpetrators
(c) Biological fathers are rarely the perpetrators
(d) When it occurs outside the home, the perpetrator is usually a stranger
(e) There is little evidence for the existence of 'sex rings'

22.8 *Regarding the effects of child abuse:*

(a) Post-traumatic stress disorder is a recognised consequence

(b) Abused children are more likely to be rejected by their peer group
(c) The majority of abused children go on to abuse their own children when they become parents
(d) Self-cutting may be a sign of sexual abuse
(e) Sexually abused boys are more likely to become sexual abusers themselves

22.9 *Regarding sexual abuse:*

(a) About one third of seriously abused girls are not believed by their mothers
(b) It is essential that the mental health professional who first hears about the abuse conducts a physical examination before the signs disappear
(c) A negative physical examination does not rule out the possibility of sexual abuse
(d) Reflex anal dilatation is pathognomonic
(e) Denial by the perpetrator is routine and does not influence the likelihood of successful rehabilitation

22.10 *When parents bring injured children to casualty, the following elements should increase suspicion of physical abuse:*

(a) Delay in seeking medical help
(b) The parents describe how the injury was sustained with a lot of circumstantial detail
(c) The child is tearful and frightened of the hospital staff
(d) The parents do not show much concern or anxiety
(e) The parents attempt to leave hospital before investigations are complete

22.11 *Interventions for child abuse are more likely to be successful when:*

(a) The child has non-organic failure to thrive
(b) The child presented with Munchausen syndrome by proxy
(c) The parents were themselves abused in childhood
(d) There is access to good local child care
(e) The parents are able to put the child's needs before their own

23 Mental Retardation

23.1 *Concerning mental retardation (MR):*

(a) For legal and administrative purposes, MR is defined by the combination of low intelligence and educational disability
(b) About half of all children with an IQ under 50 are never identified by medical, educational or social services.
(c) Mild MR is defined by an IQ between 50 and 79
(d) The prevalence of mild MR is much greater than would be expected if IQ were normally distributed (the second 'hump')
(e) Severe MR affects around 0.4 individuals per 1000

23.2 *In severe mental retardation:*

(a) An identifiable organic cause is more likely than in mild MR
(b) Polygenic effects are of greater aetiological significance than in mild MR
(c) Males substantially outnumber females

(d)   The child needs to attend a training centre rather than a school
(e)   The ability to learn new skills is markedly impaired

23.3   *In normal-variant (subcultural) mental retardation:*

(a)   The child's head circumference is usually below the third centile
(b)   Siblings are often of borderline intelligence
(c)   There is commonly an identifiable enzyme defect
(d)   There is a steep socioeconomic gradient
(e)   The modal IQ is in the 35–45 band

23.4   *Concerning Down's syndrome:*

(a)   Present in around 1 in 600 births to mothers aged 45 or more
(b)   95% are due to translocations of chromosome 21
(c)   Accounts for over 20% of all mental retardation (IQ under 70)
(d)   Associated with atrial septal defects
(e)   Associated with congenital duodenal atresia

23.5   *Common features of Down's syndrome include:*

(a)   Tall stature
(b)   Single palmar crease
(c)   Low-set simple ears
(d)   Hypertonia
(e)   Epicanthic folds

23.6   *The fragile X syndrome:*

(a)   Affects around 1 per 170 births
(b)   Involves an excess of tripeptide repeats
(c)   Reduces IQ in affected males but not in affected females
(d)   Testicular enlargement is rarely evident before puberty
(e)   Laboratory diagnosis requires cell culture in folate-deficient media

23.7   *The fetal alcohol syndrome:*

(a)   Height, weight and head circumference are usually low from birth onwards
(b)   Accounts for about 20% of severe mental retardation
(c)   Typically involves prominent ears
(d)   Typically involves short palpebral fissures
(e)   Upper lip typically forms a prominent 'Cupid's bow'

23.8   *The following syndromes are inherited in an autosomal recessive fashion:*

(a)   Neurofibromatosis
(b)   Galactosaemia
(c)   Hurler's
(d)   Tay–Sachs
(e)   Hunter's

23.9   *The following syndromes are inherited in an autosomal recessive fashion:*

(a)   Sturge–Weber
(b)   Homocystinuria

(c) Phenylketonuria
(d) Lesch–Nyhan
(e) Tuberous sclerosis

23.10 *Tuberous sclerosis:*

(a) Cutaneous and subcutaneous nodules in the distribution of cutaneous nerves appear in late childhood
(b) Adenoma sebaceum is usually evident by 2 years of age
(c) Hypopigmented patches are rarely evident until school age
(d) Associated with axillary freckling
(e) Commonest associated seizure type is petit mal

23.11 *The following maternal infections during pregnancy may be related to subsequent mental retardation in the child:*

(a) Rubella
(b) Measles
(c) Toxoplasmosis
(d) Cytomegalovirus
(e) Gonococcus

23.12 *The following have a role to play in the prevention of mental retardation:*

(a) Folic acid supplementation around the time of conception
(b) Neonatal screening for hypothyroidism
(c) Neonatal screening for galactosaemia
(d) Polio immunisation
(e) Traffic calming in residential areas

23.13 *Mental retardation is associated with an increased risk of the following disorders:*

(a) Conduct disorders
(b) Hyperactivity disorders
(c) Emotional disorders
(d) Autistic disorders
(e) Sleep disorders

23.14 *Self-injurious behaviour in children with mental retardation is:*

(a) Commoner when the MR is severe rather than mild
(b) Commoner when children are bored or isolated
(c) Reinforced whenever caregivers respond with extra attention
(d) Best treated with behavioural approaches
(e) Usually helped by stimulant medication

23.15 *The following pairings of physical syndromes and behavioural phenotypes are correct:*

(a) Prader–Willi syndrome and cocktail party speech
(b) Lesch–Nyhan syndrome and severe self-injury
(c) Fragile X syndrome and social anxiety with gaze avoidance
(d) Congenital rubella and insatiable overeating
(e) Fetal alcohol syndrome and autism

24   Brain Disorders

24.1 *Psychiatric problems in children with epilepsy or cerebral palsy:*

(a) Are much commoner than among comparably disabled children with non–cerebral disorders
(b) Are mainly conduct and emotional problems
(c) Often involve deliberate aggression or antisocial behaviour, e.g. bullying or vandalism
(d) Episodic outbursts of rage are usually epileptic in origin
(e) Hyperactivity and autistic disorders are particularly over-represented

24.2 *In childhood:*

(a) Human immunodeficiency virus (HIV) infections can present with loss of established skills and additional emotional or behavioural problems
(b) Sexual abuse can present with loss of established skills and additional emotional or behavioural problems.
(c) Rolandic seizures are particularly likely to be misdiagnosed as hysterical pseudo-seizures
(d) Severe closed head injury can result in lasting social disinhibition
(e) Left hemisphere lesions are substantially more likely than right hemisphere lesions to result in depression

25   Language Disorders

25.1 *Different aspects of language:*

(a) Prosody refers to the production of speech sounds
(b) Syntax refers to the production and comprehension of grammatically correct sentences
(c) Phonology refers to communication via tone of voice and inflexion
(d) Pragmatics refers to communication via signs
(e) Semantics refers to the encoding and decoding of meaning in words

25.2 *Concerning childhood language disorders:*

(a) Under 1% of children of normal intelligence have language disorders that are severe, persistent, and socially impairing
(b) Boys are much more often affected than girls
(c) In semantic–pragmatic disorder the main abnormalities are in the use and content of language, not in its form
(d) Expressive language disorder is rarer than receptive language disorder
(e) Even when children outgrow language problems, they remain at a substantially increased risk of specific reading and spelling difficulties

25.3 *Psychiatric problems in children with language disorders:*

(a) Are mostly conduct problems
(b) Are no commoner than expected once low IQ has been taken into account
(c) Are often more obvious in older children than in younger children

(d)   Are commoner with articulation problems than with receptive language difficulties
(e)   May include autistic-like problems in social relationships

26 Reading Disorders

26.1 *Specific reading disorder (developmental dyslexia) is:*

(a)   Present in 15–25% of children
(b)   Commoner in girls than boys
(c)   More frequent in only children
(d)   Particularly common in deprived areas of the inner city
(e)   Accompanied by left-handedness in over 50% of cases

26.2 *Specific reading disorder (developmental dyslexia):*

(a)   Should not usually be diagnosed without testing a child's intelligence
(b)   Usually involves severe spelling as well as reading problems
(c)   Cannot be present if the child's reading age is less than a year below his or her chronological age
(d)   Is not usually associated with any arithmetical difficulties
(e)   Is associated with strephosymbolia (mirror writing)

26.3 *Routine investigations of a child with reading problems should include:*

(a)   CT scan
(b)   Audiometry
(c)   EEG
(d)   Psychometry
(e)   Chromosomes

26.4 *Specific reading disorder (developmental dyslexia) is associated with:*

(a)   Above-average intelligence
(b)   Epilepsy or cerebral palsy
(c)   Non-verbal intelligence lower than verbal intelligence
(d)   Conduct disorders and delinquency
(e)   High parental pressure for academic success

26.5 *Specific reading disorder (developmental dyslexia) is more likely with:*

(a)   A family history of reading problems
(b)   Middle class parents
(c)   Hyperactivity
(d)   Impaired phonological awareness
(e)   A tendency to muddle left and right

26.6 *Specific reading disorder (developmental dyslexia) is associated with:*

(a)   School refusal
(b)   Poor coordination
(c)   A family history of left-handedness
(d)   Myopia
(e)   Musical or artistic talent

26.7 *Children with specific reading disorder (developmental dyslexia):*

(a) Usually continue to have reading or spelling problems despite remedial teaching
(b) Are unlikely to develop new psychiatric problems in adolescence if they are free from psychiatric problems in middle childhood
(c) Usually end up with above-average educational qualifications because of their tendency to over-compensate
(d) Are at high risk of adult depression
(e) Are disproportionately likely to have a manual occupation in adult life

27   Insecure Attachment

27.1 *Regarding children's attachments to caregivers:*

(a) Children first become attached to their parents because they associate parents with food and play
(b) Smiling, crying and angry outbursts can all function as attachment behaviours
(c) The proximity of an attachment figure inhibits a young child's exploratory behaviour
(d) Selective attachments are not usually evident before 11 months of age
(e) Attachment behaviour tends to increase if the child is ill

27.2 *The Strange Situation Procedure:*

(a) Was devised by John Bowlby
(b) Usually involves children aged 24–30 months
(c) Involves an unfamiliar adult staying in the same room as the child throughout the procedure
(d) Involves two separations from a parent (or other caregiver) and two reunions
(e) Is usually carried out in the child's own home

27.3 *Rating attachment security from the Strange Situation Procedure:*

(a) When rating attachment security, the amount of distress on separation is not as good a guide as the child's response to reunion
(b) When parents of securely attached children leave and re-enter the room, their children generally continue playing as though nothing had happened
(c) Children with resistant-ambivalent attachments are very distressed by separation and hard to settle on reunion
(d) Children with disorganised attachments behave in a way that suggests fear or confusion in the caregiver's presence
(e) Avoidantly attached children welcome the separation and respond to the reunion with anger and tears

27.4 *Regarding attachment security:*

(a) Less than half of all children from community samples are securely attached
(b) Most children from maltreating families show a disorganised attachment pattern
(c) Maternal depression is associated with a higher rate of insecure attachment
(d) It is very unusual for a child who is securely attached to one parent to be insecurely attached to the other

(e) In community samples, the relative proportion of the different attachment categories is almost constant across cultures

27.5 *The Adult Attachment Interview (AAI):*

(a) Was developed by Mary Ainsworth
(b) Applies discourse analysis to establish the respondent's current state of mind with respect to attachment
(c) The criteria for autonomous attachment insist on convincing narrative evidence that the individual experienced emotionally supportive relationships in childhood
(d) A dismissing attachment typically involves many affectively charged memories of childhood rejection, leaving respondents highly critical of the parenting they received
(e) A pregnant woman's AAI classification is a good predictor of her unborn child's future attachment classification

27.6 *Concerning the predictive value of early attachment classification:*

(a) Attachment security predicts the quality of social impairment with unfamiliar adults better than it predicts the quality of close relationships
(b) With early and extensive day care, a child's future development is better predicted by the quality of attachment to day-care staff than by the quality of attachment to parents
(c) Secure attachment to parents predicts better relationships with siblings, teachers and classmates too
(d) Young children with resistant-ambivalent attachments are substantially more likely to be aggressive to other children in nursery school
(e) Most adults with mental illnesses or personality disorders have unresolved-disorganised attachments

28 Nature, Nurture and Family Adversities

28.1 *Regarding genes, shared environment and non-shared environment:*

(a) If a trait is influenced by shared environment, this will result in monozygotic ('identical') twins being more alike than dizygotic ('fraternal') twins.
(b) The resemblance between adoptees and their adoptive relatives is a measure of the strength of shared environmental effects
(c) If genetic factors are important, adoptees will resemble their biological relatives
(d) If a trait is particularly influenced by non-shared environment, the correlation between monozygotic ('identical') twins will be low.
(e) Variance not explained by genes or shared environment could be due to measurement error or the role of chance in brain development

28.2 *Regarding genes, shared environment and non-shared environment:*

(a) For most psychological traits, heritability is around 50%
(b) Liability to autism has an exceptionally low heritability
(c) Shared environment accounts for around 30% of the variance for most psychological traits

(d) Current evidence suggests that conduct problems run in families largely as a result of shared environment rather than shared genes

(e) If favouritism affects child development, this is an example of a non-shared environmental effect

28.3 *Hospital admissions:*

(a) A child admitted alone for a long period is likely to go through phases of protest, despair and detachment

(b) Admission is particularly upsetting for infants under 6 months of age

(c) Multiple but not single admissions are associated with higher rates of subsequent conduct disorder and delinquency

(d) The long-term effects of hospital admissions are particularly marked for children coming from discordant families

(e) The harmful effects of hospital admissions are decreased if parents can be persuaded to visit less often, thereby reducing the number of painful reunions and separations

28.4 *When a child loses a parent through death:*

(a) This often results in severe depressive withdrawal

(b) This may result in persistent disinterest in school

(c) It is not uncommon for the child's distress to be manifested in aggressive, disruptive or defiant behaviour

(d) The individual is at substantially greater risk of depression in later adult life

(e) The individual is less liable to long-term psychiatric problems than after loss of a parent through divorce

28.5 *When a child loses a parent through separation or divorce:*

(a) Mothers are often more inconsistent subsequently, particularly with sons

(b) The child typically responds by being more positive towards teachers and other adults

(c) A girl is typically more distressed than a boy by the initial separation

(d) A girl is typically more distressed than a boy by the mother remarrying

(e) The younger the child, the greater the chance of a good relationship with a stepfather

28.6 *Psychiatric problems in the children of mentally ill parents are:*

(a) More often emotional disorders than conduct disorders

(b) Largely attributable to exposure to parental hostility and marital discord

(c) More likely when parents have psychotic disorders than when parents have personality disorders

(d) More likely when the child has a difficult temperament

(e) Commoner among girls than boys

28.7 *Concerning family size and birth order:*

(a) Only children are more likely to have psychiatric problems than children from two-child families

(b) Children from large families are at an increased risk of autism

(c) The risk of juvenile delinquency is more related to the number of brothers than to the number of sisters

(d) As a group, 'middle' children come from larger families than last-born children

(e) School refusal is commoner in first-born than in last-born children

29   School and Peer Factors

29.1   *Regarding bullies and their victims:*

(a) Most bullies are boys

(b) Most victims are girls

(c) The use of social exclusion or whispering campaigns is more characteristic of female bullies than male bullies

(d) Bullies and their victims are usually in different school years

(e) Well planned interventions can reduce the rate of bullying in schools by up to 50%

29.2   *Regarding victims of bullying:*

(a) Children with sensitive high-strung personalities are more likely to be victims

(b) Boys who are physically weak are more likely to be victimised

(c) Children with hyperkinesis are particularly likely to be victimised

(d) Some children are victimised because they provoke others by taunting them or getting them into trouble

(e) Most victims have normal friendships

29.3   *Bullies are:*

(a) Usually submissive and well behaved with parents and teachers

(b) More likely than other children to have experienced hostile and critical parenting

(c) Usually anxious and insecure children

(d) Generally rejected by their classmates

(e) At increased risk of criminality and alcohol abuse in adulthood

29.4   *Regarding peer popularity and unpopularity:*

(a) The technique of asking all the children in a class to say who they most like to play with ('positive nominations') and who they least like to play with ('negative nominations') is known as anthropometry

(b) Some children attract high numbers of both positive and negative nominations

(c) Rejected children have many negative nominations and few positive nominations, whereas neglected children have few nominations of either sort

(d) Physical factors, such as obesity or wearing glasses, are by far the commonest identifiable reason for peer rejection

(e) Neglected and rejected children are almost equally likely to have long-term mental health problems

29.5   *Regarding school influences on behaviour:*

(a) Much of the variation between schools in rates of delinquency and truancy is explained by differences in catchment area and intake

(b) Behavioural problems are more common in larger schools

(c) Behavioural problems are less common in schools where children are frequently praised and given responsibility

(d) Behavioural problems are more common when the school is housed in old buildings with cramped playgrounds

(e) Behavioural problems are less common in schools that set high standards

30   Treatment: First Principles

30.1   *A diagnostic label:*

(a) May fuel the family's sense of inadequacy and despair

(b) May relieve the family's fear of the unknown

(c) Should only be given when a specific treatment for that condition is available

(d) Should be accompanied or followed by information on the relevant parents' group for that condition

(e) Often facilitates access to suitable services

30.2   *Regarding treatment:*

(a) It is bad practice to embark on two or more treatment approaches simultaneously

(b) 'Masterly inactivity' may be the most appropriate approach for good-prognosis disorders

(c) Provided symptoms are adequately treated, the social impairments that resulted from those symptoms can be relied on to melt away

(d) Biological disorders need biological treatments; psychosocial disorders need psychosocial treatments

(e) Helping parents, teachers and children understand the aetiology of a condition can be a powerful intervention in its own right

30.3   *There is extensive and sound evidence for the effectiveness of:*

(a) Tricyclic antidepressants for childhood depression

(b) Behavioural treatments for soiling and enuresis

(c) Parent training for childhood conduct disorder

(d) Family therapy for anorexia nervosa

(e) Social work for delinquency

30.4   *Concerning treatment effectiveness:*

(a) Some intuitively appealing psychosocial treatments can be significantly more harmful than no treatment at all

(b) When evaluating treatment trials or meta-analyses, it is important to remember that statistically significant findings are not necessarily clinically significant

(c) If a trial shows that a treatment has an effect size of 1.0, that treatment moved the average trial patient one standard deviation closer to the population mean

(d) Successful psychological therapies typically have effect sizes of around 1.3 to 1.5 when administered in research settings

(e) In ordinary clinical settings, the average effect size of psychological therapies is around 0.6 to 0.8

30.5   *The following factors probably account for psychological therapies for children being less effective in routine clinical practice than in research trials:*

(a) Clinics make less use of family therapy

(b) Clinics have to treat many cases with multiple disorders and hard-to-engage families
(c) Clinics make less use of structured therapy with treatment manuals
(d) Clinicians are less effective than research therapists
(e) Research trials are more likely to involve mixed and eclectic therapy methods

30.6 *Concerning the limitations of current 'evidence based' treatment recommendations:*

(a) These often impose unethical restrictions on clinical freedom
(b) Many clinic cases have mixed or partial syndromes that have never been the subject of formal trials
(c) The evidence on efficacy is largely derived from white middle-class American samples and has been shown not to apply to other groups
(d) The child or family's circumstances may make standard protocols unworkable
(e) Research trials often establish the best first-choice treatment without examining what to do next if this fails or is impractical

31 Medication and Diet

31.1 *Concerning pharmacokinetic differences between children and adults:*

(a) Children have lower stomach acidity, thereby accelerating the absorption of acidic drugs such as tricyclics
(b) Allowing for body size, children's livers are less metabolically active, thereby reducing the 'first pass' clearance of drugs that are metabolised by the liver
(c) Children have a relatively high proportion of extracellular fluid, increasing the volume of distribution
(d) Children have more permeable blood-brain barriers
(e) To adjust for pharmacokinetic differences, the weight-for-weight doses of psychotropic drugs is often 25–50% lower for children than for adults

31.2 *Concerning stimulant drugs:*

(a) The most effective stimulants have mixed serotonergic and anti-cholinergic effects
(b) When stimulants are used to treat hyperactivity, the effect size rarely exceeds 1.0
(c) When a hyperactive child responds to stimulants, adding in behavioural therapy only rarely produces worthwhile additional benefits
(d) The hyperactivity of autistic children may be helped by stimulants, but sometimes at the cost of a worsening of repetitive behaviours
(e) Stimulants are very unlikely to reduce restlessness or inattention if the child also has a tic disorder

31.3 *In children and adolescents, neuroleptics have an established role in:*

(a) The acute treatment of schizophrenic relapses
(b) The acute treatment of anorexia nervosa
(c) The long-term treatment of Tourette's syndrome
(d) The long-term treatment of aggressive behaviour in individuals who are mentally retarded
(e) The long-term treatment of hyperactivity or stereotypies in individuals who are mentally retarded

31.4   *Concerning the side-effects of neuroleptics:*

(a)   Sedation can interfere with learning
(b)   Sulpiride and risperidone are more likely than haloperidol to produce early dystonic reactions
(c)   Antimuscarinic drugs for parkinsonian side-effects can usually be discontinued after about six weeks
(d)   Pimozide can trigger potentially fatal cardiac arrhythmias
(e)   The likelihood of late-onset dyskinesias is related to the lifetime dose of neuroleptics

31.5   *Regarding the neuroleptic malignant syndrome:*

(a)   Body temperature falls progressively as the individual becomes increasingly immobile
(b)   Signs of autonomic dysfunction include pallor, sweating or shivering
(c)   Blood tests may show raised creatinine phosphokinase and a high white count
(d)   The syndrome usually progresses from early symptoms to circulatory collapse and multiple organ failure in less than 12 hours
(e)   Once the syndrome has developed, neuroleptics need to be discontinued gradually, not abruptly

31.6   *Concerning tricyclic antidepressants for children and adolescents:*

(a)   Imipramine is of proven value in the treatment of hyperactivity
(b)   Clomipramine is of proven value in the treatment of obsessive–compulsive disorder
(c)   Imipramine can reduce the frequency of bed wetting
(d)   Desipramine has been particularly associated with cardiac arrhythmias and sudden deaths
(e)   Warning signs of tricyclic-induced cardiotoxicity include prolongation of the P-R and Q-T intervals

31.7   *Clonidine:*

(a)   Has mixed adrenergic and dopaminergic actions
(b)   Even on a constant dose, therapeutic effects may go on increasing for several months
(c)   Is used in the treatment of hyperactivity
(d)   Is used in the treatment of depression
(e)   Alerts children and interferes with them getting to sleep

31.8   *Regarding the use of lithium for children and adolescents:*

(a)   Lithium is widely used in the treatment or prophylaxis of bipolar affective disorder
(b)   Lithium can be used to control oppositional behaviour that has not responded to psychological approaches
(c)   Monitoring plasma lithium levels is of little or no use in children and adolescents
(d)   Thirst and fine tremor are warning signs of impending lithium toxicity
(e)   Regular thyroid function tests are needed because of the risk of lithium-induced hypothyroidism

31.9 *Regarding medication for children and adolescents:*

(a) Short courses of benzodiazepines or other hypnotics are usually sufficient treatment for children's sleep problems

(b) Selective serotonin reuptake inhibitors (SSRIs) are proven treatments for obsessive-compulsive disorder

(c) Common side effects of SSRIs include gastrointestinal disturbance and restlessness

(d) Monoamine oxidase inhibitors (MAOIs) are of demonstrated value in the treatment of hyperactivity

(e) Selective MAOIs such as moclobemide need to be used with particular caution since they are more likely than nonselective MAOIs to interact badly with dietary amines

31.10 *When children's behaviour problems are affected by food, the dietary components that are commonly responsible include:*

(a) Artificial colours, flavours and preservatives

(b) Sugars

(c) Dairy products

(d) Citrus fruits

(e) Foods the child particularly craves

31.11 *When children's behaviour problems are affected by food:*

(a) Skin patch testing is usually able to identify correctly which dietary components are responsible

(b) Blood tests (IgE) are usually able to identify correctly which dietary components are responsible

(c) The 'few foods' technique identifies dietary intolerance by excluding most foods and then progressively reintroducing them

(d) Controlled trials have confirmed that a Feingold diet free from additives and natural salicylates is usually particularly effective

(e) An exclusion diet that reduces hyperactivity is unlikely to bring about much reduction in any associated irritability or oppositionality

32   Behaviourally-Based Treatments

32.1 *Regarding operant conditioning:*

(a) The principles were first described by Watson

(b) 'Positive reinforcement' refers to the rewarding of desired behaviour

(c) 'Negative reinforcement' refers to the withdrawal of rewards after undesired behaviour

(d) 'Extinction' refers to a behaviour becoming less frequent when formerly rewarding consequences are taken away

(e) Operant conditioning can be used to increase desired behaviours as well as decreasing undesired behaviours

32.2   *In behavioural treatment:*

(a) 'ABC' analysis refers to affects, behaviours and cognitions
(b) 'Time out' refers to a reward for good behaviour when the child is allowed to have a brief break from adult-imposed activities
(c) 'Response cost' can include making a child pay back pocket money after undesired behaviour
(d) Rewards should be given as soon as possible after the desired behaviour has occurred
(e) Unless undesired behaviours are abolished entirely, they usually rebound in the medium term

32.3   *In behavioural treatment:*

(a) Rewards should not be switched every few days
(b) Using the child's preferred free-time activities as a reward is known as the Premack principle
(c) Adolescents should not be allowed to negotiate about house rules
(d) Effectiveness is enhanced if the beliefs and mood states of parents and children are addressed
(e) Classical conditioning involves linking a physiological response to a new stimulus

32.4   *Behaviourally-based treatments:*

(a) Are particularly useful for eating, sleeping and elimination disorders in younger children
(b) Are more effective for hyperactivity than for antisocial behaviour
(c) Parental attention is not a useful reward for antisocial children since they refuse to pay attention to their parents
(d) When using extinction, the undesired behaviour may initially worsen while the child tries to restore the previous status quo ('extinction burst')
(e) Have been validated by many single-case studies but few randomised controlled trials

33   Cognitive and Interpersonal Therapies

33.1   *Cognitive therapy:*

(a) Should not be used in combination with behaviour therapy
(b) Addresses specific distortions in the content of thought
(c) Does not influence behaviour
(d) Is concerned with the cognitive accompaniments of emotions rather than with emotions per se
(e) Is generally more useful with adolescents than with young children

33.2   *Cognitive therapy:*

(a) Is far less effective than tricyclic antidepressants for depression in adolescents
(b) Only leads to a convincing response in around half of depressed adolescents, of whom many relapse
(c) Helps less than a third of children with anxiety symptoms

(d) Is less effective than medication for hyperactivity
(e) Is more effective than behavioural management for hyperactivity

33.3 *Social problem-solving skills programmes:*

(a) Were pioneered by Myrna Shure and George Spivack
(b) Are always delivered in one-to-one settings
(c) Require the child to generate a number of alternative solutions to the problem
(d) Teach children to ignore their own anger in conflictual situations
(e) Help children focus on the precise behaviour of others rather than their motives

33.4 *Interpersonal psychotherapy:*

(a) Developed from the work of Melanie Klein
(b) Focuses on the role of past upbringing in influencing current relationships
(c) Can involve seeing the parents together with the patient in a session
(d) Specifically addresses issues related to growing up in a single parent family
(e) The therapist predicts that depressive feelings will worsen immediately after termination of treatment

33.5 *In psychodynamic psychotherapy with children:*

(a) It is usual to get the child's signed consent before starting
(b) Advice is not given
(c) The main aim is the relief of symptoms
(d) Interpretation may focus primarily on a child's drawings or play rather than on what the child says
(e) Once therapy is successfully focusing on the child's inner realities, neither the therapist nor any other member of the team should work with the child or family on changing outer realities

34 Family Therapies

34.1 *In family therapy:*

(a) Behaviour is seen as substantially determined by the interactional context in which it occurs
(b) By definition, family rules are explicit and known to all members
(c) Some ideas are drawn from cybernetics and general systems theory
(d) The processes governing how family members communicate are often more important than the content of what they say to each other
(e) Models based on Heisenberg's uncertainty principle are frequently used

34.2 *In family therapy, important stages in the family life cycle include:*

(a) Leaving home
(b) Realignment of members of the extended family following marriage
(c) Moving from one house to another
(d) Granting adolescents increasing autonomy so they can move in and out of the system
(e) Adjusting the marital relationship following retirement

34.3 *In structural family therapy:*

(a) The authority of parents over children is emphasised
(b) An undifferentiated boundary may result in enmeshment
(c) An impermeable boundary may result in disengagement
(d) An alliance between two family members is unhealthy
(e) Triangulation of a child with its parents is desirable

34.4 *In structural family therapy:*

(a) Circular questioning is a key part of assessment
(b) The therapist is directive
(c) The therapist accommodates to the family style so as to feel what it is like
(d) The therapist may deliberately try to unbalance the family system by exposing the way it is dysfunctional
(e) The boundary between sibling and parental sub-systems may be reinforced by getting siblings to carry out a joint task

34.5 *In strategic family therapy:*

(a) All behaviour may be seen as communication
(b) The focus is often on times when the problem behaviour was absent
(c) It is important to determine how a problem arose
(d) The therapist may encourage the family member with the problem behaviour to exhibit it more often
(e) It is important to show respect for the family and their concerns by avoiding humour or light-hearted comments

34.6 *In Milan systemic family therapy:*

(a) The focus is on behaviour not beliefs
(b) Circular questioning reveals inter-relationships amongst family members
(c) The therapist offers solutions
(d) The symptoms may be reframed as a helpful attempt by the child to keep the family in balance
(e) Hypothesising is carried out before the family are seen

34.7 *Regarding family therapy methods:*

(a) Externalising the problem is sometimes a helpful way to unite the family in the 'battle' against the problem
(b) Narrative therapies acknowledge the power of the stories people tell themselves to account for their lives
(c) Salvador Minuchin is associated with structural family therapy
(d) The main schools of family therapy expect the child to be seen alone at least once before family work begins
(e) There are several randomised controlled trials demonstrating the efficacy of family therapy for problems in middle childhood

Answers to the MCQs

Each answer is marked T for True or F for False, followed by a relevant page, box or chapter number where appropriate. Longer comments are appended when necessary.

1 Assessment

1.1 (a) T, p. 4 (b) F, p. 8 (c) F, p. 8 (d) T, p. 10 (e) T, p. 11
There are often identifiable risk factors for child psychiatric disorders, but only rarely is there a single sufficient cause.

1.2 (a) F, p. 13 (b) T, p. 13 (c) T, p. 13 (d) F (e) F

1.3 (a) F, p. 15 (b) F, p. 15 (c) T, p. 16 (d) T, p. 16 (e) T, p. 16

1.4 (a) F, p. 17 (b) T, p. 17 (c) F (d) F (e) T, p. 18
A physical examination is essential but may be restricted to observation; measuring height and weight (and head circumference) is desirable, whereas cardiac auscultation is rarely necessary. Most dysmorphic syndromes include abnormalities of the head, face or hands that can be seen without undressing the child. Having seen some dysmorphic signs, it is then appropriate to go on to a fuller examination.

2 Classification

2.1 (a) F, p. 23 (b) T, p. 24 (c) F, p. 27: Table 2.1 (d) F, p. 28 (e) T, p. 23
Anorexia nervosa and schizophrenia are examples of adolescent disorders that do not fit into one of the three groupings.

2.2 (a) T, p. 26 (b) F, p. 26 (c) T, p. 26 (d) T, p. 26 (e) T, p. 8

2.3 (a) T, p. 28: Table 2.2 (b) F, p. 28: Table 2.2 (c) T, p. 28: Table 2.2
(d) F (e) T, p. 28: Table 2.2

2.4 (a) T, p. 24 (b) F, p. 24 (c) F (d) F, p. 24: Box 2.1 (e) T, p. 25: Box 2.2
Eigenvalues may be used to help decide on the number of dimensions to retain in factor analyses.

3 Epidemiology

3.1 (a) F, p. 32 (b) F, p. 41 (c) F, pp. 27, 34 (d) F, p. 35 (e) F, p. 38

3.2 (a) T, p. 36: Box 3.2; Ch.17 (b) F, p. 36: Box 3.2; Ch.5 (c) F, p. 36: Box 3.2; Ch.25 (d) T, p. 36: Box 3.2; Ch.21 (e) F, p. 36: Box 3.2; Ch.11

3.3 (a) F, p. 36: Box 3.2; Ch.9 (b) F, p. 36: Box 3.2; Ch.8 (c) F, p. 36: Box 3.2; Ch.11 (d) F, p. 36: Box 3.2; Ch.15 (e) T, p. 36: Box 3.2; Ch.6

3.4   (a) F, p. 36: Box 3.3; Ch.17   (b) T, p. 36: Box 3.3; Ch.21   (c) T, p. 36: Box 3.3; Ch.10   (d) F, p. 36: Box 3.3; Ch.4   (e) F, p. 36: Box 3.3; Ch.15

3.5   (a) T, p. 76   (b) F, p. 41   (c) T, p. 174: Table 23.1   (d) F, p. 74   (e) T, p. 69

4   Autistic Disorders

4.1   (a) T, p. 42   (b) F   (c) F   (d) T, p. 42   (e) T, p. 41
Specific fears or self-injurious behaviour are relatively common but are not characteristic.

4.2   (a) F, p. 42   (b) T, p. 42   (c) F   (d) T, p. 47   (e) T, p. 41
Autistic children are often resistant to change, not indifferent to it. The poor eye contact of autistic children is often referred to as gaze avoidance, though it is often gaze indifference rather than active avoidance (whereas children with the fragile X syndrome are more likely to be truly gaze avoidant).

4.3   (a) F, p. 44; p. 150: Box 21.2   (b) T, p. 42   (c) T, p. 41   (d) T, p. 43
(e) T, p. 43

4.4   (a) F, p. 44   (b) F, p. 43   (c) F, p. 150: Box 21.2   (d) F, p. 43   (e) T, p. 43

4.5   (a) F   (b) T, p. 45   (c) T, p. 44   (d) F   (e) T, p. 44; Ch.25

4.6   (a) F, p. 41   (b) F, p. 41   (c) F, p. 41   (d) F, p. 46   (e) F, p. 46
The prevalence of all autistic disorders is around 2 per 1000, with infantile autism accounting for around a quarter of this, i.e. around 5 per *10 000*.

4.7   (a) T, p. 48   (b) F   (c) F   (d) T, p. 48   (e) F
Paradoxically, the prognosis of autism may be better in the presence of some associated disabilities: clumsiness, tics and a history of delayed visual maturation.

4.8   (a) T, p. 48   (b) F   (c) F, p. 48   (d) F, p. 48   (e) T, p. 48
Roughly 10% lose cognitive skills in adolescence. Roughly 10% hold a paid job, and far fewer marry.

4.9   (a) T, p. 43   (b) F   (c) T   (d) F   (e) T, p. 47; Box 4.1
If autistic individuals do lose cognitive skills, this is usually at onset (under 3 years) or in adolescence. Islets of normal or superior ability may include the following: the ability to do puzzles, artistic or musical talents, or the ability to work out what day of the week particular dates fall on, e.g. Christmas Day 1887 ('calendrical calculators').

4.10   (a) T, p. 44   (b) T, p. 44   (c) T, p. 44   (d) T, p. 44   (e) F, p. 44

5   Hyperactivity (Hyperkinesis/ADHD)

5.1   (a) T   (b) F, p. 50   (c) F, p. 50   (d) F, p. 50   (e) T, p. 51

5.2   (a) T, p. 50   (b) F   (c) T, p. 50   (d) F   (e) F
Hand flapping and mannerisms is a pointer to autism or mental retardation. Some hyperactive children seem 'high' in mood, but this is not characteristic.

5.3   (a) T, p. 51   (b) T, p. 51   (c) T, p. 51   (d) F   (e) T, p. 51
Sudden repetitive stereotyped purposeless movements are tics.

5.4   (a) T, p. 51   (b) T, p. 51   (c) F, p. 51   (d) F   (e) F, pp. 56, 237
Some hyperactive children need very little sleep while others sleep long and hard; sleep problems are not characteristic.

5.5   (a) F, p. 52   (b) T, p. 52   (c) F, p. 52   (d) T, p. 52   (e) T, p. 52
5.6   (a) F   (b) F   (c) T, p. 54; Ch.24   (d) T, p. 52   (e) T, p. 50
Parental neglect and other adverse family factors are more likely to be associated with conduct disorder. Only a minority of hyperactive children have overt neurological disorders, and the suspicion that most of the rest have covert neurological problems remains a suspicion rather than an established fact.
5.7   (a) T, p. 51   (b) T, p. 51   (c) T, p. 56   (d) T, p. 56   (e) T, p. 56
5.8   (a) F   (b) F   (c) T, p. 54   (d) F, pp. 56, 237   (e) T, pp. 55, 234
There is no convincing research or clinical evidence that the restlessness and inattentiveness of severely hyperactive children is helped by psychodynamic psychotherapy. Hyperactive children do best in quiet, non-distracting classrooms.
5.9   (a) F, p. 55   (b) T, p. 55   (c) T, p. 55   (d) F, p. 55   (e) T, p. 55

6 Conduct Disorder

6.1   (a) F, p. 62   (b) T, p. 62   (c) T, p. 61   (d) T, pp. 34, 62   (e) F, p. 35
Commoner in boys at all ages. Typically more persistent than emotional disorders.
6.2   (a) T, p. 52   (b) T, pp. 60, 180   (c) T, pp. 60, 196   (d) T, p. 183   (e) T, p. 63
6.3   (a) T, pp. 63, 215   (b) F   (c) T, pp. 63, 215   (d) T, p. 64   (e) F
6.4   (a) F   (b) F   (c) T, p. 63   (d) T, pp. 62, 216   (e) F
It is lack of supervision and inconsistent discipline that is associated with more conduct disorder.
6.5   (a) F, p. 60: Box 6.1   (b) T, p. 60: Box 6.1   (c) T, p. 60: Box 6.1   (d) T, p. 60: Box 6.1   (e) F, p. 60: Box 6.1
Theft and truancy are features of conduct disorder (Box 6.2).
6.6   (a) T   (b) T, p. 214   (c) T   (d) T   (e) F !
6.7   (a) T, p. 66   (b) T, p. 66   (c) T, p. 66   (d) F, p. 66   (e) F, p. 66
6.8   (a) T, p. 66   (b) F, p. 66   (c) F, p. 60   (d) T, p. 63   (e) T, pp. 35, 66
6.9   (a) F, p. 76   (b) F, p. 76   (c) T, p. 76   (d) T, p. 76   (e) F, p. 76
Physical illness is the main cause of absence from school at most ages.

7 Juvenile Delinquency

7.1   (a) F, p. 68   (b) T, p. 68   (c) F, p. 69   (d) F, p. 69   (e) T, p. 69
7.2   (a) F, p. 68   (b) T, p. 70   (c) F, p. 70   (d) F, p. 70   (e) F, p. 71
The majority of juvenile delinquents are one-time offenders, and most of these are free from psychiatric disorders. By contrast, the minority of recidivist delinquents are likely to be behaviourally disordered before, during and after adolescence (p. 147).
7.3   (a) T, p. 71   (b) F, p. 71   (c) T   (d) F, p. 71   (e) T, p. 71
In the Cambridge longitudinal study of delinquent development, a teacher report of troublesome behaviour at age 8 was predictive of later delinquency.
7.4   (a) T, p. 70   (b) T, p. 70   (c) F   (d) T, p. 70   (e) T, p. 70

8   School Refusal

8.1   (a) T, p. 74   (b) F, p. 74   (c) F   (d) F, p. 74   (e) F, p. 76
8.2   (a) F   (b) F, p. 74   (c) T, p. 75   (d) F, p. 76   (e) F, p. 76
      Most often starts when the child has to return to school after some time off, so
      more common at the beginning of the school year than towards the end. School
      refusal accounts for less school non-attendance than do physical illnesses or
      truancy.
8.3   (a) F, p. 77   (b) F, p. 77   (c) T, p. 75   (d) T, p. 77   (e) T, p. 77
8.4   (a) T, p. 75   (b) F, p. 75   (c) F   (d) F   (e) F
      School refusal is primarily associated with emotional disorders, not with
      hyperkinesis, conduct disorder or delinquency. Most parents of school refusers
      consider education important and are very worried that their child is out of
      school. The view that school is unimportant is more likely to accompany
      deliberate parental withholding (p. 76).
8.5   (a) T, p. 77   (b) T, p. 77   (c) T, p. 75   (d) F   (e) F, p. 78
      There is no particular link with stealing from home or other conduct problems.
      Only a small minority become agoraphobic subsequently.
8.6   (a) F, p. 77   (b) T, p. 78   (c) F, p. 78   (d) F, p. 78   (e) F, p. 78
8.7   (a) T, p. 78   (b) T, p. 78   (c) F   (d) F, p. 78   (e) F, p. 78
      Roughly a third have persisting emotional disorders.

9   Anxiety Disorders

9.1   (a) T, pp. 34, 80   (b) T, pp. 34, 80   (c) F   (d) F   (e) T, p. 80
      Reading disorders are primarily associated with conduct not emotional disorders
      (p. 196).
9.2   (a) F, p. 82   (b) T, p. 77   (c) F   (d) F, p. 82   (e) F, p. 82
      Common in prepubertal schoolchildren. Reluctance to speak except at home
      points towards selective mutism (Ch.15).
9.3   (a) F, p. 83   (b) T, p. 82   (c) T, p. 83   (d) T, p. 83   (e) T, p. 83
9.4   (a) F, p. 83   (b) T, p. 83   (c) F, p. 83   (d) T, p. 84   (e) F, p. 84

10   Depression and Mania

10.1   (a) F, p. 87   (b) T, p. 87   (c) T, pp. 77, 87   (d) F, p. 87   (e) F, p. 88
10.2   (a) F, p. 88   (b) F, p. 88   (c) T, p. 90; Ch.33   (d) F, p. 90   (e) F, p. 90
10.3   (a) T, p. 91   (b) F, p. 91   (c) F, p. 91   (d) T, p. 91   (e) F, p. 91

11   Suicide and Deliberate Self-Harm

11.1   (a) T, p. 92   (b) F, p. 92   (c) F, p. 92   (d) T, p. 93   (e) F, p. 92
11.2   (a) T, p. 93   (b) T, p. 92   (c) T, p. 92   (d) T, p. 93   (e) T, p. 93
11.3   (a) F, p. 94   (b) T, p. 94   (c) F, p. 94   (d) F, p. 94   (e) F, p. 95
      Roughly 100 times commoner than completed suicide.
11.4   (a) T, p. 94   (b) T, p. 94   (c) T, p. 94   (d) T, p. 94   (e) T, p. 94

11.5   (a) T, p. 96   (b) T, p. 96   (c) T, p. 96   (d) F, p. 96   (e) F, p. 96
About 1% of young people who harm themselves do subsequently kill themselves, usually within the next 2 years.

12   Reactions to Stress

12.1   (a) T, p. 98   (b) T, pp. 98, 214   (c) F, p. 98   (d) F, p. 98   (e) T, p. 98
12.2   (a) T, p. 99   (b) T, p. 99   (c) T, p. 99   (d) F   (e) T, p. 99
Although peer problems can have psychiatric consequences such as depression or self-harm, rejection by friends is not likely to involve the sort of intensely arousing and frightening experience that results in PTSD.
12.3   (a) T, p. 99   (b) F   (c) T, p. 99   (d) T, p. 99   (e) F
12.4   (a) T, p. 99   (b) T, p. 99   (c) F   (d) F   (e) T, p. 99

13   Obsessive-Compulsive Disorder

13.1   (a) F, p. 102   (b) T, p. 102   (c) T, p. 102   (d) T, p. 102   (e) F, p. 102
13.2   (a) F   (b) T, p. 104   (c) F   (d) F   (e) T, p. 104
OCD may be associated with increased oxytocin levels in CSF or with evidence of basal ganglia abnormalities.
13.3   (a) F   (b) F   (c) T, p. 104   (d) T, p. 104   (e) F
Though sex and death are common themes of obsessional worries – which might seem to make them particularly suitable for Freudian approaches – there is no convincing research evidence that psychodynamic psychotherapy is an effective treatment for OCD. Fenfluramine is a serotonergic stimulant that has been used, without much success, in the treatment of autism (p. 44).

14   Tourette's Syndrome and Other Tic Disorders

14.1   (a) T, p. 106   (b) T, p. 106   (c) T, p. 106   (d) T, p. 106   (e) T, p. 106
14.2   (a) T, p. 106   (b) F, p. 106   (c) T, p. 106   (d) T, p. 106   (e) F, p. 106
14.3   (a) F, p. 106   (b) T, p. 106   (c) F, p. 106   (d) F, p. 106   (e) F
Epilepsy is unusual.
14.4   (a) F   (b) T, p. 107   (c) F   (d) T, p. 107   (e) F, p. 108
Mental retardation and focal neurological signs are unusual.
14.5   (a) F   (b) T, pp. 104, 107   (c) T, p. 108   (d) F, p. 108   (e) F, p. 108
Imipramine may be used to treat associated hyperactivity.

15   Selective Mutism

15.1   (a) F, p. 110   (b) F, p. 110   (c) T, p. 111   (d) F   (e) T, p. 110
15.2   (a) T, p. 110   (b) T, p. 110   (c) T, p. 110   (d) F   (e) T, p. 113
Sudden onset after a definite stress is more characteristic of hysterical muteness, involving loss of speech in all settings.

16 Attachment Disorders

16.1   (a) F, p. 115   (b) F, p. 115   (c) F, p. 115   (d) F, p. 115   (e) F
16.2   (a) F, p. 114   (b) T, p. 114   (c) T, p. 114   (d) T, p. 114   (e) F, p. 114
         Clinginess in infancy and a willingness to approach unfamiliar adults for comfort
         are features of children with a disinhibited type of attachment disorder.
16.3   (a) T, p. 114   (b) F, p. 114   (c) F   (d) T, p. 114   (e) F, p. 114
         Aggression in response to their own or another person's distress is a feature of
         children with a reactive-inhibited type of attachment disorder. Sleep dis-
         turbance is not a characteristic feature of attachment disorders.

17 Enuresis

17.1   (a) T, p. 120: Table 17.2   (b) T, p. 120: Table 17.2   (c) F, p. 120   (d) T, p.
         120: Table 17.2   (e) T, p. 120
17.2   (a) T, p. 120   (b) F, p. 121   (c) F   (d) T, p. 120   (e) F, p. 121
         Maturational lags do not seem likely to be relevant to children who become dry
         at the normal time and only start wetting again years later.
17.3   (a) T, p. 120   (b) F, p. 121   (c) F   (d) F, p. 121   (e) T, p. 121
         There are good (humanitarian) reasons for avoiding harsh toilet training, but
         reducing the risk of subsequent enuresis is not one of them.
17.4   (a) F, p. 121   (b) F, p. 121   (c) T, p. 121   (d) F, p. 121   (e) F, p. 121
         Enuresis is associated with an increase in both emotional and conduct problems.
         The increase in psychiatric problems occurs to the same extent whether the
         enuresis is primary or secondary enuresis.
17.5   (a) F, p. 122   (b) F, p. 121   (c) F, p. 121   (d) T, p. 122   (e) F, p. 121
17.6   (a) T, p. 124   (b) F   (c) T, p. 124   (d) F, p. 124   (e) F
         Stimulants are used for hyperactivity. Carbamazepine is an anticonvulsant that
         can also be used as an alternative to lithium as prophylaxis for bipolar affective
         disorder.
17.7   (a) F, p. 124   (b) F, p. 123   (c) T, p. 123   (d) F, p. 123   (e) F, p. 124
17.8   (a) F, p. 122   (b) F, p. 122   (c) F, p. 122   (d) T, p. 122   (e) T, p. 122

18 Faecal Soiling

18.1   (a) F, p. 141: Box 20.1   (b) T, p. 141: Box 20.1   (c) F, p. 126   (d) F, p.
         126   (e) T, p. 126
18.2   (a) T, p. 127   (b) F, p. 126   (c) T, p. 127   (d) T, p. 128   (e) T, p. 128
18.3   (a) T, p. 126   (b) T, p. 127   (c) F   (d) T, p. 127   (e) F
18.4   (a) T, p. 127   (b) F, p. 127   (c) F   (d) T, p. 127   (e) F
         Imipramine may be used as a symptomatic treatment for enuresis.
18.5   (a) F   (b) T, p. 128   (c) F, p. 128   (d) T, p. 128   (e) T, p. 128
         Prognosis is independent of gender.

19 Psychosomatics

19.1   (a) F, p. 130   (b) T, p. 133   (c) T, p. 134   (d) T, p. 133   (e) T, p. 130: Box
         19.1

19.2 (a) F, p. 135   (b) F, p. 135   (c) F, p. 135   (d) F, p. 136   (e) F, p. 136
19.3 (a) F, p. 136   (b) T, p. 136   (c) F, p. 136   (d) F, p. 136   (e) T, p. 137
19.4 (a) F, p. 137   (b) F, p. 137   (c) T, p. 138   (d) F, p. 138   (e) T, p. 138

20 Preschool Problems

20.1 (a) F, p. 141: Box 20.1   (b) T, p. 141: Box 20.1   (c) F, Ch.4   (d) T, p. 141: Box 20.1   (e) T, p. 141: Box 20.1
20.2 (a) F   (b) T, p. 141: Box 20.1   (c) T, p. 141: Box 20.1   (d) T, p. 141: Box 20.1   (e) T, p. 141: Box 20.1
20.3 (a) F, p. 141: Box 20.1   (b) F, p. 141: Box 20.1   (c) F, p. 141: Box 20.1   (d) T, p. 141: Box 20.1   (e) T, p. 141: Box 20.1

21 Disorders of Adolescence

21.1 (a) T, p. 147: Box 21.1   (b) T, p. 147: Box 21.1   (c) F, p. 147: Box 21.1   (d) F, p. 147: Box 21.1   (e) F, p. 147: Box 21.1
Whether long-standing or new-onset, most adolescent disorders are emotional or conduct disorders.
21.2 (a) F, p. 148   (b) F, p. 148   (c) T, p. 148   (d) T, p. 148   (e) F
21.3 (a) F   (b) T, p. 149   (c) T, p. 149   (d) F   (e) T, p. 149
Erosion of dental enamel can be a sign of repeated deliberate vomiting in anorexia or bulimia nervosa.
21.4 (a) T, p. 149   (b) F   (c) T, p. 149   (d) F, p. 149   (e) F, p. 149
21.5 (a) T, p. 149   (b) F, p. 149   (c) F, p. 149   (d) T, p. 149   (e) T, p. 149
21.6 (a) T, p. 149   (b) T, p. 149   (c) F   (d) F   (e) T, p. 149
Insistence on sameness and pronominal reversal are pointers to autism.
21.7 (a) F, p. 150   (b) F, p. 150   (c) F, p. 151   (d) F, p. 151   (e) T, p. 151
21.8 (a) F, p. 151   (b) F, p. 151   (c) F, p. 151   (d) T, p. 151   (e) T, p. 151: Box 21.3
21.9 (a) T, p. 152   (b) T, p. 152   (c) F, p. 152   (d) F, p. 153   (e) T, p. 153
21.10 (a) T, p. 153   (b) F, p. 153   (c) F, p. 153   (d) T, p. 153   (e) F, p. 153

22 Maltreatment of Children

22.1 (a) F, p. 156   (b) F, p. 156   (c) F, p. 156   (d) T, p. 157   (e) F, p. 157
22.2 (a) T, p. 157   (b) T, p. 157   (c) T, p. 158   (d) T, p. 158   (e) F, p. 158
22.3 (a) T, p. 162: Box 22.1   (b) T, p. 162: Box 22.1   (c) F   (d) T, p. 162: Box 22.1   (e) T, p. 162: Box 22.1
Although alcohol dependence is associated with child abuse, 4 units per week is a modest intake (about two pints of beer or half a bottle of wine per week).
22.4 (a) F   (b) F   (c) T, p. 156   (d) T, p. 162: Box 22.1   (e) F
22.5 (a) F, p. 159   (b) F, p. 159   (c) F   (d) T, p. 160   (e) T, p. 159
Emotional abuse usually accompanies other forms of abuse.
22.6 (a) F, p. 160   (b) T, p. 160   (c) F, p. 161   (d) T, p. 161   (e) F, p. 161
22.7 (a) T, p. 161   (b) T, p. 161   (c) F, p. 161   (d) F, p. 161   (e) F, p. 161
22.8 (a) T, pp. 99, 165   (b) T, p. 164   (c) F, p. 164   (d) T, p. 165   (e) T, p. 165

22.9   (a) T, p. 165   (b) F, p. 167   (c) T, p. 167   (d) F   (e) F, p. 169: Table 22.1
22.10 (a) T, p. 156   (b) F, p. 156   (c) F   (d) T, p. 156   (e) T, p. 157
Many children attending casualty with injuries unrelated to abuse are tearful and apprehensive about what hospital staff are going to do to them.
22.11 (a) F, p. 169: Table 22.1   (b) F, p. 169: Table 22.1   (c) F, p. 169: Table 22.1   (d) T, p. 169: Table 22.1   (e) T, p. 169: Table 22.1

23   Mental Retardation

23.1   (a) F, p. 173   (b) F, p. 174   (c) F, p. 173   (d) F, p. 173   (e) F, p. 174
23.2   (a) T, p. 174: Table 23.1   (b) F   (c) T, p. 174: Table 23.1   (d) F, p. 178
(e) T
'Ordinary' polygenes are probably more important in mild mental retardation, whereas single major genes are more important in severe mental retardation. Marked problems learning new skills is a direct consequence of very low IQ.
23.3   (a) F   (b) T, p. 174: Table 23.1   (c) F   (d) T, p. 174: Table 23.1   (e) F
Microcephaly and enzyme defects are much more characteristic of severe mental retardation. As normally defined, mild mental retardation involves an IQ in the 50–69 band.
23.4   (a) F, p. 175   (b) F, p. 175   (c) F   (d) T, p. 176   (e) T, p. 176
Down's syndrome accounts for a substantial portion of severe mental retardation, but a much lower portion of all mental retardation (when the large number of mildly mentally retarded children are included too).
23.5   (a) F, p. 175   (b) T, p. 175   (c) T, p. 175   (d) F, p. 176   (e) T, p. 175
Hypotonia not hypertonia.
23.6   (a) F, p. 19   (b) F   (c) F, p. 19   (d) T, p. 19   (e) F
With direct DNA testing, cell culture is no longer routinely necessary. The pathology is an excess of trinucleotide repeats, not tripeptide repeats. Remember to read questions carefully – examiners may resort to mean tricks on occasions!
23.7   (a) T, p. 19   (b) F   (c) F   (d) T, p. 20   (e) F
The fetal alcohol syndrome is a commoner cause of mild than severe mental retardation. Large ears may be due to the fragile X syndrome. The upper lip in the fetal alcohol syndrome is usually thin and turned in; hypoplasia of the philtrum often obliterates the 'Cupid's bow' shape of normal upper lips.
23.8   (a) F, pp. 20, 176   (b) T   (c) T, p. 176   (d) T   (e) F, p. 176
Neurofibromatosis is dominant. Hunter's is X-linked recessive.
23.9   (a) F, p. 20   (b) T   (c) T   (d) F, p. 176   (e) F, pp. 20, 176
Sturge-Weber is usually sporadic. Lesch-Nyhan is X-linked recessive. Tuberous sclerosis is a dominant condition that is often a new mutation.
23.10 (a) F, p. 20   (b) F, p. 20   (c) F, p. 20   (d) F   (e) F
Axillary freckling is a pointer to neurofibromatosis. There can be various sorts of seizures, but infantile spasms are the most characteristic.
23.11 (a) T   (b) F   (c) T   (d) T   (e) F
23.12 (a) T, p. 177   (b) T, p. 177   (c) T, p. 177   (d) F   (e) T, p. 177
23.13 (a) T, p. 179   (b) T, p. 179   (c) T, p. 179   (d) T, p. 179   (e) T, p. 179

23.14 (a) T, p. 179   (b) T, p. 179   (c) F   (d) T, p. 181   (e) F

Although extra attention will reinforce the self-injurious behaviour of some children, it will have the opposite effect when the primary function of the behaviour is to drive people away and reduce unwanted demands and intrusions. Stimulants may help the hyperactivity of children with mild and moderate retardation, but sometimes at the cost of exacerbating ritualistic and repetitive behaviours.

23.15 (a) F   (b) T, pp. 8, 179   (c) T, pp. 19, 179   (d) F   (e) F

Williams syndrome (idiopathic infantile hypercalcaemia) is associated with 'cocktail party speech', involving fluent speech with an excess of clichés, stock phrases and irrelevancies. The Prader-Willi syndrome is associated with insatiable overeating. The fetal alcohol syndrome is associated with hyperactivity.

24   Brain Disorders

24.1   (a) T, p. 182   (b) T, p. 183   (c) F, p. 183   (d) F, p. 183   (e) T, p. 183
24.2   (a) T, p. 185   (b) T, p. 185   (c) F   (d) T, p. 185   (e) F, p. 183

Frontal rather than Rolandic seizures are particularly likely to be misdiagnosed as pseudoseizures.

25   Language Disorders

25.1   (a) F, p. 188: Box 25.1   (b) T, p. 188: Box 25.1   (c) F, p. 188: Box 25.1
(d) F, p. 188: Box 25.1   (e) T, p. 188: Box 25.1
25.2   (a) T, p. 187   (b) T, p. 187   (c) T, p. 188   (d) F, p. 188   (e) F, p. 189
25.3   (a) F, p. 189   (b) F, p. 189   (c) T, p. 189   (d) F, p. 189   (e) T, p. 189

26   Reading Disorders

26.1   (a) F, p. 193   (b) F, p. 193   (c) F   (d) T, p. 193   (e) F, p. 193

Specific reading disorder is associated with large rather than small family size.

26.2   (a) T   (b) T, p. 193   (c) F, p. 192: Box 26.1   (d) F, p. 193   (e) T, p. 193

Without measures of both intelligence and reading ability, it is not generally possible to be sure if there is a significant discrepancy between the two. There are exceptions, e.g. an articulate 14 year old who is very good at solving orally presented problems, but who has never learned to read despite much effort, can confidently be said to have specific reading problems without formal tests of intelligence (though these tests would still be of interest).

26.3   (a) F   (b) F   (c) F   (d) T   (e) F

As mentioned above, psychometric measures of intelligence and reading ability are almost always necessary for the diagnosis of specific reading disorder.

26.4   (a) F, p. 193   (b) T, p. 195   (c) F, p. 193   (d) T, p. 196   (e) F
26.5   (a) T, p. 195   (b) F, p. 193   (c) T, p. 196   (d) T, p. 195   (e) T, p. 193
26.6   (a) F, p. 76   (b) T, p. 193   (c) F   (d) F   (e) F
26.7   (a) T, p. 196   (b) T, p. 197   (c) F, p. 196   (d) F, p. 197   (e) T, p. 196

27   Insecure Attachment

27.1   (a) F, p. 199   (b) T, p. 200   (c) F, p. 200   (d) F, p. 200   (e) T, p. 200
27.2   (a) F, p. 201   (b) F, p. 201   (c) F, p. 202: Box 27.1   (d) T, p. 202: Box
27.1   (e) F, p. 201
Mary Ainsworth devised the Strange Situation Procedure.
27.3   (a) T, p. 201   (b) F, p. 203: Table 27.1   (c) T, p. 203: Table 27.1
(d) T, p. 203: Table 27.1   (e) F, p. 203: Table 27.1
27.4   (a) F, p. 203: Table 27.1   (b) T, p. 204   (c) T, p. 204   (d) F, p. 204
(e) F, p. 203
27.5   (a) F, p. 205   (b) T, p. 205   (c) F, p. 205   (d) F, p. 205   (e) T, p. 206
Mary Main developed the Adult Attachment Interview.
27.6   (a) F, p. 206   (b) T, p. 204   (c) T, p. 206   (d) F, p. 207   (e) F, p. 207

28   Nature, Nurture and Family Adversities

28.1   (a) F, p. 211: Box 28.1   (b) T, p. 211: Box 28.1   (c) T, p. 211: Box 28.1
(d) T, p. 211: Box 28.1   (e) T, p. 212
28.2   (a) T, p. 210   (b) F, p. 211   (c) F, p. 211   (d) T, p. 211   (e) T, p. 212
28.3   (a) T, p. 213   (b) F, p. 213   (c) T, p. 213   (d) T, p. 213   (e) F, p. 213
28.4   (a) F, p. 214   (b) T, p. 214   (c) T, p. 214   (d) F, p. 214   (e) T, p. 213
28.5   (a) T, p. 214   (b) F, p. 214   (c) F, p. 214   (d) T, p. 214   (e) T, p. 214
28.6   (a) F, p. 215   (b) T, p. 215   (c) F, p. 215   (d) T, p. 215   (e) F
28.7   (a) F, p. 216   (b) F   (c) T, p. 216   (d) T, p. 216   (e) F, p. 216

29   School and Peer Factors

29.1   (a) T, p. 219   (b) F, p. 219   (c) T, p. 219   (d) F, p. 218   (e) T, p. 219
29.2   (a) T, p. 219   (b) T, p. 219   (c) T, p. 219   (d) T, p. 219   (e) F, p. 219
29.3   (a) F, p. 219   (b) T, p. 219   (c) F, p. 219   (d) F, p. 219   (e) T, p. 219
29.4   (a) F, p. 220   (b) T, p. 220: Box 29.1   (c) T, p. 220: Box 29.1
(d) F, p. 220   (e) F, p. 220
29.5   (a) T, p. 221   (b) F, p. 221   (c) T, p. 221   (d) F, p. 221   (e) T, p. 221

30   Treatment: First Principles

30.1   (a) T, p. 225   (b) T, p. 226   (c) F   (d) T, p. 226   (e) T, p. 226
Even if a diagnosis does not lead on to a specific treatment, families may be
pleased to know the diagnosis since it may help them understand the aetiology,
the prognosis, or the likelihood that another family member will be similarly
affected.
30.2   (a) F, p. 227   (b) T, p. 226   (c) F, p. 227   (d) F, p. 228   (e) T, p. 226
30.3   (a) F, p. 90; p. 229: Box 30.1   (b) T, p. 123; Ch.18; p. 229: Box 30.1   (c) T, p.
65; p. 229: Box 30.1   (d) T, p. 152; p. 229: Box 30.1   (e) F, p. 228; p. 229: Box
30.1
30.4   (a) T, p. 228   (b) T, p. 228   (c) T, p. 228   (d) F, p. 228   (e) F, p. 229

30.5   (a) F, p. 229: Box 30.2   (b) T, p. 229: Box 30.2   (c) T, p. 229: Box 30.2   (d) F, p. 229: Box 30.2   (e) F, p. 229: Box 30.2

30.6   (a) F   (b) T, p. 230   (c) F   (d) T, p. 230   (e) T, p. 230

It is unethical for clinicians to abuse their clinical freedom by administering treatments without due regard to relevant evidence on efficacy.

31   Medication and Diet

31.1   (a) F, p. 231   (b) F, p. 231   (c) T, p. 231   (d) T, p. 231   (e) F, p. 232

31.2   (a) F, p. 233   (b) F, p. 233   (c) F, pp. 55, 233   (d) T, p. 233   (e) F, p. 233

Drugs other than stimulants are usually the first choice for treating hyperactivity in children with tics – not because stimulants are typically ineffective, but because they may worsen the tics.

31.3   (a) T, p. 150   (b) F, p. 153   (c) T, p. 108   (d) F, p. 181   (e) T, p. 181

31.4   (a) T, p. 235   (b) F, p. 235   (c) T, p. 235   (d) T, p. 108   (e) T, p. 235

31.5   (a) F, p. 235   (b) T, p. 235   (c) T, p. 235   (d) F, p. 235   (e) F, p. 235

The neuroleptic malignant syndrome is characterised by pyrexia, not hypothermia. Early symptoms can progress to circulatory collapse and multiple system failure in under 48 hours. Neuroleptics should be discontinued at once if there is good reason to suspect the syndrome is developing.

31.6   (a) T, p. 234   (b) T, p. 234   (c) T, p. 234   (d) T, p. 90   (e) T, p. 234

31.7   (a) F, p. 233   (b) T, p. 233   (c) T, p. 233   (d) F, p. 233   (e) F, p. 233

31.8   (a) T, p. 235   (b) F   (c) F, p. 235   (d) F, p. 235   (e) T, p. 235

Lithium may be used to treat children who have severe aggressive outbursts that are triggered with minimal provocation, and who have not been helped by appropriate psychological approaches, i.e. for a much more serious indication than simple oppositionality.

31.9   (a) F, p. 236   (b) T, p. 234   (c) T, p. 234   (d) T, p. 234   (e) F, p. 234

31.10   (a) T, p. 237   (b) F, p. 237   (c) T, p. 237   (d) T, p. 237   (e) T, p. 237

31.11   (a) F, p. 237   (b) F, p. 237   (c) T, p. 237   (d) F, p. 236   (e) F, p. 237

32   Behaviourally-Based Treatments

32.1   (a) F, p. 239   (b) T, p. 239   (c) F, p. 239   (d) T, pp. 239, 242   (e) T, p. 239

Operant conditioning was described by Skinner. Negative reinforcement is when a behaviour is reinforced because its allows the individual to escape from unpleasant consequences, e.g. temper outbursts may be very effective at discouraging parents from asking a child to do chores or homework.

32.2   (a) F, p. 240: Box 32.1   (b) F, p. 243   (c) T, p. 243   (d) T, p. 244   (e) F, p. 241

32.3   (a) F, p. 244   (b) T, p. 244   (c) F, p. 244   (d) T, p. 245   (e) T, p. 239

32.4   (a) T, p. 246   (b) F, p. 246   (c) F   (d) T, p. 242   (e) F, p. 246

33   Cognitive and Interpersonal Therapies

33.1   (a) F, p. 247   (b) T, pp. 247–9   (c) F, p. 247   (d) T, p. 247   (e) T, p. 247

33.2   (a) F, p. 248   (b) T, p. 248   (c) F, p. 248   (d) T, p. 249   (e) F, p. 249

33.3   (a) T, p. 249   (b) F, p. 249   (c) T, p. 249   (d) F, p. 250   (e) F, p. 250

33.4   (a) F   (b) F, p. 250   (c) T, p. 252   (d) T, p. 251   (e) T, p. 252

Developed by Gerald Klerman and Myrna Weissman.

33.5   (a) F, p. 253   (b) T, p. 252   (c) F, p. 252   (d) T, p. 253   (e) F, p. 253

34   Family Therapies

34.1   (a) T, p. 256   (b) F, p. 256   (c) T, p. 255   (d) T, p. 255   (e) F

34.2   (a) T, p. 257: Box 34.1   (b) T, p. 257: Box 34.1   (c) F   (d) T, p. 257: Box 34.1   (e) T, p. 257: Box 34.1

34.3   (a) T, p. 259   (b) T, p. 260   (c) T, p. 260   (d) F, p. 260   (e) F, p. 260

34.4   (a) F   (b) T, p. 261   (c) T, p. 261   (d) T, p. 261   (e) T, p. 261: Box 34.2

Circular questioning is a key component of Milan systemic therapy.

34.5   (a) T, p. 262   (b) T, p. 265   (c) F, p. 262   (d) T, p. 263   (e) F, p. 263

34.6   (a) F, p. 265   (b) T, p. 265   (c) F, p. 266   (d) T, p. 268   (e) T, p. 266

34.7   (a) T, p. 263   (b) T, p. 269   (c) T, p. 259   (d) F, p. 270   (e) F, p. 270

Seeing the child alone at least once is good practice, even if it is not a standard family therapy recommendation.

Index

WITHDRAWN